UPDATE IN

This book should be returned by the last date stamped
above. You may renew the loan for a further period
if the book is not required by another reader.

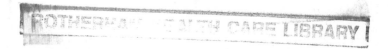

UPDATE IN INTENSIVE CARE MEDICINE

Springer

New York
Berlin
Heidelberg
Hong Kong
London
Milan
Paris
Tokyo

MECHANICAL VENTILATION

Volume Editors:

Arthur S. Slutsky, MD
Professor of Medicine, Surgery
and Biomedical Engineering
University of Toronto
Vice-President, Research
St. Michael's Hospital
Toronto, Canada

Laurent Brochard, MD
Department of Intensive Care
Hospital Henri Mondor
University Paris XII
Créteil, France

Series Editor:

Jean-Louis Vincent, MD, PhD
Head, Department of Intensive Care
Erasme University Hospital
Brussels, Belgium

With 73 Figures and 34 Tables

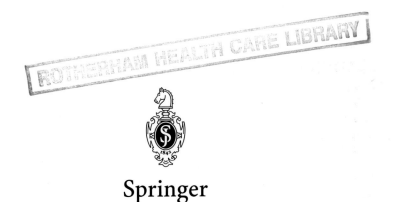

Springer

Prof. Arthur S. Slutsky, MD
Professor of Medicine, Surgery and
Biomedical Engineering
Director, Interdepartmental Division
of Critical Care Medicine
University of Toronto
Vice-President (Research)
St. Michael's Hospital
Queen Street Wing, Room 4-042
30 Bond Street, Toronto, ON M5B 1W8, Canada

Prof. Laurent Brochard
Department of Intensive Care
Hospital Henri Mondor
University Paris XII
94010 Créteil, France

Series Editor
Prof. Jean-Louis Vincent
Head, Department of Intensive Care
Erasme University Hospital
Route de Lennik 808
B-1070 Brussels
Belgium

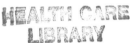
Cataloging-in-Publication Data applied for

A catalog record for this book is available from the Library of Congress.

Bibliographic information published by Die Deutsche Bibliothek
Die Deutsche Bibliothek lists this publication in the Deutsche Nationalbibliografie;
detailed bibliographic data is available in the Internet at http://dnb.ddb.de

Printed on acid-free paper.

Production managed by A. Gösling, Heidelberg, Germany
Typeset by Satz & Druckservice, Leimen, Germany
Printed and bound by Mercedes-Druck, Berlin, Germany
Printed in Germany

9 8 7 6 5 4 3 2

ISSN 1610-4056
ISBN 3-540-20267-6   SPIN 11596066

Springer-Verlag New York Berlin Heidelberg
A member of Springer Science+Business Media

Contents

Non-invasive Ventilation

ARDS/VILI: Mechanisms

ARDS/VILI: Assessment

ARDS/VILI: Therapy

Contributors

Albert R.K.
Dept of Medicine
Denver Health Medical Center
777 Bannock, MC 4000
Denver, CO 80206-4507
USA

Amato M.
Respiratory Intensive Care Unit
Hospital das Clinicas
Av Dr Eneas Carvalho de Aguiar 255
Sao Paulo
Brazil

Antonelli M.
Dept of Anesthesiology
and Intensive Care
Policlinico A. Gemelli
Largo A Gemelli 8
00168 Rome
Italy

Beck J.
Dept of Critical Care Medicine
St-Michaels Hospital
30 Bond Street
Toronto, Ontario M5B1W8
Canada

Berrios J.C.
Thoracic Diseases Research Unit
Division of Pulmonary
and Critical Care Medicine
Dept of Medicine
Mayo Clinic
200 First Street SW
Rochester, MN 55905
USA

Borges J.B.
Respiratory Intensive Care Unit
Hospital das Clinicas
Av Dr Eneas Carvalho de Aguiar 255
Sao Paulo
Brazil

Broccard A.F.
Dept of Pulmonary
and Critical Care Medicine
Regions Hospital
640 Jackson Street
St. Paul, MN 55101
USA

Brochard L.
Dept of Medical Intensive Care
Hôpital Henri Mondor
51 Avenue du Maréchal de Lattre de
Tassigny
94010 Créteil
France

Brower R.G.
Dept of Pulmonary & Critical Care
Medicine
Johns Hopkins Hospital
Baltimore, MD 21287
USA

Ceriana P.
Respiratory Intensive Care Unit
Fondazione S. Maugeri
Via Ferrata 8
27100 Pavia
Italy

Chiaia B.
Polytechnic of Turin
Department of Structural Engineering
Turin
Italy

Chiumello D.
Dept of Anesthesiology
and Intensive Care
Ospedale Maggiore Policlinico-IRCCS
Via Francesco Sforza 35
20122 Milan
Italy

Conti G.
Dept of Anesthesiology
and Intensive Care
Policlinico A. Gemelli
Largo A Gemelli 8
00168 Rome
Italy

Cortinovis B.
Institute of Anesthesia
and Intensive Care
Dept of Surgical Science
and Intensive Care
San Gerardo Hospital
Via Donizetti 106
20052 Milan
Italy

Curtis J.R.
Division of Pulmonary
and Critical Care Medicine
Harborview Medical Center
Box 359762
325 Ninth Avenue
Seattle, WA 98104
USA

de A Girardi C. R.
Dept of Surgical Intensive Care
Pierre Viars
Hôpital Pitié-Salpétrière
83 Boulevard de l'Hôpital
75013 Paris
France

Ely E.W.
Center for Health Services Research
6th Floor Medical Center East, #6109
Vanderbilt University Medical Center
Nasville, TH 37232-8300
USA

Esteban A.
Dept of Intensive Care
University Hospital
Carretera de Toledo Km 12,500
Getafe, Madrid 28905
Spain

Dreyfuss D.
Dept of Intensive Care
Hôpital Louis Mourier
92700 Colombes
France

Ferguson N.D.
Dept of Medicine
Division of Respirology
and Interdepartmental Division
of Critical Care
University of Toronto
Toronto
Canada

Frutos-Vivar F.
Dept of Intensive Care
University Hospital
Carretera de Toledo Km 12,500
Getafe, Madrid 28905
Spain

Gattinoni L.
Dept of Anesthesiology & ICU
Ospedale Maggiore Policlinico-IRCCS
Via Francesco Sforza 35
20122 Milan
Italy

Hering R.
Dept of Anesthesiology & ICU
University Hospital
Siegmund-Freud-Str. 35
53105 Bonn
Germany

Hill N.S.
Pulmonary, Critical Care
and Sleep Division
Tufts-New England Medical Center
750 Wahington St #257
Boston, MA 02111
USA

Hotchkiss J.R.
Dept of Pulmonary
and Critical Care Medicine
Regions Hospital
640 Jackson Street
St. Paul, MN 55101
USA

Hubmayr R.D.
Dept of Physiology & Biophysics
Stabile 8-18
Mayo Clinic
200 First Street SW
Rochester, MN 55905
USA

Hudson L.D.
Division of Pulmonary and Critical
Care Medicine
Harborview Medical Center
Box 359762
325 Ninth Avenue
Seattle, WA 98104
USA

Imai Y.
Interdepartmental Division
of Critical Care Medicine and Division
of Respirology
Dept of Medicine
St Michael's Hospital
30 Bond Street
Toronto, Ontario M5B1W8
Canada

Kacmarek R.M.
Respiratory Care
Ellison 401
Massachusetts General Hospital
55 Fruit Street
Boston, MA 02114
USA

Kavanagh B.P.
Dept of Anesthesia and Medicine
Hospital for Sick Children
555 University Avenue
Toronto, Ontario M5G 1X8
Canada

Kwok H.
Pulmonary, Critical Care
and Sleep Division
Tufts-New England Medical Center
750 Wahington St #257
Boston, MA 02111
USA

Lee C.M.
Division of Pulmonary and Critical
Care Medicine
Harborview Medical Center
Box 359762
325 Ninth Avenue
Seattle, WA 98104
USA

Liesching T.
Pulmonary, Critical Care
and Sleep Division
Tufts-New England Medical Center
750 Wahington St #257
Boston, MA 02111
USA

MacIntyre N.
Respiratory Care
Room 7451, Duke North
Duke University Medical Center
Box 3911
Durham, NC 27710
USA

Mancebo J.
Dept of Intensive Care
Hopsital de Sant Pau
Av. S.A.M. Claret 167
08025 Barcelona
Spain

Marini J.J.
Dept of Pulmonary
and Critical Care Medicine
Regions Hospital
640 Jackson Street
St. Paul, MN 55101
USA

Nava S.
Respiratory Intensive Care Unit
Fondazione S. Maugeri
Via Ferrata 8
27100 Pavia
Italy

Okamoto V.N.
Respiratory Intensive Care Unit
Hospital das Clinicas
Av Dr Eneas Carvalho de Aguiar 255
Sao Paulo
Brazil

Parthasarathy S.
Division of Pulmonary
and Critical Care Medicine
Edwards Hines Jr., Veterans
Administrative Hospital
Route 111N
Hines, IL 60141
USA

Patroniti N.
Institute of Anesthesia
and Intensive Care Unit
Dept of Surgical Science
and Intensive Care
San Gerardo Hospital
Via Donizetti 106
20052 Milan
Italy

Pelosi P.
Dept of Clinical
and Biological Sciences
Universita degli Studi dellInsubria
Varese
Italy

Pennisi M.A.
Dept of Anesthesiology
and Intensive Care
Policlinico A. Gemelli
Largo A Gemelli 8
00168 Rome
Italy

Pesenti A.
Institute of Anesthesia
and Intensive Care Unit
Dept of Surgical Science
and Intensive Care
San Gerardo Hospital
Via Donizetti 106
20052 Milan
Italy

Putensen C.
Dept of Anesthesiology
and Intensive Care
University Hospital
Siegmund-Freud-Str. 35
53105 Bonn
Germany

Ranieri V.M.
Dept of Anesthesiology
and Intensive Care
Ospedale S. Giovanni Battista
Corso Dogliotti 14
10126 Torino
Italy

Ricard J.D.
Dept of Intensive Care
Hôpital Louis Mourier
92700 Colombes
France

Rouby J.J.
Dept of Surgical Intensive Care
Pierre Viars
Hôpital Pitié-Salpétrière
83 Boulevard de lHôpital
75013 Paris
France

Rubenfeld G.D.
Division of Pulmonary
and Critical Care Medicine
Harborview Medical Center
University of Washington
Box 359762
325 9th Avenue
Seattle, WA 98104-2499
USA

Sakr Y.
Dept of Intensive Care
Erasme Hospital
Free University of Brussels
Route de Lennik 808
1170 Brussels
Belgium

Saumon G.
Xavier Bichat Faculty of Medicine
16 rue Henri Huchard
75018 Paris
France

Sinderby C.
Dept of Critical Care Medicine
St-Michaels Hospital
30 Bond Street
Toronto, Ontario M5B1W8
Canada

Slutsky A.S.
Interdepartmental Division
of Critical Care Medicine
and Division of Respirology
Dept of Critical Care Medicine
St Michaels Hospital
30 Bond Street
Queen Wing, Room 4-042
Toronto, Ontario M5B1W8
Canada

Spahija J.
Dept of Critical Care Medicine
St-Michaels Hospital
30 Bond Street
Toronto, Ontario M5B1W8
Canada

Terragni P.P.
Dept of Anesthesiology
and Intensive Care
Ospedale S. Giovanni Battista
Corso Dogliotti 14
10126 Torino
Italy

Thomason J.W.W.
Center for Health Services Research
6th Floor Medical Center East, #6109
Vanderbilt University Medical Center
Nasville, TH 37232-8300
USA

Tobin M.J.
Division of Pulmonary
and Critical Care Medicine
Edwards Hines Jr., Veterans
Administrative Hospital
Route 111N
Hines, IL 60141
USA

Vincent J.L.
Dept of Intensive Care
Erasme Hospital
Free University of Brussels
Route de Lennik 808
1170 Brussels
Belgium

Vlahakis N.
Thoracic Diseases Research Unit
Division of Pulmonary
and Critical Care Medicine
Dept of Medicine
Mayo Clinic
200 First Street SW
Rochester, MN 55905
USA

Wrigge H.
Dept of Anesthesiology
and Intensive Care
University Hospital
Siegmund-Freud-Str. 35
53105 Bonn
Germany

Younes M.
Dept of Medicine
St Michael's Hospital
30 Bond Steeet
Toronto, Ontario M5B 1W8
Canada

Common Abbreviations

ALI	Acute lung injury
APACHE	Acute physiology and chronic health evaluation
ARDS	Acute respiratory distress syndrome
COPD	Chronic ostructive pulmonary disease
CPAP	Continuous positive airways pressure
FRC	Functional residual capacity
HFOV	High frequency oscillatory ventilation
ICU	Intensive care unit
IMV	Intermittent mandatory ventilation
LIP	Lower inflection point
NAVA	Neurally adjusted ventilatory assist
NIV	Non-invasive ventilation
PEEP	Positive end-expiratory pressure
PSV	Pressure support ventilation
SBT	Spontaneous breathing trial
UIP	Upper inflection point
VILI	Ventilator-induced lung injury
V_T	Tidal volume

Epidemiology

The Importance of Acute Respiratory Failure in the ICU

Y. Sakr and J.L. Vincent

Introduction

Acute respiratory failure (ARF) results from a disorder in which lung function is inadequate for the metabolic requirements of the individual. ARF in critically ill patients is associated with mortality rates of between 40 and 65 % [1–13], and represents a wide spectrum of syndromes with different severities, which should be viewed in the context of the underlying pathology and associated organ dysfunction. Most of the published literature has focused on the severest forms of ARF, namely acute lung injury (ALI) and acute respiratory distress syndrome (ARDS).

Mechanical ventilation is imperative in many forms of ARF, with additional concerns about associated complications, e.g., hazards related to endotracheal intubation [14], ventilator induced lung injury (VILI) [15, 16] and ventilator associated pneumonia (VAP) [17]. Clinical and experimental evidence [15, 16, 18–20] suggest that mechanical ventilation may influence end organ function, a major determinant of outcome in this population.

The Spectrum of ARF

Failure of the respiratory system represents the final common pathway for a wide range of respiratory disorders. The spectrum of ARF varies widely (Fig. 1) from the severest form, namely ARDS, with severely impaired oxygenation ($PaO_2/FiO_2 \leq$ 200 mmHg, regardless of the level of positive end-expiratory pressure [PEEP]), bilateral pulmonary infiltrates on chest radiograph, and pulmonary-artery occlusion pressure (PAOP) $\leq$ 18 mmHg or no evidence of elevated left atrial pressure on the basis of chest radiograph and other clinical data [21]. ALI is a broader category that involves patients with a less severe form of impaired oxygenation ($PaO_2/FiO_2 \leq$ 300 mmHg) but presenting other clinical and radiographic features of ARDS [21]. Other forms of ARF are not uncommon, as for patients with respiratory failure with atypical radiographic changes requiring respiratory support. While these patients are not included in the ALI/ARDS definitions, they represent an important source of concern for intensive care unit (ICU) practitioners.

Few studies have reported the incidence of ARDS in a general ICU population. Knaus et al. [22] reported that only 2.4 % (423/17,440) of all ICU admissions met the diagnostic criteria for ARDS. However, the diagnosis was not based on respi-

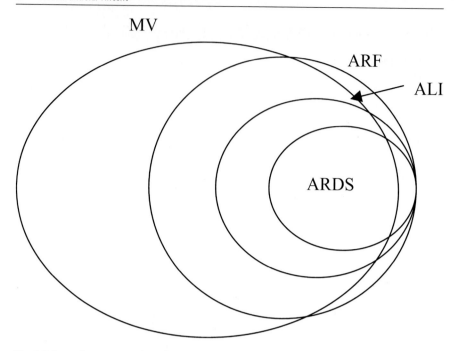

Fig. 1. Schematic representation of various ARF subpopulations and their relation to mechanical ventilation (MV mechanical ventilation, ALI acute lung injury, ARDS acute respiratory distress syndrome)

ratory variables, so this incidence is probably an underestimate. Other studies have reported an incidence of around 7 % [9, 11, 23, 24]. A cohort multicenter European study (ALIVE) reported that 7.4 % (2.8 % ALI and 5.3 % ARDS) of ICU patients were admitted with ALI/ARDS, or developed it during their stay [25], with considerable variations among countries, ranging from 1.7 % in Switzerland to 19.5 % in Portugal, although the criteria used to define ALI/ARDS were the same for all countries. Higher incidences of ARDS have been reported (11–23 %) in mechanically ventilated patients [13, 26–28].

The epidemiology of ARF in the ICU has been studied less. Lewandowski et al. [3] reported that ARF, defined as the need for intubation and mechanical ventilation > 24 hours, accounted for 69 % of all ICU bed usage in an urban population. The severity of lung disease was evaluated using the lung injury score (LIS); 3.6 % of evaluated patients had severe lung injury after 24 hours of intubation and mechanical ventilation, only 2.8 % had severe injury after 48 hours. The sequential organ failure assessment (SOFA) database of 1449 patients, excluding patients with routine postoperative surveillance, showed ARF to be present in 32 % of patients on ICU admission, with a further 24 % of patients developing ARF during their ICU stay (Fig. 2) [29]. ARF was defined as $PaO_2/FiO_2 < 200$ mmHg and the need for respiratory support, denoting a severe form of respiratory failure, and addressing the magnitude of this problem in a heterogeneous ICU population. Recently,

Esteban et al. [28], reported that 33 % (5183/15,757) of patients admitted to the participating centers received mechanical ventilation for more than 12 hours; ARDS was the cause of ARF in only 4.5% of ventilated patients.

In the recent sepsis occurrence in acutely ill patients (SOAP) study (unpublished observations) including a total of 3147 ICU patients, excluding uncomplicated postoperative patients, 58.8 % received mechanical ventilation on admission (2.6 % non-invasive ventilation), and another 5.5 % later during the ICU stay for a median of 3 days. Ventilatory days accounted for 55.6 % of total ICU days. Three hundred ninety three patients (12.5 %) had ALI/ARDS as defined by hypoxemia ($PaO_2/FiO_2 < 300$ mm Hg), bilateral chest infiltrates, and the need for mechanical ventilation in the absence of a history of chronic obstructive pulmonary disease (COPD) or manifestations of left ventricular failure.

Mortality from ARF

Reported mortality rates from ARF, ALI, and ARDS are largely influenced by the definitions used and by differences in the populations studied. The ALI and ARDS definitions proposed by the American-European Consensus Conference are widely accepted and used, but no universal definitions exist to describe the remaining part of the ARF spectrum (Fig 1).

Mortality rates from ARDS are cited within the range 40–60 % [2, 5, 6, 9–11, 13, 23, 27, 28, 30–43]. Only Ullrich et al. [35] reported a very low mortality rate of 20 %. In the SOAP study (unpublished observations), the ICU mortality of patients with ALI/ARDS was 38.9 % versus 15.6 % for patients without ALI or ARDS. The ICU mortality rate for patients with ARDS was 42.2 %. Luhr et al. [13] reported a 90 day mortality rate of 41 % in 1231 patients mechanically ventilated > 24 hours. Two other large studies reported similar mortality rates of around 40 % [4, 44]. In 615 patients mechanically ventilated > 24 hrs, Luhr et al [13] showed that mortality rates were comparable among patients who had ARDS and those who did not (44 vs. 41 %), underlining ARF as an entity with an outcome as bad as ARDS. The SOFA database [29] (Fig 2) showed a mortality rate of 31 % in patients with a severe form of ARF, an observation confirmed recently by Esteban et al. [28], although in a different population of patients with less severe ARF.

Despite increased understanding of the pathophysiology ARF related syndromes and apparent advances in respiratory support technology, there has been no clear decrease in mortality rates from ARDS over time [45]. However, there may have been changes in the case-mix of the ARDS population, with sicker patients being treated in our ICUs.

Factors Influencing Outcome from ARF

Preexisting comorbid diseases can be associated with increased mortality in ARF. In a multivariate analysis, Luhr et al. [13] reported that immunosuppression was associated with mortality in ARF patients. The SOFA database [29] identified a history of hematologic or chronic renal or liver failure as independent risk factors

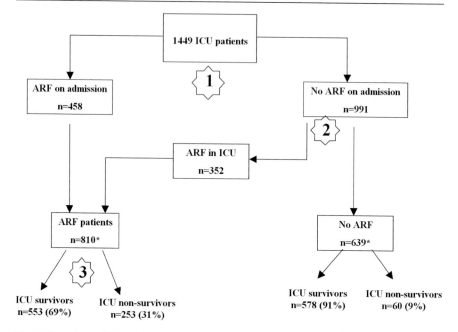

Fig. 2. Flow chart of the study and different subgroups [29]. 1 = description of the differences between ARF and non-ARF patients on ICU admission; 2 = study of risk factors for the development of ARF in the ICU; and 3 = study of the risk factors for death in the ARF patients; *outcome was undefined in four ARF patients and in one non-ARF patient. From [29] with permission

for death from ARF. Chronic liver disease has been associated with mortality from ARDS in several studies [2, 9, 13]. Zilberberg and Epstein [10] identified organ transplantation, human immunodeficiency virus (HIV) infection, cirrhosis, active malignancy, and sepsis as independent factors for hospital mortality in patients with ALI. Monchi et al. [9] reported that the length of mechanical ventilation prior to ARDS, cirrhosis, and the occurrence of right ventricular failure were associated with an increased risk of death.

Many investigators have found death from ARDS to be primarily related to the degree of organ dysfunction [24, 29, 46]. Doyle et al. [2] found that multiple organ failure (MOF), liver disease, and sepsis were the main factors contributing to death. Other important prognostic factors include age [28, 29, 47] and the development of acute renal failure [48]. The prognostic value of the degree of hypoxemia is not well established. Luhr et al. [37] emphasized that the degree of hypoxemia was unimportant in terms of mortality prediction. Likewise, Valta et al. [36] reported that the PaO_2/FiO_2 ratio at the onset of ARDS was similar in survivors and nonsurvivors.

The cause of death in ARDS patients is usually nonrespiratory, i.e., they die with, rather than from ARDS. Montgomery et al. [49] showed that only 16 % of deaths were due to refractory respiratory failure; early death (within 72 hours) was due to the underlying illness or injury whereas late death (beyond 72 hours) was due to sepsis. Ferring and Vincent [5] reported similar findings in 129 patients with ARDS of whom 67 (25 %) died: 50 % from sepsis/MOF, 16 % from respiratory failure, 15 % from cardiac failure/arrhythmia, 10 % from neurologic failure, and 8 % from other causes. Bersten et al. [23] reported that respiratory failure was the only cause of death in 9 % of patients with ARDS and contributed to death in just 24 % of ARDS patients. Recently Estenssoro and colleagues [24] noted in 217 patients with ARDS that MOF was the major cause of death in 88 patients, sepsis in 84, and refractory hypoxemia in 19; 56% of patients had more than one cause of death with 17 of the 19 patients with refractory hypoxemia also having sepsis or MOF.

The Time Course of Acute Respiratory Failure

Despite its limited prognostic value, the degree of hypoxemia can be an important predictor of disease progression in patients with ARF. As early as 1989, Bone et al [50] emphasized that survivors and nonsurvivors differed in the early response of the PaO_2/FiO_2 ratio to conventional therapy. Likewise, higher degrees of organ failure are likely to be present in nonsurvivors than in survivors, as MOF is the cause of death in the majority of patients; however, the time course of organ failure can follow different patterns before reaching this final stage.

In a prospective study of 182 patients with ARF in our institution (unpublished observations), we separated 133 patients who had early ARF (an onset < 48 hours after ICU admission) and 49 with late ARF (an onset <48 hours after ICU admission). On admission, the cardiovascular SOFA score was higher in early than in late ARF, whereas the neurologic score was higher in late than in early ARF. In early ARF, a high SOFA score and low Glasgow Coma Score were predictors of mortality, and in late ARF, a low Glasgow Coma Score at 48 hours predicted mortality. These findings suggest that there may be important differences in the epidemiology and outcome of ARF that are dependent on the time of onset.

Conclusion

ARF comprises a spectrum of diseases that includes ALI and ARDS, and importantly is a valid entity in its own right. Indeed, the severity of ARF is similar to that of ALI/ARDS and it is more easily defined. ARF is common in ICU patients and associated with considerable mortality and morbidity.

References

1. Milberg JA, Davis DR, Steinberg KP, Hudson LD (1995) Improved survival of patients with acute respiratory distress syndrome (ARDS): 1983–1993. JAMA 273:306–309
2. Doyle LA, Szaflarski N, Modin GW, Wiener-Kronish J, Matthay MA (1995) Identification of patients with acute lung injury. Predictors of mortality. Am J Respir Crit Care Med 152:1818–1824

3. Lewandowski K, Metz J, Deutschmann C, et al (1995) Incidence, severity, and mortality of acute respiratory failure in Berlin, Germany. Am J Respir Crit Care Med 151:1121–1125
4. Vasilyev S, Schaap RN, Mortensen JD (1995) Hospital survival rates of patients with acute respiratory failure in modern respiratory intensive care units. An international, multicenter, prospective survey. Chest 107:1083–1088
5. Ferring M, Vincent JL (1997) Is outcome from ARDS related to the severity of respiratory failure? Eur Respir J 10:1297–1300
6. Suchyta MR, Clemmer TP, Elliott CG, et al (1997) Increased mortality of older patients with acute respiratory distress syndrome. Chest 111:1334–1339
7. Nolan S, Burgess K, Hopper L, Braude S (1997) Acute respiratory distress syndrome in a community hospital ICU. Intensive Care Med 23:530–538
8. Squara P, Dhainaut JF, Artigas A, Carlet J (1998) Hemodynamic profile in severe ARDS: results of the European Collaborative ARDS Study. Intensive Care Med 24:1018–1028
9. Monchi M, Bellenfant F, Cariou A, et al (1998) Early predictive factors of survival in the acute respiratory distress syndrome. Am J Respir Crit Care Med 158:1076–1081
10. Zilberberg MD, Epstein SK (1998) Acute lung injury in the medical ICU: comorbid conditions, age, etiology, and hospital outcome. Am J Respir Crit Care Med 157:1159–1164
11. Roupie E, Lepage E, Wysocki M, et al (1999) Prevalence, etiologies and outcome of the acute respiratory distress syndrome among hypoxemic ventilated patients. Intensive Care Med 25:920–929
12. Garcia-Garmendia JL, Ortiz-Leyba C, Garnacho-Montero J, Jimenez-Jimenez FJ, Monterrubio-Villar J, Gili-Miner M (1999) Mortality and the increase in length of stay attributable to the acquisition of Acinetobacter in critically ill patients. Crit Care Med 27:1794–1799
13. Luhr OR, Antonsen K, Karlsson M, et al (1999) Incidence and mortality after acute respiratory failure and acute respiratory distress syndrome in Sweden, Denmark, and Iceland. The ARF Study Group. Am J Respir Crit Care Med 159:1849–1861
14. Troche G, Moine P (1997) Is the duration of mechanical ventilation predictable? Chest 112:745–751
15. Dreyfuss D, Saumon G (1993) Role of tidal volume, FRC, and end-inspiratory volume in the development of pulmonary edema following mechanical ventilation. Am Rev Respir Dis 148:1194–1203
16. Tremblay L, Valenza F, Ribeiro SP, Li J, Slutsky AS (1997) Injurious ventilatory strategies increase cytokines and c-fos m-RNA expression in an isolated rat lung model. J Clin Invest 99:944–952
17. Rello J, Ollendorf DA, Oster G, et al (2002) Epidemiology and outcomes of ventilator-associated pneumonia in a large US database. Chest 122:2115–2121
18. Ranieri VM, Suter PM, Tortorella C, et al (1999) Effect of mechanical ventilation on inflammatory mediators in patients with acute respiratory distress syndrome: a randomized controlled trial. JAMA 282:54–61
19. Ranieri VM, Giunta F, Suter PM, Slutsky AS (2000) Mechanical ventilation as a mediator of multisystem organ failure in acute respiratory distress syndrome. JAMA 284:43–44
20. Imai Y, Kajikawa O, Frevert C, et al (2001) Injurious ventilatory strategies enhance organ apoptosis in rabbits. Am J Respir Crit Care Med 163:A677 (Abst)
21. Bernard GR, Artigas A, Brigham KL, et al (1994) The American-European Consensus Conference on ARDS. Definitions, mechanisms, relevant outcomes, and clinical trial coordination. Am J Respir Crit Care Med 149:818–824
22. Knaus WA, Sun X, Hakim RB, Wagner DP (1994) Evaluation of definitions for adult respiratory distress syndrome. Am J Respir Crit Care Med 150:311–317
23. Bersten AD, Edibam C, Hunt T, Moran J (2002) Incidence and mortality of acute lung injury and the acute respiratory distress syndrome in three Australian States. Am J Respir Crit Care Med 165:443–448
24. Estenssoro E, Dubin A, Laffaire E, et al (2002) Incidence, clinical course, and outcome in 217 patients with acute respiratory distress syndrome. Crit Care Med 30:2450–2456

25. Brun-Buisson C, Minelli C, Brazzi L, et al (2000) The European Survey of acute lung injury and ARDS: Preliminary results of the ALIVE study. Intensive Care Med 26 (suppl 3):617 (Abst)
26. Trouillet JL, Chastre J, Vuagnat A, et al (1998) Ventilator-associated pneumonia caused by potentially drug-resistant bacteria. Am J Respir Crit Care Med 157:531–539
27. Markowicz P, Wolff M, Djedaini K, et al (2000) Multicenter prospective study of ventilator-associated pneumonia during acute respiratory distress syndrome. Incidence, prognosis, and risk factors. ARDS Study Group. Am J Respir Crit Care Med 161:1942–1948
28. Esteban A, Anzueto A, Frutos F, et al (2002) Characteristics and outcomes in adult patients receiving mechanical ventilation: a 28-day international study. JAMA 287:345–355
29. Vincent JL, Akca S, de Mendonca A, et al (2002) The epidemiology of acute respiratory failure in critically ill patients. Chest 121:1602–1609
30. Hudson LD, Milberg JA, Anardi D, Maunder RJ (1995) Clinical risks for development of the acute respiratory distress syndrome. Am J Respir Crit Care Med 151:293–301
31. Chastre J, Trouillet JL, Vuagnat A, et al (1998) Nosocomial pneumonia in patients with acute respiratory distress syndrome. Am J Respir Crit Care Med 157:1165–1172
32. Brochard L, Roudot-Thoraval F, Roupie E, et al (1998) Tidal volume reduction for prevention of ventilator-induced lung injury in acute respiratory distress syndrome. The Multicenter Trail Group on Tidal Volume reduction in ARDS. Am J Respir Crit Care Med 158:1831–1838
33. Weg JG, Anzueto A, Balk RA, et al (1998) The relation of pneumothorax and other air leaks to mortality in the acute respiratory distress syndrome. N Engl J Med 338:341–346
34. Stewart TE, Meade MO, Cook DJ, et al (1998) Evaluation of a ventilation strategy to prevent borotrauma in patients at high risk for acute respiratory distress syndrome. N Engl J Med 338:355–361
35. Ullrich R, Lorber C, Roder G, et al (1999) Controlled airway pressure therapy, nitric oxide inhalation, prone position, and extracorporeal membrane oxygenation (ECMO) as components of an integrated approach to ARDS. Anesthesiology 91:1577–1586
36. Valta P, Uusaro A, Nunes S, Ruokonen E, Takala J (1999) Acute respiratory distress syndrome: frequency, clinical course, and costs of care. Crit Care Med 27:2367–2374
37. Luhr OR, Karlsson M, Thorsteinsson A, Rylander R, Frostell CG (2000) the impact of respiratory variables on mortality in non-ARDS and ARDS patients requiring mechanical ventilation. Intensive Care Med 26:508–517
38. The ARDS Network (2000) Ventilation with lower tidal volumes as compared with traditional tidal volumes for acute lung injury and the acute respiratory distress syndrome. N Engl J Med 342:1301–1308
39. Esteban A, Alia I, Gordo F, et al (2000) Prospective randomized trial comparing pressure-controlled ventilation and volume-controlled ventilation in ARDS. For the Spanish Lung Failure Collaborative Group. Chest 117:1690-1696
40. Rocco Jr TR, Reinert SE, Cioffi W, Harrington D, Buczko G, Simms HH (2001) A 9-year, single-institution, retrospective review of death rate and prognostic factors in adult respiratory distress syndrome. Ann Surg 233:414–422
41. Gattinoni L, Tognoni G, Pesenti A, et al (2001) Effect of prone positioning on the survival of patients with acute respiratory failure. N Engl J Med 345:568–573
42. Nuckton TJ, Alonso JA, Kallet RH, et al (2002) Pulmonary dead-space fraction as a risk factor for death in the acute respiratory distress syndrome. N Engl J Med 346:1281–1286
43. Derdak S, Mehta S, Stewart TE, et al (2002) High-frequency oscillatory ventilation for acute respiratory distress syndrome in adults: a randomized, controlled trial. Am J Respir Crit Care Med 166:801–808
44. Kurek CJ, Dewar D, Lambrinos J, Booth FV, Cohen IL (1998) Clinical and economic outcome of mechanically ventilated patients in New York State during 1993: analysis of 10,473 cases under DRG 475. Chest 114:214–222
45. Pola MD, Navarrete-Navarro P, Rivera R, Fernandez-Mondejar E, Hurtado B, Vazquez-Mata G (2000) Acute respiratory distress syndrome: resource use and outcomes in 1985 and 1995, trends in mortality and comorbidities. J Crit Care 15:91–96

46. Gowda MS, Klocke RA (1997) Variability of indices of hypoxemia in adult respiratory distress syndrome. Crit Care Med 25:41–45
47. Dellinger RP, Zimmerman JL, Taylor RW, et al (1998) Effets of inhaled nitric oxide in patients with acute respiratory distress syndrome: Results of a randomized phase II trial. Crit Care Med 26:15–23
48. Rogers RM, Weiler C, Ruppenthal B (1972) Impact of respiratory intensive care unit on survival of patients with acute respiratory failure. Chest 62:94–97
49. Montgomery BA, Stager MA, Carrico J, et al (1985) Causes of mortality in patients with the adult respiratory distress syndrome. Am Rev Respir Dis 132:485–491
50. Bone RC, Maunder R, Slotman G, et al (1989) An early test of survival in patients with the adult respiratory distress syndrome. The PaO2/FiO2 ratio and its differential response to conventional therapy. Chest 96:849–851

The Epidemiology of Mechanical Ventilation

F. Frutos-Vivar, N. D. Ferguson, and A. Esteban

Introduction

Mechanical ventilation is a commonly used technique in the intensive care unit (ICU) [1]. Newer modes of ventilation are continually incorporated into daily practice, however it is most often the case that these new methods do not have any associated studies demonstrating advantages over older methods, especially in terms of morbidity or mortality. In most cases we are only able to find studies that assessed the effects of different ventilator modes on physiological variables. There appears to be an incongruity between the amount of resources used in the development and introduction of new modes of ventilation and the paucity of information that exists regarding the use and outcomes of mechanical ventilation as well as the description of what modes or settings should be considered standard or conventional mechanical ventilation.

In 1993 a Mechanical Ventilation Consensus Conference [2] analyzed the benefits and complications associated with mechanical ventilation, focusing on the management of patients with acute respiratory failure (ARF). Due to a lack of clinical trials comparing the efficacy of different modes of ventilation and different settings, the recommendations of the Consensus Conference were based on 'expert opinion', which is of course a low level of evidence. Since the publication of this consensus conference, however, a number of observational studies have been published that attempt to answer a number of important questions regarding the use mechanical ventilation and its associated outcomes. In this chapter, we will summarize the prevalence, indications, method of use, and outcomes related to mechanical ventilation.

Prevalence of Mechanical Ventilation

The first studies published on the use of mechanical ventilation coincide with the development of the first ICUs [2–5]. In 1972, Rogers et al. [6] published an analysis of the application of mechanical ventilation during the first 5 years of their ICU. They observed a very high mortality rate of 63 % in the 212 mechanically ventilated patients studied [6]. Seven years later, Nunn et al. [7] analyzed the outcome of 100 consecutive patients requiring mechanical ventilation. This cohort of patients accounted for 23.5 % of the patients admitted to their ICU and had a hospital survival rate of 47 %.

The first study with information about the incidence of mechanical ventilation in a large population of patients admitted to the ICU was published by Knaus et al. in 1991 [8]. These authors reported that 49 % of the 3884 patients included in the APACHE III database had received mechanical ventilation, but also noted that a significant percentage (64 %) of these patients were in the postoperative period and therefore needed mechanical ventilation for less than 24 hours. In contrast, an observational study performed in 48 Spanish medical-surgical ICUs found that 46 % of patients were mechanically ventilated at least for 24 hours [9]. In 1996, a one-day point prevalence study was carried out with 4,153 patients admitted in 412 ICUs from 8 countries, showing that 39% of patients required mechanical ventilation [10]. More recently, it has been reported, in a prospective study including 15,757 patients from 20 countries, that 5183 patients (33 %) required mechanical ventilation [11].

Characteristics of Mechanically Ventilated Patients

There are a few studies that analyze the characteristics of patients receiving mechanical ventilation. Most of these studies are focused on specific pathologies such as chronic obstructive pulmonary disease (COPD) and acute respiratory distress syndrome (ARDS). In the past decade, however, the Spanish Lung Failure Collaborative Group has coordinated three epidemiological studies [9–11] that help to better illustrate the profile of the patient requiring mechanical ventilation.

Demographic Data

In our international studies, the median age of mechanically ventilated patients was 61 years in 1996 [10] (interquartile range: 44–71), and 63 years (interquartile range: 48–73) in 1998 [11]. Interestingly, in both studies approximately 25 % of the patients were older than 75. This finding seems to indicate that many physicians do not consider this age to be a contraindication to ICU admission and the use of mechanical ventilation.

Distribution by gender was equal and similar in the observational studies [10, 11]. This is in contrast to several clinical trials of patients with ARDS [12], sepsis [13], or myocardial infarction [14], which all enrolled almost twice as many males as females.

Reason for the Initiation of Mechanical Ventilation

Pathophysiological indications (hypoxemic respiratory failure or hypercapnic respiratory failure) for mechanical ventilation are well known [15] but there are fewer reports about the diseases that cause the respiratory distress. Again, most of these studies attempt to address the incidence of only one specific disease like COPD or

Table 1. Indications for mechanical ventilation in three observational studies.

	1992	1996	1998
	Esteban et al. [9]	Esteban et al. [10]	Esteban et al. [11]
Acute on chronic PD	21%	13%	13%
COPD	21%	13%	10%
Asthma	n.a.	n.a.	1.5%
Other	n.a.	n.a.	1%
Acute respiratory failure	42%	66%	69%
ARDS	n.a.	12%	4.5%
Postoperative	n.a.	15%	21%
Aspiration	n.a.	3%	2.5%
Pneumonia	n.a.	16%	14%
Sepsis	n.a.	16%	9%
Trauma	n.a.	12%	8%
CHF	n.a.	12%	10%
Cardiac arrest	n.a.	n.a.	2%
Neurological	20%	18%	19%
Coma	20%	15%	17%
NMD	n.a.	3%	2%

PD: pulmonary disease; COPD: chronic obstructive pulmonary disease; ARDS: acute respiratory distress syndrome; CHF: congestive heart failure; NMD: neuromuscular disease; n.a.: not available

ARDS. Table 1 shows the reasons for the initiation of mechanical ventilation reported in three studies that have included an unselected population of mechanically ventilated patients [9–11].

Management of Mechanical Ventilation

Airway Management

The decision to place an oral or nasal tracheal tube rests with the practitioner and is based on a variety of considerations [16]. The major reasons for placing nasal tubes include improved patient comfort, better oral hygiene, and perhaps a decreased risk of laryngeal injury and self-extubation. On the other hand, the oral route is preferable in many patients with high minute ventilation, copious secretions or a need to undergo fiberoptic bronchoscopy due to the advantages of the larger tube that can be placed orally rather than nasally. The smaller lumen and the smaller radius of the curvature of nasal tubes result in higher resistance. Finally, nasal tubes have the added disadvantage of occluding the ostia of the maxillary sinus, leading to fluid accumulation in the sinuses, and an increased risk of the development of sinusitis and nosocomial pneumonia [17].

For the reasons outlined above, the preferable intubation route for most physicians is orotracheal. In the 1996 study [10], airway access for the delivery of mechanical ventilation consisted of (on the day of study) an endotracheal tube in 75% of patients, a tracheostomy in 24% and a facial mask in 1%. Of the endotracheal tubes, 96% were passed through the mouth and 4% through the nose. The type of this study, a one-day point prevalence study, is one of the most likely reasons for the high percentage of patients with tracheostomy and the low proportion of patients with facial mask. This explanation is borne out when the results of the prospective cohort study that followed patients from the first day of mechanical ventilation to discharge from the unit [11] are examined. In this study [11], the proportion of patients with an endotracheal tube was 93% (89% orotracheal and 4% nasotracheal), 5% of patients were initially ventilated with facial mask, and 2% had a previous tracheostomy.

Despite decades of clinical investigations into the risks and benefits of various techniques of airway management, no reasonable consensus exists as to the ideal timing of the performance of the tracheostomy. A consensus conference on weaning and discontinuing ventilatory support [18], therefore, again recommended a guideline based upon expert opinion. Kollef et al. [19] performed a prospective cohort study including 521 patients requiring mechanical ventilation for more than 12 hours. In this study about 10% of patients received a tracheostomy at a mean time of 9.7 ± 6.4 days from beginning mechanical ventilation. Esteban et al. [10] showed that a tracheostomy was performed in 24% of patients. The frequency of tracheostomy varied significantly depending on the patient's underlying condition and the time from initiation of mechanical ventilation. Over the initial 3 weeks, a tracheostomy was performed more frequently in patients with neuromuscular disease (31.3%) compared to those with COPD (14.8%, $p < 0.05$) or with acute respiratory failure (9.1%, $p < 0.001$). After the third week, the proportion of patients with a tracheostomy (among patients still requiring mechanical ventilation) did not differ among the diagnostic categories. Two years later in the Mechanical Ventilation International Study [20], the incidence of tracheostomy was 11% and the median number of days to tracheostomy was 12 (P_{25}: 7; P_{75}: 17). Similar to the observations from 1996, early tracheostomy was performed in patients with neurological disease (coma or neuromuscular disease) but by the third week there were no differences in tracheostomy rate between pathologies (Fig. 1). The variables associated with a higher probability for tracheostomy were duration of mechanical ventilation, reintubation, coma and neuromuscular disease.

Modes of Ventilation

Until the publication of our studies [9–11], there were limited data on physicians' preferences for different modes of mechanical ventilation. Venus et al. [21] reported the results of an American survey of hospital-based respiratory care departments. Seventy-two percent of the responders indicated that intermittent manda-

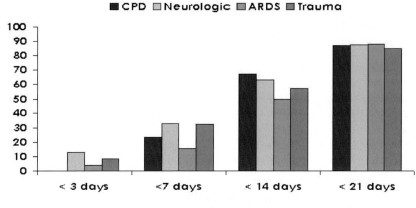

	N	< 3 days	< 7 days	< 14 days	< 21 days
CPD	63	-	23%	67%	87%
Neurological	147	13%	33%	63%	87.5%
ARDS	26	4%	15%	50%	88%
Trauma	72	8,5%	32%	57%	85%

Fig. 1. Timing of tracheostomy according to the indication for mechanical ventilation (data from [20]). CPD: Acute on chronic pulmonary disease; ARDS: acute respiratory distress syndrome.

tory ventilation (IMV) was the primary mode of ventilatory support. In contrast with this study that was based upon the expressed preferences of the physicians, our studies reflect the clinical use of each mode of ventilation, as shown in Table 2.

A lack of evidence for the superiority of one mode over another [22] together with a larger experience in the use of assist-control ventilation are likely the main reasons explaining why this method is the most commonly used in the ICU. This predominance of assist-control ventilation is independent of the reason for initiation of mechanical ventilation (Table 3) and is maintained over the entire course of mechanical ventilation (Fig. 2).

Because invasive mechanical ventilation is obviously not free of complications [23], in the last several years there has been a significant increase in the study and use of non-invasive ventilation (NIV). In the Mechanical Ventilation International Study [11] the proportion of patients who were initially ventilated with NIV was 4%; a significantly lower percentage than the 35% reported in a French multicenter study [24]. One of the reasons for this difference is that in the study by Esteban et al. [11] only patients with a duration of mechanical ventilation longer than 12 hours were included, and this criteria could have led to the exclusion of patients who received NIV for a short time.

A recent meta-analysis comparing traditional invasive versus non-invasive ventilation [25] showed a significant reduction in mortality in patients receiving NIV.

Table 2. Modes of mechanical ventilation used in three observational studies[a]

	1992	1996	1998
	Esteban et al. [9]	Esteban et al. [10]	Esteban et al. [11]
AC	55%	47%	53%
PCV	1%	–	5%
SIMV	26%	6%	8%
SIMV-PS	8%	25%	15%
PS	8%	15%	4%

AC: assist-control ventilation; PCV: pressure control ventilation; SIMV: synchronized intermittent mandatory ventilation; PS: pressure support
[a]In the two first studies, the percentage corresponds to the mode used on the day of the study, whereas in the last study, it corresponds to the mode used on the first day of mechanical ventilation

Table 3. Comparison of the modes of ventilation used in patients with COPD and ARDS (modified from [12]).

	COPD			ARDS		
	Day1	Day 3	Day 7	Day1	Day 3	Day 7
AC	66%	64%	67%	67%	64%	61%
SIMV	5%	3.5%	2%	4%	25%	2%
SIMV-PS	10%	11%	11%	10%	11%	10%
PS	8%	8.5%	12%	1%	3%	4%
PCV	45%	4%	2%	10%	13%	16%

AC: Assist-control ventilation; PC: Pressure control ventilation; SIMV: Synchronized intermittent mandatory ventilation; PSV: Pressure support

However, when the patients and studies were separated according to the primary disease process studied (COPD vs. hypoxemic respiratory failure) the reduction in mortality appeared to be due almost entirely to the beneficial effect observed in the COPD patients. In contrast, patients with hypoxemic respiratory failure who received NIV did not appear to have a reduced mortality. Table 4 shows the evolution of the patients who were non-invasively ventilated in the Mechanical Ventilation

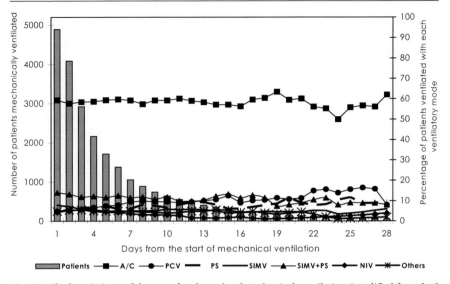

Fig. 2. Daily descriptions of the use of each mode of mechanical ventilation (modified from [11] with permission). AC: Assist/control ventilation; PCV: pressure controlled ventilation; PS: pressure support; SIMV: synchronized intermittent mandatory ventilation; NIV: non invasive ventilation

Table 4. Outcomes of patients who received non-invasive ventilation (NIV) (data from [11])

	COPD	Hypoxemic respiratory failure
% Patients with non-invasive ventilation	16%	4%
% Patients who failed NIV	26%	36,5%
Mortality with failure of NIV	27%	48%

International Study [11]. A cautionary finding of this part of the study was that patients successfully managed with NIV had a mortality rate of 17%, while those patients that required intubation after the failure of NIV had a mortality of 48%. This rate of death among patients who failed NIV was significantly higher than that seen in patients with respiratory failure who were intubated primarily without a trial of NIV. One may speculate, therefore, that the delay in the intubation of patients with acute respiratory failure caused by an attempt of NIV may be associated with a significant increase in their risk of death.

Ventilator Settings

Tidal volume

For many years, physicians have chosen ventilator tidal volumes (V_T) between 10 and 15 ml/kg. This practice in the past could be justified by the fact that early experience with mechanical ventilation came from anesthesiology, where the aim of the mechanical ventilation was to avoid atelectasis and maintain good oxygenation during the surgical intervention [26].

In recent years, however, several clinical and experimental studies have been performed investigating the concept of ventilator-induced lung injury (VILI) [27]. Findings from both animal studies and early non-controlled human trials suggested that certain ventilator settings (high V_T and low levels of positive end-expiratory pressure [PEEP]) could affect the extent of lung injury and even influence outcome. A number of randomized trials have now been performed that have evaluated the influence of the ventilatory settings (predominantly V_T), on the outcome of the mechanically ventilated patient with ARDS.

Initial retrospective and prospective uncontrolled trials using low-pressure-limited ventilation and allowing the use of permissive hypercapnia demonstrated a significantly lower hospital mortality rate than predicted by the APACHE II score [28, 29]. These promising results led to five prospective randomized controlled studies comparing conventional ventilation to a lung protective ventilatory approach [12, 30–33]. Three of these studies [31–33] demonstrated no advantage from this protective strategy, and in fact all three studies showed non-significant increases in mortality in the protective ventilation group. These studies were characterized by only moderate increases in plateau pressure in the control ventilation arms (compared to the recommended maximum plateau pressure of 30–40 cmH$_2$O suggested by the Consensus Conference [2]) resulting in only moderate differences in both V_T and plateau pressures between the two groups. Levels of PEEP were moderate (approximately 8–10 cmH$_2$O) and by design were equivalent in both the treatment and control arms. During both conventional and protective ventilation, PEEP levels only reached the lower limits of the Consensus Conference recommended levels of 10–15 cmH$_2$O. These characteristics could explain why these trials showed negative results.

On the other hand, there are two studies that show that a protective ventilation strategy can improve the outcome of ARDS patients. Amato et al. [30] used a comprehensive ventilatory management strategy consisting of setting PEEP levels above the inflection point of the static pressure-volume (PV) curve, using frequent recruitment maneuvers, as well as limiting V_T and plateau pressure. In this study the mortality of the experimental group was 38% but the mortality of the control group was higher than that described in most observational studies (71%). The ARDS Network study [12] also found a reduced mortality (31 vs. 40%) in the group ventilated with low V_T. This study certainly showed that the V_T employed has an impact on the outcome of patients with ARDS. Debate continues, however, regarding whether the low V_T strategy was protective, or the high volume strategy harmful. In the ARDS Network study the possible bias of these studies could be that the control group was ventilated with a V_T (12 ml/kg) that, at this moment, cannot be considered as conventional. In observational studies we have observed that the mean V_T used to ventilate patients with ARDS was 8.7 ± 2 ml/kg in 1996 [10] and 8.5 ± 2 ml/kg in 1998 [11]. This finding is similar to a recent report by Thompson et al. [34] who analyzed the ventilatory settings used prior to the initiation of the protocol in the patients included in the ARDS Network study. At that moment the mean V_T set was 8.6 ml/kg.

Positive End-expiratory Pressure

Determining the effect of PEEP on different physiological variables has been the aim of several studies. From the initial favorable experience of Petty and Asbaugh [35], extensive research has been undertaken to evaluate both the hemodynamic effects of PEEP and its effects on the distribution of V_T and alveolar recruitment [36]. Although clinical [30] and experimental [37–40] studies have shown a protective effect associated with a high level of PEEP, the findings of the observational studies [10, 11] suggest that physicians make little effort to look for 'optimal' PEEP and show that there are a high number of patients who are ventilated without PEEP (Fig. 3). In the observational studies [10, 11], however, a significant difference was

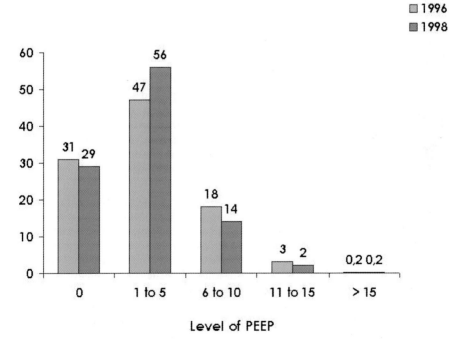

Fig. 3. Levels of PEEP observed in two epidemiological studies. (Date from 1996 [10] is the level of PEEP set on day of study and data from 1998 [11] is the level of PEEP set on first day of the mechanical ventilation)

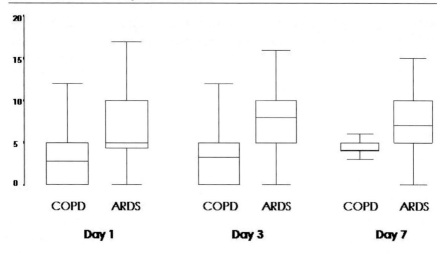

Fig. 4. Comparison of the levels of PEEP employed in COPD and ARDS patients [11]. (Box plots showing median and interquartile ranges. Bars show the range of the applied PEEP)

observed between the level of PEEP applied to patients with ARDS and that applied to patients with COPD (Fig. 4).

Weaning

Weaning from mechanical ventilation is an aspect that has been subjected to several randomized controlled trials. Brochard et al. [41] reported a difference in the rate of successful weaning between patients weaned with pressure support ventilation (PSV) and patients weaned with either synchronized intermittent mandatory ventilation (SIMV) or with a T-tube. In contrast, the Spanish Lung Failure Collaborative Group [42] found that a single daily trial of spontaneous breathing achieved a threefold and twofold increase in the rate of successful weaning compared with IMV and PSV, respectively. Likely stemming from this extensive research, important changes in the current clinical practice of weaning may be observed (Table 5). The demonstration of the superiority of the spontaneous breathing trial (SBT) may account for the increase in the use of this approach over time (4% in 1996 and 46% in 1998) as well as the decrease in the use of SIMV from 18% in 1992, 5% in 1996, and 5% in 1998. We were somewhat surprised to find a significant use of SIMV combined with PSV as this method, to our knowledge, has only been evaluated in one study with 19 difficult to wean COPD patients [43]. In this study, SIMV with PSV did not significantly decrease the time of weaning. Interestingly, the time devoted to weaning has remained constant at around 40% of total ventilator time from 1992 to 1998 [9, 11].

Table 5. Changes over time seen in the utilization of the methods for weaning from mechanical ventilation.

	1992	1996	1998
	Esteban et al. [9]	Esteban et al. [10]	Esteban et al [11]
PS	15%	36%	12%
SIMV	18%	5%	5%
SIMV-PS	9%	28%	12%
Intermittent SBT trials	24%	17%	4%
Once daily SBT trial	–	4%	46%
Combination of two or more methods	33%	9%	31%

PS: pressure support; SIMV: synchronized intermittent mandatory ventilation; SBT: spontaneous breathing trial

Complications Associated with Mechanical Ventilation

Barotrauma

Barotrauma is a frequent complication of mechanical ventilation and is associated with increased morbidity and mortality [45,46]. Investigators have reported incidences of barotrauma as low as 0.5% in postoperative patients [47] and as high as 87% in patients with ARDS [45]. These variations in the reported incidence of ventilator-associated barotrauma may relate to differences in the patients' underlying disease. Barotrauma is increased in patients with severe underlying lung disease, especially in patients with ARDS [30–32, 45, 46, 48, 49, 51], aspiration pneumonia [50], *Pneumocystis carinii* pneumonia [51], and pre-existing COPD [46, 52–55].

Barotrauma has been reported at variable time intervals after the start of mechanical ventilation. In a cohort of 5183 mechanically ventilated patients Anzueto et al. [55] observed that 80% of the barotrauma appeared within the first 3 days of mechanical ventilation. These results are similar to the report of Gammon et al. [48] in patients with ARDS and of Schnapp et al. [56] in patients with multiple underlying conditions.

The development of barotrauma has been associated with ventilator mode [57], high airway pressures [52], high PEEP [40], high V_T [30], and increased end-expiratory lung volume [58]. However, in a large series of patients with ARDS [49] and in a cohort of patients mechanically ventilated for more than 24 hours [48], the development of barotrauma was not related to the use of conventional pressures and volumes. In the study by Anzueto et al. [55] there were no differences in the measured pressures and V_T among patients with and without barotrauma. Amato et al. [30] reported a statistically significant relationship with both V_T and PEEP to the frequency of barotrauma. These investigators found that 42% of patients with ARDS who were ventilated with a V_T of 12 ml/kg developed barotrauma compared to only 7% of patients ventilated with a V_T of 6 ml/kg (p< 0.001). In larger studies, however, the incidence of barotrauma did not differ between patients ventilated with and without strategies designed to limit airway pressures and V_T [12, 31, 32].

Ventilator-associated Pneumonia

Ventilator associated pneumonia (VAP), defined as pneumonia occurring more than 48 hours after endotracheal intubation and initiation of mechanical ventilation, complicates the course of 8–28% of the patients receiving mechanical ventilation [59]. Accurate data on the epidemiology of VAP are limited by the lack of standardized criteria for its diagnosis.

Prolonged mechanical ventilation, defined as that lasting for more than 48 hours, is the most important factor associated with nosocomial pneumonia. A prospective Italian study [60] found that the frequency of VAP rose from 5% for patients receiving mechanical ventilation for one day to 69% for patients who required mechanical ventilation for more than 30 days. Fagon et al. [61] estimated the cumulative risk of pneumonia as 7% at 10 days and 19% at 20 days after the initiation of mechanical ventilation. In this study, the incremental risk of pneumonia was constant over the course of respiratory support, with a mean rate of 1% per day. Recently Cook et al. [62] observed, in a study involving 1014 mechanically ventilated patients, that although the cumulative risk for developing VAP increased over the time, the daily hazard rate decreased after day 5, so the risk per day was evaluated as 3% on day 5, 2% on day 10 and 1% on day 15.

Outcomes Following Mechanical Ventilation

In our large study of mechanically ventilated patients [11], the median duration of mechanical ventilation was 3 days (P_{25}: 2; P_{75}: 7). It is interesting to note that only 3% of patients had a duration of mechanical ventilation longer than 21 days. In this study significant differences (p <0.001) were found between two of the more clinically relevant pathologies, namely ARDS and COPD. The COPD patients had a median duration of ventilation of 4 days (P_{25}: 2; P_{75}: 6) while the ARDS patients had a median duration of 6 days (P_{25}: 3; P_{75}: 11). These differences in the duration of ventilatory support between underlying diseases are similar to those reported previously by other authors. Stauffer et al. [64] found that patients with pneumonia had a longer duration of mechanical ventilation (11.4 days) than other diseases (3.7 to 7.4 days). Troché and Moine [64] showed that the duration of mechanical ventilation was dependent on the underlying disease with values ranging from 2 days for postoperative status to 15 days for acute lung injury (ALI).

Table 6. Mortality rates in observational studies of the general population of mechanically ventilated patients

Author	Patients (N)	Mortality (%)	
		ICU	Hospital
Papadakis et al. [65]	612		64
Esteban et al. [9]	290	34	
Douglas et al. [66]	57		44
Esteban et al. [11]	5183	31	39

The mortality rates of mechanically ventilated patients have been described with widely varying results, likely due to heterogeneity of the populations included in the studies. Table 6 shows the mortality rates reported in recent observational studies that included a general and unselected population of patients. This mortality has been associated with baseline factors including age; severity of disease or previous functional status; coma, sepsis or ARDS as the reason of mechanical ventilation; with factors related to the management of the patient such as the use of vasoactive drugs, use of neuromuscular blockers, peak pressure higher than 50 cmH$_2$O, plateau pressure higher than 35 cmH$_2$O; and with complications developed over the course of mechanical ventilation such as barotrauma, ARDS, sepsis, hypoxemia and multiple organ failure [11].

Cost-effectiveness of Mechanical Ventilation

Mechanical ventilation and intensive support of patients with respiratory failure or multiple organ dysfunction have grade I level of evidence according to their efficacy (US Preventive Service Task Force [67]). There are a few of studies evaluating the cost-effectiveness of mechanical ventilation, but these are generally focused on particular diseases like ARDS [68], COPD [69, 70], non-traumatic coma [71], stroke [72], or acquired-immune deficiency syndrome (AIDS) [73]. There are, however, fewer studies examining cost-effectiveness in a general population of mechanically ventilated patients. Schmidt et al. [74] retrospectively studied 137 consecutive patients who required at least 48 h of ventilatory support. The mean total hospital cost was $16,930/patient (U.S. dollars, 1976–1977). The average cost-benefit was $1826 per life-year gained. More recently, Rodríguez-Roldán et al. [75] studied marginal cost-effectiveness ratios in 101 consecutive patients who required mechanical ventilation for at least 72 hours. They found that total costs for the mechanically ventilated patients amounted to 3,288,608 €. When these results were linked to quality-adjusted life years (QALYs) gained through the use of utilities, they found a marginal cost of 5552 € per QALY gained. This cost-effectiveness ratio places mechanical ventilation and intensive care among the intermediate-priority techniques, quite close to the $5000/QALY high priority threshold, according to criteria of the Advisory Group In Health Technology Assessment [76].

Conclusion

In conclusion, when one examines the available data and considers a typical medical-surgical ICU, it appears that approximately one third of the patients admitted to the ICU will receive mechanical ventilatory support for more than 12 hours. The reason for initiating mechanical ventilation will be acute respiratory failure in 2 out of every 3 cases. The average age of the ventilated patients will likely be close to 62 years of age and in 65% of cases they will be male. Most typically they will be ventilated using an assist-control (A/C) volume based ventilator mode throughout their course on the ventilator. The average V_T and PEEP levels employed are likely to be around 8.5 ml/kg and ≤ 5 cmH$_2$O, respectively. Finally, the average duration of mechanical ventilation will be approximately 5 days with a probability of survival to hospital discharge of about 61%. These estimates are based largely on the multicenter international observational study performed in 1998. Clearly the data presented here may not be applicable to every ICU, and it is possible that practice patterns may have changed in the last few years. Nevertheless, these data represent the most up to date and comprehensive information available at the current time. Further studies will be needed in the future to determine how (if at all) these figures are changing over time.

References

1. Snider GL (1989) Historical perspective on mechanical ventilation; from simple life support system to ethical dilemma. Am Rev Respir Dis 140:52–57
2. Slutsky AS (1993) ACCP Consensus Conference Mechanical Ventilation. Chest 104:1833–1859
3. Linton RC, Walker FW, Spoerel WE (1965) Respiratory care in a general hospital: a five-year survey. Can Anaesth Soc J 12:451–457
4. Bigelow DB, Petty TL, Ashbaugh DG, Levine BE, Nett LM, Tyler SW (1967) Acute respiratory failure. Experiences of a respiratory care unit. Med Clin North Am 51:323–40
5. Noehren TH, Friedman I (1968) A ventilation unit for special intensive care of patients with respiratory failure. JAMA 203:641–3.
6. Rogers RM, Weiler C, Ruppenthal B (1972) Impact of the respiratory intensive care unit on survival of patients with acute respiratory failure. Chest 62:94–97
7. Nunn JF, Milledge JS, Singaraya J (1979) Survival of patients ventilated in an intensive therapy unit. Br Med J 1:1525–1527
8. Knaus WA (1989) Prognosis with mechanical ventilation: the influence of disease, severity of disease, age, and chronic health status on survival from an acute illness. Am Rev Respir Dis 140: S8–S13
9. Esteban A, Alía I, Ibañez J, Benito S, Tobin MJ and the Spanish Lung Failure Collaborative Group (1994) Modes of mechanical ventilation and weaning. A national survey of Spanish hospitals. Chest 106:1188–1193
10. Esteban A, Anzueto A, Alía I, et al, for the Mechanical Ventilation International Study Group (2000) How is mechanical ventilation employed in the Intensive Care Unit? An international utilization review. Am J Respir Crit Care Med 161:1450–1458.

11. Esteban A, Anzueto A, Frutos F, et al., for the Mechanical Ventilation International Study Group (2002) Characteristics and outcomes in adult patients receiving mechanical ventilation. JAMA 287:345–355

12. The Acute Respiratory Distress Syndrome Network (2000) Ventilation with lower tidal volumes as compared with traditional tidal volumes for acute lung injury and the acute respiratory distress syndrome. N Engl J Med 342:1301–1308

13. Bernard GR, Vincent JL, Laterre PF, et al. (2001) Recombinant human protein C Worldwide Evaluation in Severe Sepsis (PROWESS) study group. N Engl J Med 344:699–709

14. The Global Use of Strategies to Open Occluded Coronary Arteries (GUSTO III) Investigators (1997) A comparison of reteplase with alteplase for acute myocardial infarction. N Engl J Med 337:1118–23

15. Aldrich TK, Prezant DJ (1994) Indications for mechanical ventilation. In: Tobin MJ (ed) Principles and Practice of Mechanical Ventilation. McGraw-Hill, New York, pp 155–189

16. Bishop MJ (1994) Airway management. In: Tobin MJ (ed) Principles and Practice of Mechanical Ventilation, McGraw-Hill, New York, pp 695–709

17. Holzapfel L, Chastang C, Demingeon G, Bohe J, Piralla B, Coupry A (1999) A randomized study assessing the systematic search for maxillary sinusitis in nasotracheally mechanically ventilated patients. Influence of nosocomial maxillary sinusitis on the occurrence of ventilator-associated pneumonia. Am J Respir Crit Care Med 159:695–701

18. MacIntyre NL, Cook DJ, Ely EW, et al. (2001) Evidence-based guidelines for weaning and discontinuing ventilatory support. Chest 120:375S–395S

19. Kollef MH, Ahrens TS, Shannon W (1999) Clinical predictors and outcomes for patients requiring tracheostomy in the intensive care unit. Crit Care Med 27:1714–1720

20. Esteban A, Frutos F, Anzuelo A, et al. (2001) Impact of tracheostomy on outcome of mechanical ventilation. Am J Respir Crit Care Med 163:A129

21. Venus B, Smith RA, Mathru M (1997) National survey of methods and criteria used for weaning from mechanical ventilation. Crit Care Med 15:530–533

22. Leung P, Jubran A, Tobin MJ (1997) Comparison of assisted modes on triggering, patient effort and dyspnea. Am J Respir Crit Care Med 155:1940–1948

23. Pingleton SK (1994) Complications associated with mechanical ventilation. In: Tobin MJ (ed) Principles and Practice of Mechanical Ventilation. McGraw-Hill, New York, pp 775–792

24. Carlucci A, Richard J, Wysocki M, Lepage E, Brochard L, and the SRLF collaborative group on mechanical ventilation (2001) Noninvasive versus conventional mechanical ventilation. An epidemiological survey. Am J Respir Crit Care Med 163:874–880

25. Peter JV, Moran JL, Phillips-Hughes J, Warn D (2002) Noninvasive ventilation in acute respiratory failure – A meta-analysis update. Crit Care Med 30:555 562

26. Lutch JS, Murray JF (1972) Continuous positive pressure ventilation: effects on systemic oxygen transport and tissue oxygenation. Ann Intern Med 76:193–202

27. Dreyfuss D, Saumon G (1998) Ventilator-induced lung injury. Lessons from experimental studies. Am J Respir Crit Care Med 157:294323

28. Hickling KG, Henderson SJ, Jackson R (1990) Low mortality associated with low volume pressure limited ventilation with permissive hypercapnia in severe adult respiratory distress syndrome. Intensive Care Med 16: 372–377

29. Hickling KG, Walsh J, Henderson S, Jackson R (1994) Low mortality rate in adult respiratory distress syndrome using low-volume, pressure-limited ventilation with permissive hypercapnia: a prospective study. Crit Care Med 22:1568–1578

30. Amato MB, Barbas CS, Medeiros DM, et al. (1998) Effect of a protective-ventilation strategy on mortality in the acute respiratory distress syndrome. N Engl J Med 338:347–354

31. Stewart TE, Meade MO, Cook DJ, et al. (1998) Evaluation of a ventilation strategy to prevent barotrauma in patients at high risk for acute respiratory distress syndrome. Pressure- and Volume-Limited Ventilation Strategy Group. N Engl J Med 338:355–361

32. Brochard L, Roudot-Thoraval F, Roupie E, et al. (1998) Tidal volume reduction for prevention of ventilator-induced lung injury in acute respiratory distress syndrome. Am J Respir Crit Care Med 158:1831–1838
33. Brower RG, Shanholtz CB, Fessler HE, et al. (1999) Prospective, randomized, controlled trial comparing traditional versus reduced tidal volume ventilation in acute respiratory distress syndrome patients. Crit Care Med 27:1492–1498
34. Thompson BT, Hayden D, Matthay MA, Brower R, Parsons PE (2001) Clinicians´ approaches to mechanical ventilation in acute lung injury and ARDS. Chest 120:1622–1627
35. Petty TL, Ashbaugh DG (1971) The adult respiratory distress syndrome: clinical features, factors influencing prognosis and principles of management. Chest 60:273–279
36. Rossi A, Ranieri MV (1994) Positive end-expiratory pressure. In: Tobin MJ (ed) Principles and Practice of Mechanical Ventilation, McGraw-Hill, New York, pp 259–303
37. Dreyfuss D, Saumon G (1993) Role of tidal volume, FRC, and end-inspiratory volume in the development of pulmonary edema following mechanical ventilation. Am Rev Respir Dis 148:1194–1203
38. Bshouty Z, Ali J, Younes M (1988) Effect of tidal volume and PEEP on rate of edema formation in in situ perfused canine lobes. J Appl Physiol 64:1900–1907
39. Sandhar BK, Niblett DJ, Argiras EP, Dunnill MS, Sykes MK (1988) Effects of positive end-expiratory pressure on hyaline membrane formation in a rabbit model of the neonatal respiratory distress syndrome. Intensive Care Med 14:538–546
40. Argiras EP, Blakeley CR, Dunnill MS, Otremski S, Sykes MK (1987) High PEEP decreases hyaline membrane formation in surfactant deficient lungs. Br J Anaesth 59:1278–1285
41. Brochard L, Rauss A, Benito S, et al. (1994) Comparison of three methods of gradual withdrawal from ventilatory support during weaning from mechanical ventilation. Am J Respir Crit Care Med 150:896–903
42. Esteban A, Frutos F, Tobin MJ, et al. for the Spanish Lung Failure Collaborative Group (1995) A comparison of four methods of weaning patients from mechanical ventilation. N Engl J Med 332:345–350
43. Jounieaux V, Duran A, Levi-Valensi P (1994) Synchronized intermittent mandatory ventilation with and without pressure support ventilation in weaning patients with COPD from mechanical ventilation. Chest 105:1204–1210
44. Gattinoni L, Bombino M, Pelosi P, Lissoni A, Pesenti A, Fumagalli R, Tagliabue M (1994) Lung structure and function in different stages of severe adult respiratory distress syndrome. JAMA 271:1772–1779
45. Gammon RB, Shin MS, Buchalter SE (1992) Pulmonary barotrauma in mechanical ventilation. Patterns and risk factors. Chest 102:568–572
46. Schnapp LM, Chin DP, Szaflarski N, Matthay MA (1995) Frequency and importance of barotrauma in 100 patients with acute lung injury. Crit Care Med 23:272–278
47. Cullen DJ, Caldera DL (1979) The incidence of ventilator-induced pulmonary barotrauma in critically ill patients. Anesthesiology 50:187–190
48. Gammon RB, Shin MS, Groves RH, Hardin JM, Hsu C, Buchalter SE (1995) Clinical risk factors for pulmonary barotrauma: A multivariate analysis. Am J Respir Crit Care Med 152:1235–1240
49. Weg JG, Anzueto A, Balk RA, Wiedemann HP, Pattishall EN, Schork MA, Wagner LA (1998) The relation of pneumothorax and other air leaks to mortality in the acute respiratory distress syndrome. N Engl J Med 338:341–346
50. de Latorre FJ, Tomasa A, Klamburg J, Leon C, Soler M, Rius J (1977) Incidence of pneumothorax and pneumomediastinum in patients with aspiratoryaspiration pneumonia requiring ventilatory support. Chest 72:141–144
51. Sepkowitz KA, Telzak EE, Jonathan W, et al (1991) Pneumothorax in AIDS. Ann Intern Med 114:458–459
52. Petersen GW, Baier H (1983) Incidence of pulmonary barotrauma in a medical ICU. Crit Care Med 11:67–69

53. Kumar A, Pontoppidam H, Falke KJ, Wilson RS, Laver MD (1973) Pulmonary barotrauma during mechanical ventilation. Crit Care Med 4:181–186
54. Zwillich CW, Pierson DJ, Creagh CE, et al. (1974) Complications of assisted ventilation: a prospective study of 354 consecutive patients. Am J Med 57:161–170
55. Anzueto A, Frutos F, Esteban A, et al. (2003) Incidence, risk factors and outcome of barotrauma in mechanically ventilated patients. (In press)
56. Schnapp LM, Chin DP, Szaflarski N, Matthay MA (1995) Frequency and importance of barotrauma in 100 patients with acute lung injury. Crit Care Med 23:272–278
57. Mathru M, Rao TLK, Venus B (1983) Ventilator-induced barotrauma in controlled mechanical ventilation versus intermittent mandatory ventilation. Crit Care Med 11:359–361
58. Williams TJ, Tuxen DJ, Scheindestel CD (1992) Risk factors for morbidity in mechanically ventilated patients with severe asthma. Am Rev Respir Dis 146:607–615
59. Chastre J, Fagon JY (2002) Ventilator-associated pneumonia. Am J Respir Crit Care Med 165:1618–1623
60. Langer M, Mosconi P, Cigada M, Mandelli M (1989) Long-term respiratory support and risk of pneumonia in critically ill patients. Am Rev Respir Dis 140:302–305
61. Fagon JY, Chastre J, Domart Y, et al. (1989) Nosocomial pneumonia in patients receiving continuous mechanical ventilation. Prospective analysis of 52 episodes with use of a protected specimen brush and quantitative culture techniques. Am Rev Respir Dis 139:877–884
62. Cook DJ, Walter SD, Cook RJ, et al. (1998) Incidence of and risks factors for ventilator-associated pneumonia in critically ill patients. Ann Intern Med 129:433–440
63. Stauffer JL, Fayter NA, Graves B, et al. (1993) Survival following mechanical ventilation for acute respiratory failure in adult men. Chest 104:1222–1229
64. Troché G, Moine P (1997) Is the duration of mechanical ventilation predictable? Chest 112:745–751
65. Papadakis MA, Lee KK, Brower WS, et al. (1993) Prognosis of mechanically ventilated patients. West J Med 159:659–664
66. Douglas SL, Daly BJ, Brennan PF, Harris S, Nochowitz M, Dyer MA (1997) Outcomes of long-term ventilator patients: a descriptive study. Am J Crit Care 6:99–105
67. US Preventive Services Task Force (1989) An assessment of the effectiveness of 169 interventions. Williams and Wilkins, Baltimore
68. Hamel MB, Phillips RS, Davis RB, et al. (2000) Outcomes and cost-effectiveness of ventilator support and aggressive care for patients with acute respiratory failure due to pneumonia or acute respiratory distress syndrome. Am J Med 109:614–620
69. Ely EW, Baker AM, Evans GW, Haponik EF (2000) The distribution of costs of care in mechanically ventilated patients with chronic obstructive pulmonary disease. Crit Care Med 28:408–413
70. Añón JM, García de Lorenzo A, Zarazaga A, Gómez-Tello V, Garrido G (1999) Mechanical ventilation of patients on long-term oxygen therapy with acute exacerbations of chronic obstructive pulmonary disease: prognosis and cost-utility analysis. Intensive Care Med 25:452–457
71. Hamel MB, Phillips R, Teno J, et al. (2002) Cost effectiveness of aggressive care for patients with nontraumatic coma. Crit Care Med 30:1191–1196
72. Mayer SA, Copeland D, Bernardini GL, et al. (2000) Cost and outcome of mechanical ventilation for life-threatening stroke. Stroke 31:2346–2353
73. Wachter RM, Luce JM, Safrin S, Berrios DC, Charlebois E, Scitovsky AA (1995) Cost and outcome of intensive care for patients with AIDS, Pneumocystis carinii pneumonia, and severe respiratory failure. JAMA 273:230–235
74. Schmidt CD, Elliott CG, Carmelli D, et al. (1983) Prolonged mechanical ventilation for respiratory failure: a cost-benefit analysis. Crit Care Med 11:407–411
75. Rodríguez Roldán JM, Alonso Cuesta P, López Martínez J, Del Nogal Sáez F, Jiménez Martín MJ, Suárez Saiz J (2002) Análisis de coste-efectividad de la ventilación mecánica y del tratamiento intensivo de pacientes en situación crítica. Med Intensiva 26:391–398

76. Advisory Group in Health Technology Assessment (1993) Assessing the effects of health technologies, principles, practice, and proposals. Department of Health, London

Long-term Outcomes of Mechanical Ventilation

L. D. Hudson, C. M. Lee, and J. R. Curtis

Introduction

Traditionally, outcomes of mechanical ventilation for acute respiratory failure reported by investigators have been physiologic changes, mortality, duration of mechanical ventilation, and length of stay in both intensive care unit (ICU) and hospital. Various definitions for a mortality outcome have been used, often either an arbitrary period from acute disease onset such as 28 day mortality, or mortality at hospital discharge. Occasionally costs of the hospitalization have been included.

In recent years reports of longer term outcomes in patients with acute respiratory failure (and especially in acute lung injury [ALI]/acute respiratory distress syndrome [ARDS]) have been published. These outcomes have included long-term survival, pulmonary function, and – more recently – quality of life and conditions or complications of acute respiratory failure that could affect quality of life. These complications or conditions include neurocognitive and neuropsychological abnormalities and neuromuscular complaints and impairments.

The subject of this chapter is long-term outcomes after mechanical ventilation. For the most part, we are unable to differentiate which outcomes in survivors of acute respiratory failure are related to the use of mechanical ventilation and which are due either to the underlying condition for which mechanical ventilation was being performed or a variety of other factors including co-morbidity and the effects of other therapies. We will approach this issue by first describing long-term outcomes associated with mechanical ventilation for acute respiratory failure in a general way. We will describe survival, emphasizing when available data on long term follow-up of these patients, and also quality of life and complications occurring in survivors. Mechanical ventilation may allow the occurrence or development of complications – but not be directly responsible for them. After a description of outcomes we will briefly discuss possible etiologic factors whenever data exist to allow this, including whether mechanical ventilation could be implicated. Most of the data will be reported separately for the differing underlying conditions or types of acute respiratory failure, mainly since the original papers most frequently report outcomes for particular disease cohorts, but also because the underlying condition is likely such an important determinant of outcome.

Why is it important that we know the long-term outcomes after mechanical ventilation for acute respiratory failure? The answers vary depending on the category of the outcomes being considered. Survival is important in order to know prognosis, which could play a role in decision making for both the patient and his or her surrogates and the caregivers during the ICU admission. Knowledge of long-term survival may also be important in resource development and utilization planning. Objectively measured physiologic outcomes such as pulmonary function can help connect events and therapy during the acute illness with other more patient-centered outcomes. These measurements may provide information about mechanisms and also may have predictive value. Patient-centered outcomes such as quality of life and symptoms are what patients care about. Also, by understanding the prevalence and severity of these outcomes, we can begin to link them with possible etiologic factors during the critical illness that are potentially modifiable. In this way we can begin to develop strategies for patient management both during the critical illness and in follow-up that may be able to prevent or minimize these adverse long-term outcomes.

Survival/Mortality

Hospital Mortality for Patients Receiving Mechanical Ventilation

Esteban and colleagues conducted an international prospective cohort study of adult patients admitted to ICUs and receiving mechanical ventilation for more than 12 consecutive hours during March, 1998 and reported their results in 2002 [1]. The study included 5183 patients in 361 ICUs in 20 countries. Mean duration of mechanical ventilation was 5.9 days and mean ICU length of stay was 11.2 days. Overall mortality was 31%, 52% in patients receiving mechanical ventilation for ARDS and 22% receiving mechanical ventilation for an exacerbation of chronic obstructive pulmonary disease (COPD). This large study confirmed previous reports of higher mortality rates in patients with ARDS and lower mortality for COPD patients with acute respiratory failure.

Analysis of the types of patients and their conditions included in this cohort provides important information about the practice of mechanical ventilation in the broad international critical care community. It also helps inform us about the relative magnitude of those populations in which long-term outcomes may be of interest. Of the 5183 patients, 17% were being ventilated for coma, 2% for neuromuscular disease, 13% for acute respiratory failure or chronic pulmonary disease, and 69% for acute respiratory failure without previous lung disease. Of those patients with acute respiratory failure, about a third (21% of the total of mechanically ventilated patients) were post-operative. Ten percent of the total had congestive heart failure, 2% were post cardiac arrest. Thirty-eight percent had either pneumonia (14%) or some other cause known to be associated with ALI (sepsis, trauma, aspiration) although whether criteria for ALI were met is not known. Only 4.5% of the total carried a diagnosis of ARDS. In this chapter we will deal with long-term outcomes in patients with acute respiratory failure superimposed on chronic pulmonary disease (mainly COPD), ALI/ARDS, and will briefly mention available data for mechanically ventilated patients with acute cardiogenic pulmonary edema.

Hospital Mortality in Patients with COPD and Acute Respiratory Failure

Most series of patients with COPD and acute respiratory failure include both non-ventilated (usually the majority) and ventilated patients. Overall mortality rates are usually lower than or similar to the 22% in the Esteban study for ventilated patients. For example, Connors et al., in data from the multi-center SUPPORT study, found an 11% overall mortality rate for 1016 patients with exacerbations of COPD , of whom 348 were treated with mechanical ventilation [2]. They did not report hospital mortality rates stratified by mechanical ventilation. Seneff et al., in a prospective multi-center inception cohort study of 362 admissions to ICUs for an acute exacerbation of COPD, found an overall hospital mortality of 24% with the mortality in ventilated patients (n=170) being 31.8% compared to 16.7% in non-ventilated patients (n=192) [3]. When a multivariate analysis of potential variables to explain mortality was performed, the physiological measurements contained in the acute physiology score of the APACHE III score and the pre-ICU hospital length of stay were the two most important predictors of hospital mortality. After accounting for these, the use of mechanical ventilation was not a statistically significant predictor of hospital mortality. Hospital mortality rates in these two multicenter studies are similar to those in previous reports since 1975 through the early 1990s [4].

Long-term Mortality Rates in Patients with COPD and Acute Respiratory Failure

Studies from the 1970s and 1980s suggested that once patients with COPD survive an episode of acute respiratory failure, their subsequent survival is similar to patients with the same degree of pulmonary dysfunction without an acute exacerbation of COPD [5, 6]. In other words, the prognosis of a patient with COPD was dependent on their severity of COPD and was unaffected by a previous history of an episode of acute respiratory failure. Most patients in these studies were not treated with mechanical ventilation.

The studies by Connors et al. [2] and Seneff et al. [3] described above for hospital mortality also reported mortality at 6 months and one year (and two years for the Connors study). For the SUPPORT study cohort of 1016 patients reported by Connors, mortality rates increased from the 11% hospital mortality to 33%, 43%, and 49% respectively for 6 months, one and two years of follow-up. Approximately one-third of patients received mechanical ventilation (348/1016). Reduced survival was observed in patients who required mechanical ventilation – 43% mortality at 6 months compared to 28% in patients who were not ventilated.

In the study by Seneff and co-workers, specific longer-term survival data are limited to those patients aged 65 years or older. Two hundred and sixteen of the 362 patients met these age criteria and complete data were available for 167 of those 216. Overall mortality was 30% at hospital discharge, 47% at 6 months, and 59% at one year. Mortality figures for those receiving mechanical ventilation compared to those who did not were, respectively, 37% vs. 23% at hospital discharge, 54% vs.

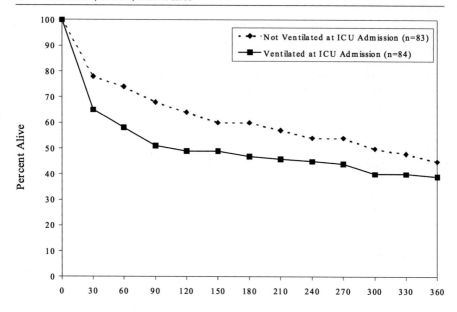

Fig. 1. Kaplan-Meier 1-year survival for 167 patients aged 65 years or older admitted to an ICU for acute exacerbation of COPD according to need for mechanical ventilation at ICU admission. Adapted from [3] with permission

42% at 6 months, and 62% vs. 56% at one year. Thus, hospital mortality but not subsequent mortality was higher in those patients receiving mechanical ventilation (Fig. 1). When a multivariate analysis was performed to assess factors associated with mortality, however, mortality was explained by the physiologic abnormalities captured in the acute physiology score and by pre-ICU hospital length of stay and mechanical ventilation was not independently significant (Fig. 2).

Almagro and colleagues in Spain followed a cohort of 135 patients hospitalized for acute exacerbation of COPD for over two years [7]. Only eight of these patients were treated with mechanical ventilation. Hospital mortality is not described; mortality at 6 months, 1, 2, and 2.5 years was 16%, 22%, 36% and 44%, respectively. Separate analysis for patients receiving mechanical ventilation is not reported.

In summary, although hospital survival for patients with COPD and acute respiratory failure is relatively good, there is a high cumulative mortality over the next year. Ventilated patients have approximately twice the hospital mortality as non-ventilated patients but mechanical ventilation did not influence subsequent mortality. The multivariate analysis finding that respiratory physiology and severity of baseline COPD predicts mortality is relatively more important for long-term than short-term outcome.

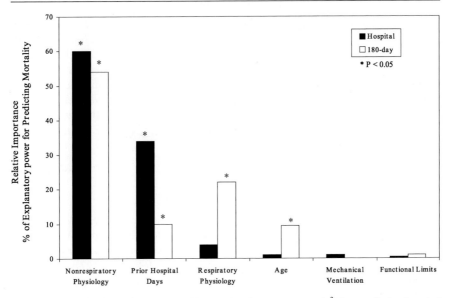

Fig. 2. Relative importance, as measured by % of explanatory power (x^2) for predicting hospital and 180-day mortality rates, of prognostic factors for 167 patients aged 65 years or older admitted to an ICU for acute exacerbation of COPD. Adapted from [3]

Hospital Mortality in ALI/ARDS

Values for 28 or 30-day mortality or hospital mortality in patients with ALI/ARDS vary considerably, ranging from about 30–60% [1, 4, 8, 9]. In the Esteban international study, the mortality listed for ARDS is 52% [1]. In a prospective cohort study from Sweden, Denmark and Iceland the 90 day mortality was 42% for ALI not fulfilling ARDS criteria and similar at 41% for ARDS [8]. In a recent one-year study of ALI in King County, Washington, USA in which all ventilated patients were systemically screened for the diagnosis of ALI, the overall mortality was 34% [9]. A number of variables affect the mortality rate including age and underlying etiology or risk condition of ALI, making comparisons between cohorts difficult without having detailed data on case-mix and comorbid states. Suntharalingam and colleagues reported a statistically insignificant trend of higher hospital mortality in patients with ARDS from a pulmonary (direct) etiology compared to those with ARDS from a non-pulmonary (indirect) etiology (47 vs. 28%, p=0.11) [10].

Our group at the University of Washington in Seattle, USA first reported on a declining hospital mortality rate for patients with ARDS in 1995 [11]. Using data from a registry of ARDS patients available since the early 1980s in which patients were prospectively screened for a diagnosis of ARDS using the same criteria, we showed a reduction in hospital mortality from greater than 60% in the 1980s to less than 40% in the early 1990s. The hospital in which the study was performed, Harborview Medical Center, is the major trauma referral center for a five state region. Trauma as a risk condition for ALI or ARDS is known to be associated with a lower mortality than other common risk conditions, particularly sepsis, which may explain our relatively lower mortality compared to other studies. The reduction in mortality rate over time, however, was related more to a decreased mortality in patients with sepsis as their ARDS risk. The severity of illness as judged by APACHE score was similar comparing the earlier years with a high mortality to later years with a lower mortality. The reduction was not affected after adjusting for frequency of risk conditions and age. Since our report, two other groups have reported a reduction in mortality rate over time, one report from England [12] and another from France [13].

Long-term Survival in ALI/ARDS

Although many have reported the hospital mortality associated with ARDS, there has only been one study that specifically investigated the effects of ARDS on long-term survival compared with a control group. Davidson and colleagues conducted a prospective, matched parallel cohort study following 127 survivors of ARDS related to trauma or sepsis, and 127 control survivors with sepsis or trauma without ARDS [14]. The control group was matched for severity of illness, using the Injury Severity Score for trauma patients, and the APACHE III score for those with sepsis. The median follow-up period for both subjects and controls was 753 days. This study found no difference in long-term mortality between the ARDS survivors and their matched controls (Fig. 3). Survival in both groups was correlated most significantly with risk factor, with a 3% late mortality in the trauma

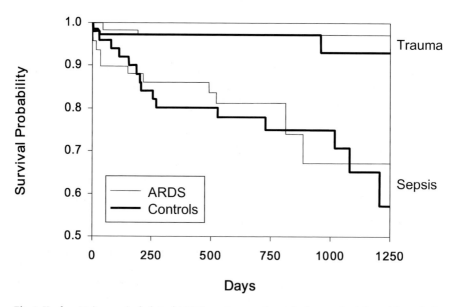

Fig. 3. Kaplan-Meier survival plot of ARDS survivors and matched controls. Adapted from [14]

group compared to 22% in sepsis. Increased age and serious comorbidities in the sepsis patients were also associated with increased late mortality.

Long-term Mortality in Patients with Acute Cardiogenic Pulmonary Edema

Wiener et al. reported survival data in 44 patients with acute cardiogenic pulmonary edema associated with coronary artery disease, of whom 26 had acute myocardial infarction (AMI) [15]. The authors do not describe the frequency of mechanical ventilation. Hospital mortality was strongly influenced by the presence of AMI; 12 of 26 patients (46%) with AMI died in hospital compared to only 1 of 18 patients (6%) in its absence (p=0.006). Of the 30 hospital survivors, 8 of 30 (27%) had died at 1 year and 21 of 30 patients (70%) had died at 6 years. There was no significant difference in subsequent survival between those with and without AMI.

Adnet and coworkers followed a cohort of 79 patients with age > 75 years requiring endotracheal intubation and mechanical ventilation for acute cardiogenic pulmonary edema [16]. Hospital mortality was 26.6%. Independent predictors of increased ICU mortality from multiple logistic regression analysis were the presence of multiple organ failure, epinephrine use, length of ICU stay, and duration of mechanical ventilation. The 58 hospital survivors were followed for a mean duration of 23 months (range 2–56 months) with 31 (53%) patients dying during the follow-up period. Overall 1 year mortality among hospital survivors was 30%. The most common cause of long-term mortality was congestive heart failure. Neither of these studies provide insight into the effect of mechanical ventilation on long-term survival from acute cardiogenic edema.

Long-term Outcome of Critically Ill Elderly Patients

Chelluri and colleagues reported long-term outcomes in critically ill patients aged 65 years and older, comparing those aged 75 years and older to those aged 65–74 years [17]: 97 patients were studied, 54 aged 75 years or older and 43 aged 65–74 years. Hospital mortality and mortality at one year did not differ between the two groups (39 vs. 40% and 63 vs. 58%, respectively). Neither did length of stay, hospital charges, and follow-up quality of life assessments. These authors concluded that age alone is not an adequate predictor of long-term survival and quality of life in critically ill elderly patients.

Long-term Follow-up of Diagnostic Studies

Serial diagnostic studies in the months after acute respiratory failure may provide insight into the process and timing of lung repair. There is limited information available about serial pulmonary function studies, and especially diagnostic imaging and morphologic studies during recovery from acute respiratory failure treated with mechanical ventilation.

Pulmonary Function Testing

Several studies have looked at the results of serial pulmonary function testing after survival from acute respiratory failure associated with ARDS or COPD. The studies of COPD patients benefit from baseline pulmonary function tests before onset of respiratory failure, and show that although recovery from mechanical ventilation is associated with an acute decrement of the forced expiratory volume in one second (FEV1), the majority of patients who survive the acute episode will return to their baseline pulmonary function [5, 6].

There have been two prospective studies of pulmonary function testing at uniform time points after recovery from ARDS [18, 19]. Unlike the studies in COPD, baseline pulmonary function tests were not available for survivors of ARDS, since most patients had no pre-morbid indication for testing. McHugh and associates enrolled 52 of 82 survivors of ARDS (63%), aiming to measure pulmonary function tests and self-perceived health scores at 2 weeks after extubation, and then again at 3 months, 6 months and one year [18]. The study showed that at extubation, forced vital capacity (FVC), total lung capacity (TLC) and diffusing capacity for carbon monoxide (DLCO) were all markedly reduced. There was significant improvement in pulmonary function tests between extubation and 3 months. Function improved a small amount more by 6 months, at which point the FVC was still reduced in 55% of patients studied, the TLC was reduced in 45%, and the DLCO was reduced in 79%. As previously reported, the degree of persisting impairment was mild in the majority of patients. There was no additional improvement between 6 and 12 months. In a more recent study, Herridge et al. enrolled 109 ARDS survivors in a 12 months follow-up study that included pulmonary function testing [19]. Of the 97 survivors at 12 months, 83 were evaluated (86% follow-up). Results were similar to those found by McHugh: patients had a mild restrictive defect and a moderate reduction in diffusion capacity at three months, with return of spirometry to the normal range in most patients by six months (median values were within 80% of predicted values) and continued improvement in diffusion capacity at between six months and one year.

Pathology

The only studies providing information on the long-term effects of mechanical ventilation on lung histology are of four survivors of ARDS. These investigations are quite limited, likely due to the invasive nature of obtaining tissue for evaluation. At 3 months, biopsies revealed interstitial fibrosis and infiltration of lymphocytes and plasma cells in one patient [20]. Biopsies taken between 9 and 10 months post-ARDS showed patchy interstitial fibrosis, hyperplasia of type II pneumocytes, and increased numbers of alveolar macrophages and interstitial lymphocytes in one subject, and relatively normal histology (except for residual alveolar wall thickening) in a second subject [21]. A report of two sequential biopsies in the same patient found that interstitial fibrosis was present early, and improved over time [22]. If these reports are generalizable, it appears that the increased cellularity, organization, and fibroblast proliferation with fibrosis described in the acute phase markedly improves in the recovery period.

Thoracic Imaging

There are few studies of the resolution of the radiographic changes coincident with acute respiratory failure in survivors of mechanical ventilation. These reports are limited to case series and prospective studies of patients recovering from ARDS. A review of 85 cases found that 19% of patients had persistent radiographic abnormalities at 3 or more months after extubation; the most common findings were bibasilar interstitial infiltrates and reticular changes [23]. In Herridge's et al. follow-up study of over 100 ARDS survivors, 20% of patients had radiographic abnormalities at 1 year, with findings of linear fibrosis, small bullous cysts, and isolated areas of pleural thickening [19].

There is only one study of the evolution of computed tomography (CT) abnormalities in survivors of ARDS. Following a protocol in which all patients with ARDS had chest CTs in the acute phase, Desai and colleagues performed follow-up CTs on 27 survivors, 110–267 days after intubation [24]. Investigators looked for four types of parenchymal changes, and visually quantified involvement to determine extent. Ground-glass opacities were identified in all patients in the acute phase of ARDS, with a median extent of 68%. Intense parenchymal opacification was also seen in all 27 patients in the acute phase, largely in dependent regions with a median extent of 13%. On follow-up CTs, ground glass opacities were seen in 17 of 27 patients but were not extensive (median extent of less than 1%). Twenty-three of 27 follow-up CTs demonstrated a coarse reticular pattern that distorted the underlying parenchyma, mainly in small anterior regions of the lung.

What have we learned from studies of diagnostic tests after recovery from acute respiratory failure and mechanical ventilation? For the most part, the abnormalities found in acute ARDS by pulmonary function testing, histology and radiology improve over time and stabilize by 6 to 12 months. It is possible that the method of mechanical ventilation may have an impact on the timing and degree of lung repair, although no data are currently available to support this hypothesis. CT imaging may provide a sensitive and non-invasive surrogate for lung histology and may become a useful tool in future studies of lung recovery after acute respiratory failure.

Patient-centered Long-term Outcomes

Health-related Quality of Life

There are an increasing number of studies that have examined the long-term effect of ARDS or other critical illnesses requiring mechanical ventilation on the quality of life and health status of survivors. McHugh and colleagues, using the Sickness Impact Profile (SIP), demonstrated a significant decrement in health status among survivors of ARDS and showed that health status improved during the first 3 months after discharge from the hospital but remained relatively stable thereafter [18]. Davidson and colleagues, using the Medical Outcomes Study Short Form-36 (SF-36) and the Saint George's Respiratory Questionnaire, showed that there were significant decrements in most domains of health status among survivors of ARDS and that these decrements were significantly worse for patients with ARDS compared to patients with a comparable severity of illness from sepsis or trauma, but who did not meet criteria for ARDS [25] (Fig. 4). This study suggested decrements in physical function might be the most severe.

Similarly, in the largest and most complete follow-up study of ARDS survivors, Herridge found severe impairment in health status using the SF-36 at 3 months, with marked improvement at 6 months that continued to one year. Despite this improvement, at one year the median scores in all but one domain remained significantly reduced compared with age and gender matched controls [19]. Weinert and colleagues studied 24 survivors of ALI with the SF-36, also showing reductions in many domains of health status and particularly severe reductions in social functioning and mental health domains [26]. Finally, Angus and colleagues used the Quality of Well Being questionnaire to assess health status in a cohort of 200 previously healthy patients who developed ARDS and showed marked decrements in many domains of health status at 6 months and no significant change from 6 to 12 months [27].

In addition to ARDS, studies have demonstrated reductions in health status for patients with other critical illnesses requiring prolonged mechanical ventilation,

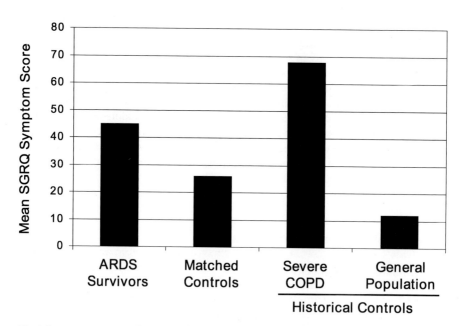

Fig. 4. Symptom scores on the St. George's Respiratory Questionnaire (SGRQ) of ARDS survivors, matched controls and historical controls. Note: lower scores denote lesser symptoms. COPD patients have a mean FEV1 of 1.3 L (45% predicted). From [23] with permission

including sepsis [28], multiple organ dysfunction [29], and general ICU patients [17, 30, 31]. Although results vary, these studies also suggest decrements in a wide range of the domains of health status.

A number of studies have attempted to define the predictors of decreased health status among survivors of ARDS or other critical illness. Several studies suggest that the health status prior to admission to the ICU is a strong predictor of the health status after discharge [32, 33]. A study by Wehler and colleagues showed that patients with the best health status prior to critical illness were more likely to have reductions in their health status while those patients with the lowest health status prior to admission to an ICU were actually more likely to improve from their baseline health status [32]. Similarly, Konopad and colleagues showed that among the very elderly, health status may actually increase from baseline after an ICU admission [34]. Severity of illness is also a significant predictor of health status after discharge from the ICU [18, 32, 33]. Increasing age predicts decreased health status after critical illness in some studies [32, 33], but other studies did not find age to be an important independent predictor of health status [17] and suggest that even those over the age of 70 who receive more than 30 days of intensive care are often satisfied with their health status and would choose to receive ICU care again if needed [30]. Schelling and colleagues showed that pulmonary function impairment predicted worse health status suggesting that treatment strategies designed to minimize lung injury may have diverse effects improving health status in ARDS survivors [35].

Exercise Tolerance

Exercise tolerance is another measure of functional ability. In the large follow-up study of ARDS survivors, Herridge evaluated the distance walked by subjects (the 6-minute walk test) at 3, 6 and 12 months post-ICU discharge [19]. Subjects' exercise tolerance improved over one year, with median distance increasing from 281 meters at 3 months, to 396 meters at 6 months, to 422 meters at 12 months. Despite this improvement, performance at one year remained markedly impaired, compared with the predicted distance of 640 meters. Most survivors assigned their exercise impairment to global muscle wasting and weakness; foot-drop, difficulty moving large joints and dyspnea were also cited.

Symptoms

Symptoms can be viewed as an additional patient-assessed outcome of import and interest to patients and their families. There have been a few studies documenting significant symptom burden for critically ill patients while in the ICU [36–38], but relatively few studies explicitly examining the symptoms of survivors of critical illness. Studies of health status among survivors of critical illness incorporate the effect that these symptoms have on individuals' lives, but it may also be important for investigators to explicitly examine the specific symptoms that are troubling to patients after a critical illness requiring mechanical ventilation as one way to understand the potential ways to decrease the symptom burden and the effect these symptoms have on patients' quality of life. For example, Angus and colleagues used the Quality of Well Being questionnaire to assess the quality of life of 132 ARDS survivors [27]. They found significant reductions in health status in the ARDS survivors and showed that the symptom domain of the Quality of Well Being questionnaire accounted for a larger decrement in quality of life than other domains including physical activity, social activity, and mobility. Symptoms accounted for approximately 70% of the reduction in health status seen in this study.

In the recent study involving comprehensive follow-up of ARDS patients, Herridge found that all subjects complained of muscle weakness and fatigue [19]. Similar to Herridge's findings, Angus et al. [27] reported that the most common symptoms were musculoskeletal, with 70% of patients describing weakness, pain and fatigue. Other bothersome symptoms included lower respiratory tract symptoms, as well as depression and anxiety, constitutional symptoms, and cognitive symptoms. These data provide some direction for investigators interested in decreasing the symptom burden experienced by survivors of ARDS.

Neuropsychological Outcomes

There has been increasing interest in examining the effect of critical illness, and especially ARDS, on the cognitive, emotional, and psychological functioning of survivors. There is mounting evidence that suggests that patients who survive critical illness may be left with decreased functioning in these realms. Hopkins and colleagues examined the cognitive functioning of 55 ARDS survivors showing that at hospital discharge all 55 patients had significant impairment in cognitive and affective functioning [39]. However, much more concerning was the finding that at 1 year after discharge from the hospital, 30% of patients still had generalized cognitive dysfunction and 78% had decrements in one or more of the following areas: attention, memory, concentration, and mental processing speed [39]. These authors attempted to identify predictors of cognitive impairment and were limited by their small sample size and by the collinearity of many of the important potential predictors such as duration of mechanical ventilation, severity of underlying lung injury, severity of desaturations in the ICU, duration of desaturations in the ICU, duration and amount of sedation. Nonetheless, their analysis did show an association between the continuous oxygen saturation measurements and the severity of cognitive deficits [39]. Another study assessed cognitive function in 46 ARDS survivors sometime between 1 and 12 years after the ARDS (with a median of 6 years) and showed that 24% had mild or moderate cognitive impairment [40]. This study suggested significant impact of this impairment on patients' lives by showing that 0 of 11 patients with cognitive impairment had returned to work while 27 of 35 patients without cognitive impairment had returned to work [40].

There has also been recent research looking at the prevalence and predictors of post-traumatic stress disorder (PTSD) after mechanical ventilation for ARDS. Schelling and colleagues used a questionnaire called the Post Traumatic Stress Syndrome 10-Questions Inventory (PTSS-10) with 80 survivors of ARDS with a median time since ARDS of 4 years and excluded patients with head trauma or pre-existing neurological or psychiatric diseases [40]. These authors found that 28% of the ARDS survivors had a PTSS-10 score above the cut-off for PTSD, a significantly higher proportion than two control groups: patients who had undergone maxillofacial surgery and German United Nations soldiers who had experienced prolonged service in Cambodia [40]. These authors showed that if patients reported memories of traumatic experiences during their ICU stay, including memories of respiratory distress, feelings of anxiety, pain, or nightmares, they were more likely to have symptoms of PTSD.

It remains unclear exactly what aspects of mechanical ventilation or ALI predispose patients to long-term neuropsychological effects. Hopkins and colleagues provide some data suggesting it may correlate with desaturations [39]. Nelson and colleagues performed a cross-sectional study of 24 survivors of ALI that showed significant correlations between both symptoms of depression and symptoms of PTSD and a number of variables including days in the ICU, days on mechanical ventilation, and days of sedation [41]. Interestingly, these authors did not show a correlation between symptoms of either depression or PTSD and APACHE III score. In an interesting preliminary study, Schelling and colleagues performed a small retrospective case-control study comparing patients who received corticosteroids for treatment of septic shock to similar patients who did not receive corticosteroids [42]. These authors found that the patients who received corticosteroids had a significantly lower incidence of PTSD (5 of 27 compared to 16 of 27) and significantly higher scores on the mental health index of the SF-36. Although all of these studies are limited by their small numbers and their observational designs, these three studies provide intriguing preliminary data to suggest that the way patients are managed in the ICU may have important effects on their long-term mental health and cognitive function. Further studies are needed to attempt to identify the components of long-term mechanical ventilation or critical illness that predispose patients to neuropsychological deficits and to tease apart the potential causes that include desaturations or decreased cerebral perfusion pressure during critical illness, inflammation and bio-trauma of sepsis and ARDS, duration and amount of sedation, and traumatic experiences during an ICU stay. Since increasing severity of illness will portend increases in many of these variables, differentiating between the importance of these collinear potential causes will be challenging. Furthermore, randomized controlled trials of different mechanical ventilation and sedation strategies should also examine the potential effects on these neuropsychological outcomes.

Return to Work after Mechanical Ventilation

For young survivors of critical illness, the ability to return to work is an important outcome. This is particularly salient for survivors of ARDS, who tend to be under age 50 (median age 39 in the Davidson study, and 45 years of age in the Herridge), compared with a median age over 65 years among COPD survivors (mean age 66 in the Seneff study [3], and median age of 70 in the Connors report [2]). Few follow-up studies have investigated return to work in ARDS survivors. At one year after hospital discharge, McHugh found that only 44% of subjects had returned to work [18]. Herridge's results were similar: at one year, 49% of survivors had returned to work, most to their original positions [19]. The reasons that were reported for not returning to previous employment included weakness and fatigue, difficulty walking due to large joint immobility (from heterotopic ossification) and foot-drop, work stress and early retirement. Rothenhausler et al. showed that decreased cognitive function was an important predictor of inability to return to work after recovery from acute respiratory failure [40].

Method of Ventilation and Outcomes

While it is likely that most of the long-term outcomes after mechanical ventilation are directly related to the disease causing acute respiratory failure, the method of ventilation and ICU supportive care have also been shown to affect morbidity and mortality. Although uncommon, upper airway trauma may develop as a result of endotracheal intubation either via translaryngeal or tracheostomy tubes [43]. This trauma may lead to tracheolaryngeal malacia or stenosis, which may present with progressive shortness of breath and may lead to respiratory failure, or the development of a tracheo-innominate artery fistula which presents as life threatening hemoptysis [44]. Endotracheal intubation is also a risk factor for nosocomial pneumonia, which has a high associated mortality. The manner of ventilation is also associated with acute patient outcomes; in ARDS, failure to use low tidal volumes is associated with increased mortality [45], multiple organ dysfunction, and pulmonary barotrauma. Additionally, most critically ill patients requiring endotracheal intubation receive significant doses of sedative and analgesic medications, drugs that are associated with hypotension, delirium, and increased ICU mortality.

Provision of ventilatory support without endotracheal intubation conceptually could reduce these complications of mechanical ventilation. There is convincing evidence from multiple randomized controlled multicenter trials of non-invasive positive pressure ventilation (NPPV) versus endotracheal intubation and mechanical ventilation in patients with acute respiratory failure from COPD that show improved mortality, morbidity, and shortened ICU and hospital stay [46]. NPPV may play a role in the support of patients with other causes of respiratory failure, including asthma, cardiogenic pulmonary edema, pneumonia, ARDS, and post-lung resection, but the data are still quite preliminary. To date, there are no studies of long-term outcomes of patients treated with NPPV, but it is conceivable that there would be a reduction in sequelae associated with intubation (airway trauma) and excessive sedation.

Conclusion

Most of the available data of long-term outcomes after mechanical ventilation deal with the survivors of ALI/ARDS. Long-term survival of these patients appears to be related more to the underlying risk condition (sepsis versus trauma) than to occurrence of ALI. Similarly, the long-term survival in patients with COPD and cardiogenic pulmonary edema is more related to the severity of the underlying condition than to the episode of acute respiratory failure itself.

In the last ten years, there has been an increasing amount of knowledge regarding long-term patient centered outcomes. Studies have revealed a significant impairment of health status, as assessed by a variety of methods, including measurements of health-related quality of life. Lung function in survivors of ALI shows substantial return towards normal function; impairment, when present, is typically mild-to-moderate and does not to appear to explain the reduced quality of life. Recent studies point to neuromuscular, neurocognitive and neuropsychologic abnormalities, which persist at one year, as being the sequelae most troublesome to survivors.

It is extremely difficult to assign causation for the long-term sequelae in survivors of critical illness who have received mechanical ventilation based on our current limited knowledge. It is likely that most of the long-term complications after recovery are caused by the underlying disease process that leads to respiratory failure, but there are many ways in which ICU management, including the method of ventilation, may affect both short and long term outcomes. For example, in addition to increasing hospital mortality, failure to use lung protective ventilation with low tidal volumes may affect lung injury and the degree of successful repair. It is also conceivable that the sustained systemic inflammation from injurious ventilation may affect end-organ function in the long-term as well as short-term, including central nervous system and neuromuscular function.

Studies are now needed to link the acute events occurring during the period of critical illness with the longer term sequelae in order to identify modifiable factors and allow strategies that will prevent or minimize these burdensome residua.

References

1. Esteban A, Anzueto A, Frutos F, et al (2002) Characteristics and outcomes in adult patients receiving mechanical ventilation: a 28-day international study. JAMA 287–345–355
2. Connors AF Jr, Dawson NV, Thomas C, et al (1996) Outcomes following acute exacerbation of severe chronic obstructive lung disease. Am J Respir Crit Care Med 154:959–967
3. Seneff Mg, Wagner DP, Wagner RP, et al (1995) Hospital and 1-year survival of patients admitted to intensive care units with acute exacerbation of chronic obstructive pulmonary disease. JAMA 274:1852–1857
4. Weiss SM, Hudson LD (1994) Outcome from respiratory failure. Crit Care Clin 10:197–215
5. Gottleib LS, Balchum OJ (1973) Course of chronic obstructive pulmonary disease following first onset of respiratory failure. Chest 63:5–8
6. Martin TR, Lewis SW, Albert RK (1982) The prognosis of patients with chronic obstructive pulmonary diseases after hospitalization for acute respiratory failure. Chest 82:310–314
7. Almagro P, Calbo E, Ochoa de Echagüen A, et al (2002) Mortality after hospitalization for COPD. Chest 121:1441–1448
8. Luhr OR, Antonsen K, Karlsson M, et al (1999) Incidence and mortality after acute respiratory failure and acute respiratory distress syndrome in Sweden, Denmark, and Iceland. Am J Respir Crit Care Med 159:1849–1861
9. Rubenfeld GD, Caldwell EC, Martin DM, Steinberg KP, Hudson LD (2002) The incidence of acute lung injury (ALI) in the US: results of the King County Lung Injury Project. Am J Respir Crit Care Med 165:A-219 (abst)

10. Suntharalingam G, Regan K, Keogh BF, Morgan CJ, Evans TW (2001) Influence of direct and indirect etiology on acute outcome and 6-month functional recovery in acute respiratory distress syndrome. Crit Care Med 29:562–566
11. Milberg J, Davis D, Steinberg K, Hudson LD (1995) Improved survival in patients with ARDS: 1983–1993. JAMA 272:306–309
12. Abel SJC, Finney SJ, Brett SJ, Keogh BF, Morgan CJ, Evans TW (1998) Reduced mortality in association with the acute respiratory distress syndrome (ARDS). Thorax 53:292–294
13. Jardin F, Fellahi J-L, Beauchet A, Vieillard-Baron A, Loubières Y, Page B (1999) Improved prognosis of acute respiratory distress syndrome 15 years on. Intensive Care Med 25:936–941
14. Davidson TA, Rubenfeld GD, Caldwell ES, Hudson LD, Steinberg KS (1999) The effect of acute respiratory distress syndrome on long-term survival. Am J Respir Crit Care Med 160:1839–1842
15. Wiener RS, Moses HW, Richeson JF, Gatewood RP Jr (1987) Hospital and long-term survival of patients with acute pulmonary edema associated with coronary artery disease. Am J Cardiol 60:33–35
16. Adnet F, LeTournelin P, LeBerre A, et al (2001) In-hospital and long-term prognosis of elderly patients requiring endotracheal intubation for life-threatening presentation of cardiogenic pulmonary edema. Crit Care Med 29:891–895
17. Chelluri L, Grenvik A, Silverman M (1995) Intensive care for critically ill elderly: mortality, costs, and quality of life: review of the literature. Arch Intern Med 155:1013–1022
18. McHugh LG, Milberg JA, Whitcomb ME, Schoene RB, Maunder RJ, Hudson LD (1994) Recovery of function in survivors of the acute respiratory distress syndrome. Am J Respir Crit Care Med 150:90–94
19. Herridge MS, Cheung AM, Tansey CM, et al (2003) One year outcomes in survivors of the acute respiratory distress syndrome. N Engl J Med 348:683–693
20. Alberts WM, Priest GR, Moser KM (1983) The outlook for survivors of ARDS. Chest 84:272–274
21. Lakshminarayan S, Stanford RE, Petty TL (1976) Prognosis after recovery from adult respiratory distress syndrome. Am Rev Respir Dis 113:7–16
22. Mittermayer C, Hassenstein J, Riede UN (1978) Is shock-induced lung fibrosis reversible? A report on recovery from "shock-lung". Pathol Res Pract 162:73–87
23. Lee CM, Hudson LD (2001) Long-term outcomes after ARDS. Semin Respir Crit Care Med 22:327–336
24. Desai SR, Wells AU, Rubens MB, Evans TW, Hansell DM (1999) Acute respiratory distress syndrome: CT abnormalities at long-term follow-up. Radiology 210:29–35
25. Davidson TA, Caldwell ES, Curtis JR, Hudson LD, Steinberg KP (1999) Reduced quality of life in survivors of acute respiratory distress syndrome compared with critically ill control patients. JAMA 281:354–360
26. Weinert CR, Gross CR, Kangas JR, Bury CL, Marinelli WA (1997) Health-related quality of life after acute lung injury. Am J Respir Crit Care Med 156:1120–1128
27. Angus DC, Musthafa AA, Clermont G, et al (2001) Quality-adjusted survival in the first year after the acute respiratory distress syndrome. Am J Respir Crit Care Med 163:1389–1394
28. Heyland DK, Hopman W, Coo H, et al (2000) Long-term health-related quality of life in survivors of sepsis. Short Form 36: a valid and reliable measure of health-related quality of life. Crit Care Med 28:3599–605
29. Pettila V, Kaarlola A, Makelainen A (2000) Health-related quality of life of multiple organ dysfunction patients one year after intensive care. Intensive Care Med 26:1473–1479
30. Montuclard L, Garrouste-Orgeas M, Timsit JF, Misset B, De Jonghe B, Carlet J (2000) Outcome, functional autonomy, and quality of life of elderly patients with a long-term intensive care unit stay. Crit Care Med 28:3389–3395
31. Welsh CH, Thompson K, Long-Krug S (1999) Evaluation of patient-perceived health status using the Medical Outcomes Survey Short-Form 36 in an intensive care unit population. Crit Care Med 27:1466–1471

32. Wehler M, Martus P, Geise A, et al (2001) Changes in quality of life after medical intensive care. Intensive Care Med 27:154–159
33. Mata GV, Fernandez RR, Carmona AG (1992) Factors related to quality of life 12 months after discharge from an intensive care unit. Crit Care Med 20:1257–1262
34. Konopad E, Noseworthy TW, Johnston R, Shustack A, Grace M (1995) Quality of life measures before and one year after admission to an intensive care unit. Crit Care Med 23:1653–1659
35. Schelling G, Stoll C, Vogelmeier C, et al (2000) Pulmonary function and health-related quality of life in a sample of long-term survivors of the acute respiratory distress syndrome. Intensive Care Med 26:1304–1311
36. Nelson JE, Meier DE, Oei EJ, et al (2001) Self-reported symptom experience of critically ill cancer patients receiving intensive care. Crit Care Med 29:277–282
37. Puntillo KA (1990) Pain experience of intensive care unit patients. Heart and Lung 19:525–533
38. The SUPPORT Principal Investigators (1995) A controlled trial to improve care for seriously ill hospitalized patients: the study to understand prognoses and preferences for outcomes and risks of treatments (SUPPORT). JAMA 274:1591–1598
39. Hopkins RO, Weaver LK, Pope D, Orme JF, Bigler ED, Larson LV (1999) Neuropsychological sequelae and impaired health status in survivors of severe acute respiratory distress syndrome. Am J Respir Crit Care Med 160:50–56
40. Rothenhausler HB, Ehrentraut S, Stoll C, Schelling G, Kapfhammer HP (2001) The relationship between cognitive performance and employment and health status in long-term survivors of the acute respiratory distress syndrome: results of an exploratory study. Gen Hosp Psychiatry 23:90–96
41. Nelson BJ, Weinert CR, Bury CL, Marinelli WA, Gross CR (2000) Intensive care unit drug use and subsequent quality of life in acute lung injury patients. Crit Care Med 28:3626–3630
42. Schelling G, Stoll C, Kapfhammer HP, et al (1999) The effect of stress doses of hydrocortisone during septic shock on posttraumatic stress disorder and health-related quality of life in survivors. Crit Care Med 27:2678–2683
43. Pingleton SK (1988) Complications of acute respiratory failure. Am Rev Respir Dis 137:1463–1493
44. Stauffer JL, Silvestri RC (1982) Complications of Endotracheal Intubation, Tracheostomy and Artificial Airways. Respir Care 27:417–434
45. The Acute Respiratory Distress Syndrome Network (2000) Ventilation with lower tidal volumes as compared with traditional tidal volumes for acute lung injury and the acute respiratory distress syndrome. N Engl J Med 342:1301–1308
46. Hill N (2001) Noninvasive mechanical ventilation for post acute care. Clin Chest Med 22:35–54

Understanding and Changing the Practice of Mechanical Ventilation in the Community

G. D. Rubenfeld

Introduction

There is a considerable body of evidence that patients frequently do not receive optimal medical care. Failure to employ thrombolytics, beta-blockers, aspirin, and angiotensin-converting enzyme inhibitors where appropriate in patients with acute myocardial infarction may cause as many as 18,000 deaths per year in the United States [1, 2]. Twenty-two to 45 percent of asthma patients in 4 European countries were treated with inappropriate beta-agonist monotherapy and 9–24% of asthma patients were on inadequate doses of inhaled corticosteroids [3]. Outpatients frequently have hypertension inadequately managed, preventive services neglected, and diagnoses such as depression missed [4, 5]. Inadequacies are not limited to failure to provide necessary treatments. Antibiotics, hysterectomies, cardiac pacemakers, and coronary angiography have all been shown to be overused in inappropriate cases [2].

These observations have led to strong responses from the academic, medical, consumer, and health care payer communities. In November 1998, the American Association of Medical Colleges and the American Medical Association convened a Clinical Research Summit devoted to establishing broad, national goals in clinical research. One of the principal recommendations of this commission was to develop a "broadened agenda of clinical research [that is], related more specifically to health outcomes and [is] designed to assess the effectiveness of methods for incorporating evidence-based practice into clinical care" [6]. Additional recommendations were to place an increased emphasis on understanding the delivery of care and the epidemiology of disease particularly as it occurs in the community outside of selected academic medical centers. A recent publication by the Institute of Medicine, "Crossing the quality chasm : a new health system for the 21st century", outlined the case that modern health care frequently fails to deliver optimal medical care even in the absence of access and financial barriers to care. This widely cited document charges the United States Department of Health and Human Services to "establish and maintain a comprehensive program aimed at making scientific evidence more useful and accessible to clinicians and patients" [7]. This chapter will review the issue of translating clinical research into clinical practice with specific emphasis on studies related to mechanical ventilation and critical care.

Table 1. Approaches to implementing behavioral change?

Approach	Theories	Focus	Intervention strategies	Example
Focus on internal processes				
Educational [65]	Adult learning theories	Intrinsic motivation of professionals	Problem based learning	Mechanical ventilation course using hands-on demonstrations
Epidemiological [66]	Cognitive theories	Rational information seeking and decision making	Evidence based guideline development and dissemination	Consensus conference on mechanical ventilation
Marketing [67]	Health promotion, innovation and social marketing theories	Attractive product adapted to needs of target audience	Needs assessment, adapting change proposals to local needs	Targeted intervention to increase use of semi-recumbent positioning based on focus groups of clinicians
Focus on external influences				
Behavioral [68]	Learning theory	Controlling performance by external stimuli	Audit and feedback, reminders, economic incentives	Physician prompt that patients have passed a trial of spontaneous breathing
Social interaction [69, 70]	Social learning and innovation theories, social influence/power theories	Social influence of significant peers/role models	Peer review in local networks, opinion leaders, academic detailing	Regionally prominent physician, nurse, and respiratory therapist who meet with local clinicians in small groups to convince them to use weaning protocol
Organizational [71]	Management theories, system theories	Creating structural and organizational conditions to improve care	Re-engineering care process, total quality management, team building, changes to systems	Development of a weaning team that consults on all patients mechanically ventilated for more than 72 hours.
Coercive [72]	Economic, power, and learning theories	Control and pressure, external motivation	Regulations, laws, budgeting, legal procedures	Hospital removes inhaled nitric oxide from formulary.

Models of Changing Clinical Practice

There are a number of conceptual models describing the processes that individuals and organizations go through as they change behavior. Not surprisingly, these models come from fields that are intimately familiar with trying to change knowledge and behavior: psychology, education, health promotion, and marketing. Understanding how to get people to write better, eat differently, stop smoking, or buy a brand of milk is not conceptually different than getting clinicians to treat myocardial infarctions or asthma correctly. Models for understanding behavioral change are important because they lead to strategies for changing behavior (Table 1). Although there is some overlap, it is useful to think of these models as falling into broad categories: educational, epidemiological, and marketing strategies (targeting an individual's internal factors) and behavioral, social, organizational, and coercive (targeting factors external to the individual).

Educational models are the ones physicians are most familiar with. Adult learning theory stresses the importance of interactive educational experiences over passive learning in lectures. Examples include Advanced Cardiac Life Support or Advance Trauma Life Support courses taught with individual skill stations [8]. Epidemiological models focus on synthesizing and presenting the evidence on optimal practice. Examples include published meta-analyses, the Cochrane reviews, and formal guideline developing activities. Large data warehouses of these resources are available on the internet [9, 10]. Marketing strategies rely on research to understand the values, concerns, aspirations, needs, and knowledge of their target audience [11]. Marketers realize that selling a product often does not rely on informing their audience about its benefits, but in convincing the target that they will be more popular if they buy it or 'left out' if they don't. Similarly, social marketers, trying to 'sell smoking cessation or appropriate antibiotic use must provide the audience with a reason to act that may have little to do with the evidence about benefits of the action.

A number of models try to influence behavior by using external factors to influence behavior. Behavioral theory uses feedback and stimulus-response to affect behavior such as automatic reminders or clinician audit and feedback reports. Social theory takes advantage of information about how individuals behave in groups. A model developed by Everett M. Rogers called the Diffusion-Adoption model has been used to study changes in use of hybrid seeds, computer technology, and magnetic resonance imaging [12]. Individuals fit into broad categories of: Innovators, Early Adopters, Early Majority, Late Majority, and Laggards based on their willingness to adopt new practices. Understanding which group a clinician fits into will let you understand the barriers to changing their practice. Organizational approaches are adapted from the Total Quality Management and other quality improvement methods used by corporations. The Institute of Healthcare Improvement (IHI) has championed these practices in healthcare [13]. Finally, coercive techniques rely on regulations, fiscal, or legal constraints or incentives to change practice.

There have been four recent extensive meta-reviews (reviews of reviews and meta-analyses) evaluating which techniques are most effective at changing clinical

Table 2. Evidence base for various behavior change strategies

Weak	Moderately or variably effective	Relatively strong or Consistently effective
Passive education by distribution of guidelines or continuing medical education lectures or unsolicited written material	Economic incentives Audit and feedback Local opinion leaders	Multifaceted interventions combining 2 or more of (feedback, reminders, education, marketing) Academic detailing Reminders or prompting

adapted from [14–17]

practice [14–17]. The authors of these reviews cite common problems with the literature: publication bias, lack of repeat studies to validate methods, and weak study designs. However, the reviews reach remarkably similar conclusions. They rank interventions to change behavior in health professionals into three categories based on the evidence of their effectiveness (Table 2). It is noteworthy that academic clinicians spend a great deal of time engaged in activities known to be only marginally effective at changing clinical practice: lectures and passive dissemination of written materials.

Implementation Research in Critical Care

Many medical specialties have responded to the observations that clinicians fail to incorporate research into their practice by creating a research program directed specifically at this issue. With the notable exception of cardiology, which has devoted extensive resources to understanding the care of patients with ischemic heart disease, most other aspects of care for critically ill patients have not been studied extensively with regard to these issues [18–20].

For example, a recent study by Cabana and colleagues systematically reviewed the extensive body of literature studying barriers to implementation of effective treatments and guidelines [21]. The authors developed a conceptual model for categorizing barriers to changing clinical behavior. A wide range of clinical topics were reviewed based on the existing literature including barriers to appropriate preventive care, obstetric care, pain control, and use of thrombolytic therapy. Similarly, studies evaluating the knowledge, attitudes, and behavior of a broad range of clinicians including general practitioners, cardiologists, radiologists, and surgeons, were reviewed. However, this extensive review did not identify a single study of the barriers to implementation of effective therapy in critical care. There is no mention of common critical illness syndromes such as sepsis, acute respiratory distress syndrome (ARDS), or acute respiratory failure. Finally, no studies of intensivists, intensive care nurses, or respiratory therapists were reported in this review. In a series of review articles published as a supplement to *Chest* titled

"Translating Guidelines Into Practice: Implementation and Physician Behavior Change", only two examples from critical care are discussed: antimicrobial prescribing in the ICU and treatment of myocardial infarction [22, 23].

There may be a perfectly acceptable reason why critical care has not produced a body of research about changing clinical practice in the ICU. Intensivists have grown used to making clinical decisions based on physiologic rationale in the absence of evidence demonstrating an improvement in outcome. Unlike our colleagues in cardiology and oncology, intensivists do not enjoy the luxury of a rich evidence base of positive clinical trials. As typical examples, consider the conclusions of recent reviews on two perennial questions in critical care: "Is colloid better than crystalloid for fluid resuscitation?" and "Is total parenteral nutrition (TPN) beneficial to critically ill patients?"

- "There is no evidence from randomized controlled trials that resuscitation with colloids reduces the risk of death compared to crystalloids in patients with trauma, burns and following surgery" [24].
- "While TPN may have a positive effect on nutritional end points and on even minor complications, the overall results of our meta-analysis fail to support a benefit of TPN on mortality or major complication rates, particularly in critically ill patients" [25].

Statements of evidence such as these allow intensivists to justify a range of therapeutic decisions. In the absence of compelling evidence of harm or benefit, physicians will base decisions on biologic rationale, experience, and personal values about cost-effectiveness [26]. If, in fact, there are very few practices in critical care of demonstrable benefit, then the question of implementing practice is moot.

Lack of compelling evidence of benefit is not the only factor that distinguishes critical care from other areas of medicine where implementation research has been studied. Although not unique in this respect, critical care relies on multiple disciplines. The intensive care unit (ICU) is essentially an organizational innovation that focuses technology and experienced clinicians into a specific location in the hospital. Intensivists rely on and work closely with primary care physicians, consulting specialists, ICU nurses, respiratory therapists, pharmacists, nutritionists, and other clinicians in the ICU. The knowledge, attitudes, and behaviors of all of these clinicians must be considered in interventions designed to implement effective ICU care. The multi-disciplinary nature of critical care must be considered in designing interventions to change behavior [27]. The SUPPORT study, a large multicenter trial designed to change clinical practice has been criticized because its intervention failed to consider the organizational structure of the ICU and interactions between clinicians [28].

Investigators studying the translation of research findings into practice in the ICU must consider the differences in barriers and facilitators likely to be encountered when evaluating interventions targeted at the system level (intensivist coverage, computerized orders, rounding pharmacist, step-down unit) versus the patient level (lung protective ventilation, activated protein C, tight glucose control). For example, identifying factors affecting structure of the ICU may require surveying the hospital chief executive officer (CEO), non-intensivist physicians who admit to the ICU, and hospital financial staff. Large capital investments, hospital-wide policy changes, and legal issues may be involved. Patient-level changes in practice may involve system factors, particularly system solutions.

Evidence and Consensus

Since evidence of benefit is the first step in translating research into practice, it is important to ask which aspects of mechanical ventilation are known to be beneficial. The amount of evidence it takes to convince individual clinicians may vary and will certainly vary with the plausibility, cost, risks, and benefits of the proposed treatment [26]. We need more compelling evidence to convince us to use inhaled nitric oxide or prone positioning in patients with ARDS than to provide oxygen supplementation to patients with acute hypoxemic respiratory failure and a PaO_2 of 40 mmHg. In fact, the purpose of this chapter is to present the current evidence for various aspects of mechanical ventilation. A number of consensus conferences on mechanical ventilation have been published over the years [29–35]. This chapter is not focused on the evidence base or consensus on the practice of mechanical ventilation but on research directed at understanding its translation into practice in the community. Research in this area includes: studies that evaluate current practice in the community, studies that explore the barriers and facilitators to changing practice, and studies that evaluate specific interventions to change the practice of mechanical ventilation.

To identify articles that address these topics the following MEDLINE search strategy was used: Artificial respiration was combined with each of the following: Guideline adherence, physician's practice patterns; questionnaires; medical audit; and surveys. This list was screened for articles that covered one of the three topics: understanding current practice, barriers to changing practice, effective strategies to change practice. It is important to note that some implementation research occurs without publication in mainstream academic research journals. For example, the Institute for Healthcare Improvement is a non-profit organization that sponsors workshops to help clinicians improve the quality of care they provide [13]. Many of these quality improvement projects have focused on critical care interventions. The projects are usually single institution, before-after studies and the results are not peer reviewed. Nevertheless, this is an important source of information about projects designed to change clinical practice at single sites or within collaborative of hospitals.

Understanding Current Practice

There are probably more data on current mechanical ventilation practice in the ICU than any other aspect of critical care. There are several techniques for measuring process of care. Clinicians can be surveyed about their attitudes about using different treatments or their practice in hypothetical case vignettes. Charts can be abstracted retrospectively by protocol by research staff. Clinicians can report on their practice prospectively. Administrative databases collected for billing or administrative purposes can be analyzed. As with all research methods each approach has specific benefits, limitations, and costs. Surveys of clinicians' behavior to measure their practice is notoriously unreliable at capturing their actual practice. Analysis of administrative data has been used to understand the outcomes of mechanical ventilation in large patient populations, but does not provide detailed data on patient management or diagnosis [36–40].

Several recent studies have explored practice in broad populations of mechanically ventilated patients or patients with acute lung injury (ALI) [41–44]. These studies used a combination of self report of practice by clinicians and survey of attitudes to describe clinical practice. The studies did not specifically compare patients' care with current practice recommendations. Despite recommendations and clinical experience that mechanical ventilation should be customized for individual diseases, patients received remarkably similar average tidal volume (V_T), positive end-expiratory pressure (PEEP), and FiO2 regardless of whether they were diagnosed with ALI, ARDS, acute hypoxemic respiratory failure, or chronic obstructive pulmonary disease (COPD) (Fig. 1). In one study, 63% of patients managed on assisted mechanical ventilation received V_T < 10 ml/kg, but patients diagnosed by their physicians with ALI were no more likely to receive low V_T than other patients [41]. Two studies have evaluated the use of long-term mechanical ventilation in the community, documenting the resources used by this population of patients with primarily neuromuscular disease and a shift from home-based care to institutional care [45, 46]. Considerable variability in the process of performing weaning parameters and in documentation of patient-ventilator system checks have been noted [47]. There is surprisingly little research documenting the penetration of non-invasive ventilation (NIV) into current practice. Doherty and Greenstone surveyed 268 hospitals in the United Kingdom and found considerable regional variation in the availability of NIV [48]. Barriers to implementation of NIV included lack of staff training, inconsistent funding to purchase equipment, and lack of training [48]. In a single site audit at a teaching hospital, Sinuff and colleagues found that NIV was used by physicians of different training levels in various settings within the hospital and found important areas for improving the quality of documentation, monitoring, and implementation of non-invasive ventilation [49].

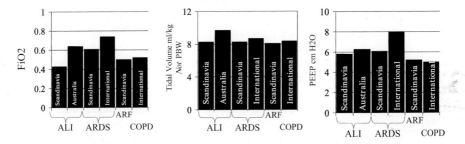

Fig. 1. Comparison of FiO2 tidal volume, and PEEP, in large cohorts of mechanically ventilated patients. ARF=acute respiratory failure. COPD = chronic obsctructive pulmonary disease. Scandinavia, Australia, and International are from [44, 43, 41], respectively.

Respondents to a physician questionnaire indicated a broad range of approaches to weaning and tracheostomy with inter-country variability [41]. Although physicians' attitudes to various weaning regimens were assessed, there was no attempt to identify how many patients received a standardized approach to weaning readiness assessment. In a study of patients with traumatic brain injury, investigators found that guideline recommendations to avoid hyperventilation were frequently violated at community hospitals and during transport to a treatment center [50]. A survey of critical care physician members of the American Thoracic Society reported a wide range of V_T used to treat patients with ARDS [51]. Wong and colleagues surveyed Canadian intensivists about their attitudes toward using oxygen in patients in the ICU. Although the study found that all responding physicians believed that oxygen contributed to complications in the ICU, there was wide variability in the tradeoffs between inspired oxygen and hemoglobin saturation [26, 52]. Finally, survey data from 1994 on withdrawal of mechanical ventilation showed significant variability in practice in withdrawing mechanical ventilation and, at least at the time of the survey, that 15% of respondents almost never withdrew mechanical ventilation when limiting life sustaining treatment in the ICU [53].

Two important Franco-Canadian studies based on a survey of ventilator circuit and secretion management practices have been performed. These showed considerable inter-country variability in physicians' stated practice regarding intubation route, ventilator circuit change frequency, humidification system, endotracheal suction system, subglottic secretion drainage, kinetic therapy beds, and body position [54, 55]. This study validated the finding that guidelines and consensus recommendations have little impact on practice even when practice is assessed by survey. Many centers reported practice that deviated from recommended evidence based standards. In a study that combined patient level data and survey data from physicians, Heyland et al. identified NIV, subglottic secretion drainage endotracheal tubes, kinetic bed therapy, small bowel feedings, and elevation of the head of the bed as effective preventive treatments for ventilator associated pneumonia (VAP) that were not being used in a set of Canadian ICUs [56].

Barriers to Changing Practice

A considerable body of literature exists evaluating why clinicians do not follow evidence based clinical practice guidelines [21]. The model proposed by Cabana and colleagues after reviewing the literature in this area identified seven categories of barriers: lack of awareness or lack of familiarity with the guidelines; lack of agreement, lack of self-efficacy, lack of outcome expectancy, or the inertia of previous practice; and external barriers (usually factors associated with the structure of the guideline or local systems of care). Relatively few studies have specifically focused on the research question about why certain ventilator practices are implemented or not. The surveys of French and Canadian intensivists asked about barriers to using the various ventilator circuit and secretion management practices across 6 domains: adverse effects, cost, patient discomfort, nurse inconvenience, not available, and other. They found that the barriers to use varied across the different treatments and noted that there were important differences between

France and Canada regarding who had decisional responsibility. In Canada, many decisions were made by respiratory therapists who have no equivalent in the French ICUs [54, 55]. Several barriers to implementing a protocol based weaning program were identified including failure to have consistent staffing of respiratory therapists in the same ICU, failure of respiratory therapists to report patient status at shift change, and individual physician reasons to exclude patients from the protocolized spontaneous breathing trial [57]. Qualitative research techniques are particularly useful to explore barriers to implementing practice. Focus groups and surveys have been used to explore barriers to implementing semi-recumbent positioning in ALI [58]. This study showed that nurses and physicians had very different perceptions of the major barriers. Nurses believed that physician failure to specify the patient's position and physicians identified nursing preference as the major barrier to using semi-recumbent positioning. It is interesting to note that most respondents identified education as the most important technique to change body positioning practice although this is known to be only marginally effective.

Effective Strategies to Change Practice

It is important to distinguish studies that demonstrate benefit of a particular approach to mechanical ventilation from studies that are primarily interested in implementing this approach. Two studies by Ely clarify this distinction. In the first, a randomized controlled trial, the value of a daily weaning screen followed by a protocolized spontaneous breathing trial and a physician prompt was shown to reduce duration of mechanical ventilation by 1.5 days [59]. In the second study, the investigators studied the effect of "graded, staged educational interventions" directed at respiratory therapists to implement the protocol found to be effective in the clinical trial [57]. Implementation research is *not* designed to identify effective treatment strategies. The research question is not whether a specific ventilator technique improves outcome this is presumed to be known. The question is whether this technique can be deployed in a larger community. The effect of the intervention on patient outcome is important, but is a secondary research question.

There have been no large scale, multicenter, community based programs to improve the quality of care to mechanically ventilated patients. A computerized decision support tool to direct mechanical ventilation in patients with ARDS was implemented in a randomized clinical trial at 10 academic sites, however, this study was directed as much at evaluating the efficacy of the ventilator strategy as the feasibility of using a computer to effect practice change [60]. Other models have been explored for changing ventilator practice. Pronovost and colleagues used a 'quality improvement' model to reduce failed extubations in a single ICU study [61]. Structural approaches including a nurse-practitioner run ICU for chronically critically ill patients and a ventilator team consult model have been explored to improve ventilator outcomes [62–64]. The evidence from other fields suggests that effective implementation studies of ventilator practices will require a multi-faceted approach that incorporates: local 'buy-in' of the treatment, local opinion leaders, staff education, audit and feedback, and timely prompts.

Conclusion

As the evidence base for clinical decisions in mechanical ventilation increases, investigators must devote attention to seeing that innovations in mechanical ventilation are translated into community practice. Evidence from other fields suggests that this will not be easy, particularly if the innovations involve protocols that use existing technology rather than new devices which will be promoted by a corporate developer. Unique barriers to implementing effective practice in mechanical ventilation are likely to be encountered. For example, differences in ICU organization mean that different clinicians have responsibility for ventilator management in each hospital. Implementing protocols for management, as opposed to simply convincing clinicians to prescribe a drug, may require more complex ongoing interventions.

An aggressive research program directed at understanding how current ventilator decisions are made, who makes them, and why effective strategies are or are not used should be started. Although several studies exist describing mechanical ventilation in broad populations, data have not been provided specifically oriented toward estimating the proportion of patients receiving care that deviates from published guidelines. Information about the use of NIV is particularly lacking. Future research directed at these questions can save lives while reducing costs and morbidity.

References

1. Chassin MR (1997) Assessing strategies for quality improvement. Health Aff (Millwood) 16:151–161
2. Chassin MR, Galvin RW (1998) The urgent need to improve health care quality. Institute of Medicine National Roundtable on Health Care Quality. JAMA 280:1000–1005
3. Veninga CC, Lagerlov P, Wahlstrom R, et al (1999) Evaluating an educational intervention to improve the treatment of asthma in four European countries. Drug Education Project Group. Am J Respir Crit Care Med 160:1254–1262
4. Wells KB, Hays RD, Burnam MA, Rogers W, Greenfield S, Ware JE Jr (1989) Detection of depressive disorder for patients receiving prepaid or fee-for-service care. Results from the Medical Outcomes Study. JAMA 262:3298–3302
5. Udvarhelyi IS, Jennison K, Phillips RS, Epstein AM (1991) Comparison of the quality of ambulatory care for fee-for-service and prepaid patients. Ann Intern Med 115:394–400
6. Heinig SJ, Quon AS, Meyer RE, Korn D (1999) The changing landscape for clinical research. Acad Med 74:726–745
7. Institute of Medicine (2001) Committee on Quality of Health Care in America. Crossing the quality chasm: a new health system for the 21st century. National Academy Press, Washington
8. Kaye W (1995) Research on ACLS training—which methods improve skill & knowledge retention? Respir Care 40:538–546
9. Ely EW, Meade MO, Haponik EF, et al (2001) Mechanical ventilator weaning protocols driven by nonphysician health-care professionals: evidence-based clinical practice guidelines. Chest 120 (6 Suppl):454S–463S
10. Meade MO, Ely EW (2002) Protocols to improve the care of critically ill pediatric and adult patients. JAMA 288:2601-2603
11. David SP, Greer DS (2001) Social marketing: application to medical education. Ann Intern Med 134:125–127

12. Gelijns A, Dawkins HV (1994) Institute of Medicine (US) Committee on Technological Innovation in Medicine. Adopting New Medical Technology. National Academy Press, Washington

13. The Institute for Healthcare Improvement. Available at: http://www.ihi.org/

14. Davis DA, Taylor-Vaisey A (1997) Translating guidelines into practice. A systematic review of theoretic concepts, practical experience and research evidence in the adoption of clinical practice guidelines. CMAJ 157:408–416

15. Bero LA, Grilli R, Grimshaw JM, Harvey E, Oxman AD, Thomson MA (1998) Closing the gap between research and practice: an overview of systematic reviews of interventions to promote the implementation of research findings. The Cochrane Effective Practice and Organization of Care Review Group. Br Med J 317:465–468

16. Smith WR (2000) Evidence for the effectiveness of techniques to change physician behavior. Chest 118 (2 Suppl):8S–17S

17. Davis D, O'Brien MA, Freemantle N, Wolf FM, Mazmanian P, Taylor-Vaisey A (1999) Impact of formal continuing medical education: do conferences, workshops, rounds, and other traditional continuing education activities change physician behavior or health care outcomes? JAMA 282:867–874

18. Krumholz HM, Radford MJ, Wang Y, Chen J, Heiat A, Marciniak TA (1998) National use and effectiveness of beta-blockers for the treatment of elderly patients after acute myocardial infarction: National Cooperative Cardiovascular Project. JAMA 280:623–629

19. O'Connor GT, Quinton HB, Traven ND, et al (1999) Geographic variation in the treatment of acute myocardial infarction: the Cooperative Cardiovascular Project. JAMA 281:627–633

20. Mehta RH, Montoye CK, Gallogly M, et al (2002) Improving quality of care for acute myocardial infarction: The Guidelines Applied in Practice (GAP) Initiative. JAMA 287:1269–1276

21. Cabana MD, Rand CS, Powe NR, et al (1999) Why don't physicians follow clinical practice guidelines? A framework for improvement. JAMA 282:1458–1465

22. Payne TH (2000) Computer decision support systems. Chest 118:47S–52S

23. Borbas C, Morris N, McLaughlin B, Asinger R, Gobel F (2000) The role of clinical opinion leaders in guideline implementation and quality improvement. Chest 118 :24S–32S

24. Alderson P, Schierhout G, Roberts I, Bunn F (2002) Colloids versus crystalloids for fluid resuscitation in critically ill patients (Cochrane Review). The Cochrane Library. Vol 1, Update Software, Oxford, CD:001208

25. Heyland DK, MacDonald S, Keefe L, Drover JW (1998) Total parenteral nutrition in the critically ill patient: a meta- analysis. JAMA 280:2013–2019

26. Rubenfeld GD (2001) Understanding why we agree on the evidence but disagree on the medicine. Respir Care 46:1442–1449

27. Curry SJ (2000) Organizational interventions to encourage guideline implementation. Chest 118 (2 Suppl):40S–46S

28. Lo B (1995) Improving care near the end of life. Why is it so hard? JAMA 274:1634–1636

29. Slutsky AS (1994) Consensus conference on mechanical ventilation—January 28-30, 1993 at Northbrook, Illinois, USA. Part 2. Intensive Care Med 20:150–162

30. Slutsky AS (1994) Consensus conference on mechanical ventilation—January 28-30, 1993 at Northbrook, Illinois, USA. Part I. European Society of Intensive Care Medicine, the ACCP and the SCCM. Intensive Care Med 20:64–79

31. Anonymous (1995) Consensus Conference III: Assessing innovations in mechanical ventilatory support. Conference held January 13-15, 1995 in Ixtapa, Mexico. Respir Care 40:926–993

32. Anonymous (1999) International consensus conferences in intensive care medicine: Ventilator-associated Lung Injury in ARDS. This official conference report was cosponsored by the American Thoracic Society, The European Society of Intensive Care Medicine, and The Societe de Reanimation de Langue Francaise, and was approved by the ATS Board of Directors, July 1999. Am J Respir Crit Care Med 160:2118–2124

33. Evans TW (2001) International Consensus Conferences in Intensive Care Medicine: non-invasive positive pressure ventilation in acute respiratory failure. Organised jointly by the

American Thoracic Society, the European Respiratory Society, the European Society of Intensive Care Medicine, and the Societe de Reanimation de Langue Francaise, and approved by the ATS Board of Directors, December 2000. Intensive Care Med 27:166–178

34. MacIntyre NR, Cook DJ, Ely EW Jr, et al (2001) Evidence-based guidelines for weaning and discontinuing ventilatory support: a collective task force facilitated by the American College of Chest Physicians; the American Association for Respiratory Care; and the American College of Critical Care Medicine. Chest 120 (6 Suppl):375S–395S

35. American Association for Respiratory Care (1992) ARC clinical practice guideline. Patient-ventilator system checks. Respir Care 37:882–886

36. Cohen IL, Lambrinos J (1995) Investigating the impact of age on outcome of mechanical ventilation using a population of 41,848 patients from a statewide database. Chest 107:1673–1680

37. Dewar DM, Kurek CJ, Lambrinos J, Cohen IL, Zhong Y (1999) Patterns in costs and outcomes for patients with prolonged mechanical ventilation undergoing tracheostomy: an analysis of discharges under diagnosis-related group 483 in New York State from 1992 to 1996. Crit Care Med 27:2640–2647

38. Kurek CJ, Dewar D, Lambrinos J, Booth FV, Cohen IL (1998) Clinical and economic outcome of mechanically ventilated patients in New York State during 1993: analysis of 10,473 cases under DRG 475. Chest 114:214–222

39. Kurek CJ, Cohen IL, Lambrinos J, Minatoya K, Booth FV, Chalfin DB (1997) Clinical and economic outcome of patients undergoing tracheostomy for prolonged mechanical ventilation in New York state during 1993: analysis of 6,353 cases under diagnosis-related group 483. Crit Care Med 25:983–988

40. Cohen IL, Lambrinos J, Fein IA (1993) Mechanical ventilation for the elderly patient in intensive care. Incremental changes and benefits. JAMA 269:1025–1029

41. Esteban A, Anzueto A, Alia I, et al (2000) How is mechanical ventilation employed in the intensive care unit? An international utilization review. Am J Respir Crit Care Med 161:1450–1458

42. Esteban A, Anzueto A, Frutos F, et al (2002) Characteristics and outcomes in adult patients receiving mechanical ventilation: a 28-day international study. JAMA 287:345–355

43. Bersten AD, Edibam C, Hunt T, Moran J, Group TA (2002) Incidence and mortality of acute lung injury and the acute respiratory distress syndrome in three Australian states. Am J Respir Crit Care Med 165:443–448

44. Luhr OR, Antonsen K, Karlsson M, et al (1999) Incidence and mortality after acute respiratory failure and acute respiratory distress syndrome in Sweden, Denmark, and Iceland. The ARF Study Group. Am J Respir Crit Care Med 159:1849–1861

45. Adams AB, Whitman J, Marcy T (1993) Surveys of long-term ventilatory support in Minnesota: 1986 and 1992. Chest 103:1463–1469

46. Gasperini M, Clini E, Zaccaria S (1998) Mechanical ventilation in chronic respiratory insufficiency: report on an Italian nationwide survey. The Italian Telethon Committee and the AIPO Study Group on Pulmonary Rehabilitation and Intensive Care. Monaldi Arch Chest Dis 53:394–399

47. Soo Hoo GW, Park L (2002) Variations in the measurement of weaning parameters: a survey of respiratory therapists. Chest 121:1947–1955

48. Doherty MJ, Greenstone MA (1998) Survey of non-invasive ventilation (NIPPV) in patients with acute exacerbations of chronic obstructive pulmonary disease (COPD) in the UK. Thorax 53:863–866

49. Sinuff T, Cook D, Randall J, Allen C (2000) Noninvasive positive-pressure ventilation: a utilization review of use in a teaching hospital. CMAJ 163:969–973

50. Thomas SH, Orf J, Wedel SK, Conn AK (2002) Hyperventilation in traumatic brain injury patients: inconsistency between consensus guidelines and clinical practice. J Trauma 52:47–52

51. Carmichael LC, Dorinsky PM, Higgins SB, et al (1996) Diagnosis and therapy of acute respiratory distress syndrome in adults: an international survey. J Crit Care 11:9–18

52. Mao C, Wong DT, Slutsky AS, Kavanagh BP (1999) A quantitative assessment of how Canadian intensivists believe they utilize oxygen in the intensive care unit. Crit Care Med 27:2806–2811
53. Faber-Langendoen K (1994) The clinical management of dying patients receiving mechanical ventilation. A survey of physician practice. Chest 106:880–888
54. Cook D, Ricard JD, Reeve B, et al (2000) Ventilator circuit and secretion management strategies: a Franco-Canadian survey. Crit Care Med 28:3547–3554
55. Ricard JD, Cook D, Griffith L, Brochard L, Dreyfuss D (2002) Physicians' attitude to use heat and moisture exchangers or heated humidifiers: a Franco-Canadian survey. Intensive Care Med 28:719–725
56. Heyland DK, Cook DJ, Dodek PM (2002) Prevention of ventilator-associated pneumonia: current practice in Canadian intensive care units. J Crit Care17:161–167
57. Ely EW, Bennett PA, Bowton DL, Murphy SM, Florance AM, Haponik EF (1999) Large scale implementation of a respiratory therapist-driven protocol for ventilator weaning. Am J Respir Crit Care Med 159:439–446
58. Cook DJ, Meade MO, Hand LE, McMullin JP (2002) Toward understanding evidence uptake: semirecumbency for pneumonia prevention. Crit Care Med 30:1472–1477
59. Ely EW, Baker AM, Dunagan DP, et al (1996) Effect on the duration of mechanical ventilation of identifying patients capable of breathing spontaneously. N Engl J Med 335:1864–1869
60. East TD, Heermann LK, Bradshaw RL, et al (1999) Efficacy of computerized decision support for mechanical ventilation: results of a prospective multi-center randomized trial. Proc AMIA Symp 251–255
61. Pronovost PJ, Jenckes M, To M, et al (2002) Reducing failed extubations in the intensive care unit. Jt Comm J Qual Improv 28:595–604
62. Daly BJ, Rudy EB, Thompson KS, Happ MB (1991) Development of a special care unit for chronically critically ill patients. Heart Lung 20:45–51
63. Daly BJ, Phelps C, Rudy EB (1991) A nurse-managed special care unit. J Nurs Adm. 21:31–38
64. Cohen IL, Bari N, Strosberg MA, et al (1991) Reduction of duration and cost of mechanical ventilation in an intensive care unit by use of a ventilatory management team. Crit Care Med 19:1278–1284
65. Slotnick HB (2000) Physicians' learning strategies. Chest 118:18S–23Se
66. Weingarten S (2000) Translating practice guidelines into patient care: Guidelines at the bedside. Chest 118:4S–7S
67. Kotler P, Roberto N (1989) Social Marketing: Strategies for Changing Public Behavior. Free Press, New York
68. Pervin LA (1970) Personality: Theory, Assessment, and Research. Wiley & Sons, New York
69. Rogers EM (1995) Diffusion of innovations. 4th ed. Free Press, New York
70. Soumerai SB, McLaughlin TJ, Gurwitz JH, et al (1998) Effect of local medical opinion leaders on quality of care for acute myocardial infarction – A randomized controlled trial. JAMA 279:1358–1363
71. Deming WE (2000) Out of the Crisis. 1st MIT Press ed. MIT Press, Cambridge
72. Yamamoto LG, Wiebe RA, Matthews WJ Jr, Sia CC (1992) The Hawaii EMS-C project data: I. Reducing pediatric emergency morbidity and mortality; II. Statewide pediatric emergency registry to monitor morbidity and morality. Pediatr Emerg Care. 8:70–78
73. Grol R (1997) Personal paper: Beliefs and evidence in changing clinical practice. Br Med J 315:418–421

Patient-ventilator Interactions, Weaning, and Monitoring

Control of Breathing During Mechanical Ventilation

M. Younes

Introduction

The respiratory control system achieved its current state through eons of evolution. It is a system that is adapted to ideally meet the stresses of natural living. The addition of a ventilator introduces new and overwhelming challenges to the control system, challenges it has not faced before, and for which it has not developed appropriate and specific responses. The onset of flow may be considerably delayed relative to onset of muscle activation (trigger delay). Air may continue to flow in when the respiratory center are expecting it to flow out (cycling off delays), or may stop flowing when it is supposed to continue flowing (premature termination of inflation). Even more challenging is the fact that the relation between respiratory muscle activation and ventilatory output (flow/volume) is no longer predictable. An increase in muscle activation may no longer result in an increase in flow or volume (volume cycled ventilation, VCV), or the change may be much less than expected (pressure support ventilation, PSV), or even opposite to what is expected; an increase in activation resulting in a smaller tidal volume (V_T, as in some cases during PSV, see below). In response to these unaccustomed challenges the respiratory center are constrained to using the built-in mechanisms developed for other reasons. The response to mechanical ventilation is an integration of these built-in stereotyped responses that may or may not be appropriate.

To the extent that the challenges posed by mechanical ventilation are new to respiratory control, the study of control of breathing on mechanical ventilation is a new science. This science is still in its infancy. It was reviewed in 1998, covering the literature to 1996 [1]. Because of the extreme shortage of real data at the time, this account was largely speculative and theoretical. Since then, the study of control of breathing during mechanical ventilation has acquired some momentum. The current chapter will focus primarily on respiratory control aspects in which new developments and insights have been generated.

Response of Respiratory Motor Output to Changes in Ventilator Settings

Immediate Responses

The immediate (first 1–2 breaths) responses to changes in ventilator settings are useful in that they define the operation of fast mechanisms, namely reflex changes in respiratory muscle activity (which have a latency of a fraction of a second), and purely mechanical effects related to changes in muscle length, which cause the muscle to generate a different pressure for the same activity through the force-length relation. This latter response is immediate [2, 3]. Responses related to changes in blood gas tensions occur after a latency of several seconds and, hence, are not a factor in mediating these immediate responses.

Timing responses: Immediate responses are generally examined by suddenly changing ventilator settings, beginning from a steady state. In VCV, an increase in flow, while keeping V_T constant, results in an increase in respiratory rate (RR), and vice versa, both in normal subjects [4–6] and in ventilator dependent patients [7, 8]. These changes in RR are the result of reciprocal changes in neural inspiratory time (nT_I decreases when flow increases, and vice versa) while neural expiratory time (nT_E) remains, on average, unchanged [8, 9]. When V_T is increased at the same flow (i.e., ventilator T_I is increased), RR decreases, and vice versa, both in normal subjects [5, 6] and in ventilator dependent patients [8]. This response is the result of an increase in neural T_E while neural T_I is unaffected [8]. A simple extension of ventilator T_I into neural expiration, by imposing brief end-inspiratory occlusions (plateau), results in respiratory slowing in normal subjects [6], ambulatory patients with chronic obstructive pulmonary disease (COPD) [10] and ventilator dependent patients [11]. This response is clearly the result of prolongation of nT_E since there was no change in ventilator output during inspiration. When flow is increased but V_T is concurrently increased to keep ventilator T_I constant, changes in RR are small and inconsistent [6, 12]. Although the changes in nT_I and nT_E have not been directly determined, it can be safely assumed, based on the response to the other interventions, that when V_T is increased at constant ventilator T_I, nT_I decreases while nT_E increases, and vice versa.

The above timing responses can all be explained by two basic neural responses. A faster rate of increase in volume (i.e., flow) during inspiration shortens nT_I, while an extension of the inflation phase into neural expiration lengthens nT_E. What happens to RR following a change in ventilator settings depends on the balance of these two responses [1]. Increasing flow at the same V_T can only increase RR because nT_I is shortened while the effect on nT_E is either nil (in the event ventilator cycle did not extend into nT_E before the change) or shortening (in the event ventilator cycle extended into nT_E before the change and this extension is reduced when ventilator T_I decreased). Increasing V_T at the same flow can only reduce RR; since nothing changes during nT_I, nT_I does not change while the increase in ventilator T_E causes further extension of inflation into nT_E, thereby lengthening it. Combined changes in flow and V_T, keeping ventilator T_I constant, produces mixed effects. nT_I shortens because of the increase in flow. Since ventilator T_I is unchanged, the reduction in nT$_I$ necessarily causes further extension of inflation into nT$_E$, thereby lengthening it. The net effect depends on the balance of these two opposing responses [1]. The change in RR may be bi-directional but, because of the presence of opposing changes, is clearly smaller than the RR response with the two other 'purer' perturbations.

The neural mechanisms by which these two timing responses are produced are unclear. The most obvious mechanism is via the Hering-Breuer inspiratory-inhibitory, expiratory-prolonging reflexes. In experimental animals, faster inflations during inspiration shorten nT$_I$ while inflations (or delayed emptying) during expiration lengthen nT$_E$ (for review see [13,14]). These reflexes are mediated by vagal, slowly adapting mechanoreceptors in pulmonary airways [15]. There are difficulties in accepting this as the sole, or even main, mechanism. Only a few of these are mentioned briefly here (see [9,11] for more details):

a. With the Hering-Breuer inspiratory inhibitory reflex, when nT$_I$ is reduced by an accelerated inflation rate, volume at the end of the abbreviated nT$_I$ is higher [16]. The same is not true in the above-cited human studies; volume at the end of the abbreviated nT$_I$ is similar, or even lower than at the end of nT$_I$ during slower inflations [9].

b. The Hering-Breuer reflexes in animals are not attenuated by sleep and anesthesia [16–18]. In fact they tend to be stronger (e.g., compare [16] with [19]). The human responses on mechanical ventilation are much stronger during wakefulness than during sleep. For example, the gain of the RR response to flow is considerably attenuated during sleep [20]. Furthermore, in awake subjects, introducing an end-expiratory plateau of 2 sec prolongs nT$_E$ by about the same amount [6, 10]. During sleep, nT$_E$ is not prolonged by inflations that are even greater than eupneic V$_T$, sustained throughout nT$_E$ [21, 22].

c. The strength of the expiratory prolonging response in ventilator dependent patients is substantially less than in normal subjects (compare [11] and [6]). This would not fit with a simple pulmonary mechanoreceptor response since these receptors respond to transpulmonary pressure [15] and, in view of the decreased compliance in patients, mechanoreceptor responses to volume should be enhanced.

These observations suggest that, while the Hering-Breuer reflexes may contribute, the responses observed after manipulation of ventilator settings are primarily mediated by reflexes that are enhanced by consciousness. The nature of these reflexes is not clear. It would be of considerable interest and practical relevance to study the gain of these responses in patients with different levels of consciousness.

To my knowledge, there have been no studies on the immediate response to different levels of pressure support on respiratory timing in normal subjects, and there is very limited information in ventilator dependent patients [8, 23]. Nonetheless, the observed responses are in keeping with those made during VCV. Thus, RR tends to decrease at higher PSV due to prolongation of nT$_E$ [8, 23]. This prolongation is related to the tendency, during PSV, for inflation to extend further into nT$_E$ as PSV is increased [8, 23–25]. The observed changes in nT$_I$ with PSV were small and less consistent but were in the same general direction; nT$_I$ tended to increase with lower PSV [8]. The small effects may be related to the fact that with PSV flow is highest early in inspiration. In many cases, nT_I is terminated very soon after triggering, even at modest levels of PSV, illustrating the powerful effect of flow on nT_I (personal observations; see also Fig. 1 in [26]). This makes it difficult to obtain further reductions in nT_I with increases in PSV and hence initial flow. Under these conditions, changes in nT_I can be observed only if PSV is reduced enough to avoid this early termination, and this was observed in one of the studies [8].

Effects on respiratory muscle activity: The changes in timing, described above, impact directly on respiratory muscle activity. Because inspiratory muscle activation progresses in a ramp-like fashion, changes in nT_I will, all else being the same, result in corresponding changes in peak inspiratory activity [16]. Changes in RR will, likewise, result in corresponding changes in muscle activation if the latter is calculated per minute. These changes in activation produced by the timing responses may be enhanced or mitigated by associated changes in the rate of rise of inspiratory activity. For the same nT_I, an increase in rate of rise will increase peak (and, hence, mean) activity per breath, and vice versa.

The immediate effect of changes of ventilator setting on rate of rise of inspiratory muscle activation has not been studied as extensively. Recently, Corne et al. [3] found an increase in rate of rise of diaphragmatic electromyogram (EMG) response (Edi), with a latency of 50–200 msec, in response to transiently increasing inspiratory flow in normal subjects. The excitatory response outlasted the increase in flow. If an excitatory response exists in ventilated patients, it would tend to mitigate the effect of flow on peak inspiratory activity produced by the timing response. There is no useful information in this respect. Imsand et al. [27] found no difference in peak Edi, or in nT_I, between assisted and unassisted breaths in synchronized intermittent mandatory ventilation (SIMV). This indicates that the rate of rise of Edi also did not change. The lack of any differences in electrical activation between assisted and unassisted breaths in this study has lead to the notion that activation is 'pre-programmed' prior to the onset of the breath and cannot be altered by intra-breath changes in assist. This concept (i.e., pre-programmed activation) is clearly untenable in view of the extensive documentation of immediate changes in inspiratory output with changes in ventilator setting, as summarized above. It is, therefore, more likely that the negative results of Imsand et al. [27] were related to factors that minimized the development of responses. For example, differences in flow between assisted and unassisted breaths in SIMV are not always large (e.g., [28]). Furthermore, all patients had severe COPD. Reflexes mediated by mechano-receptors are attenuated in these patients [11, 29, 30]. In addition, in patients with COPD, a substantial fraction of nT_I is spent before flow becomes inspiratory, due to the presence of dynamic hyperinflation. When ventilator trigger delay is added to this, the ventilator is often triggered near the very end of nT_I. Under these conditions there is no reason to expect any difference between neural output in assisted and unassisted breaths since in both cases virtually all of nT_I is unassisted. Viale et al. [31] also reported no difference in peak E_{di} between assisted and unassisted breaths during biphasic positive airway pressure. This finding is not very compelling for the same reasons outlined in relation to the study of Imsand et al.; all patients had COPD. In addition, they did not report nT_I, so that the unchanged peak E_{di} may have represented a combination of decreased nT_I and increased rate of rise in assisted breaths. From the above, it is clear that the immediate effect of ventilator settings on rate of rise of inspiratory EMG in ventilator dependent patients needs to be studied in more detail.

In experimental animals, delaying the onset of expiratory flow, for example by end-inspiratory occlusions or inflations during expiration, results in recruitment of expiratory muscle activity in the first delayed expiration (e.g., see [18]). This response is linked to prolongation of nT_E [18]. It is a compensatory response in that it would speed lung emptying once expiratory flow starts and, in this fashion, mitigate dynamic hyperinflation. In a recent study on a heterogeneous group of ventilator dependent patients, Younes et al. [11] found no evidence of increase in expiratory muscle pressure in the first expiration after introducing a delay in onset of expiratory flow. This indicates that this immediate compensatory response is lacking in these patients and suggests that when expiratory muscle activity is observed under other circumstances during mechanical ventilation (e.g. [32, 33]), it is due to behavioral responses, to reflexes that require a high degree of alertness, or to slower mechanisms that also result in recruitment of expiratory muscle activity (e.g., high chemical drive).

Immediate effects on pressure output: The immediate effect of a change in ventilator settings on pressure output will necessarily mirror the immediate effects on electrical activity, produced via timing and rate of rise in electrical activity, as outlined above. However, in addition, if the change in ventilator settings results in a different volume during nT_I, as occurs, for example, with a change in flow in VCV, or airway pressure (Paw) in PSV, pressure output will be modified further because of the operation of the intrinsic properties of respiratory muscles; at a given activity pressure output is lower if volume, or flow, is higher (force-length and force-velocity relations (see [2] for review). The magnitude of these relations during mechanical ventilation has recently been estimated [3]. In agreement with previous predictions [2], the effect of the force-velocity relation was minimal over the flow range encountered during mechanical ventilation (i.e., instantaneous pressure output is not appreciably affected by instantaneous flow). The effect of volume, however, was substantial: 11.2 ± 2.5 cmH$_2$O/l. Thus, at the same activity, pressure output of the respiratory muscles (e.g. transdiaphragmatic pressure [Pdi], respiratory muscle pressure [Pmus]) will be lower by 1.1 cmH$_2$O for every 0.1 l difference in volume.

Effect of trigger delay on immediate responses: Immediate inspiratory responses to ventilator settings can only be exerted on the inpiratory output that exists after ventilator triggering. When trigger delay (defined here as the interval between onset of inspiratory effort and triggering) is a large fraction of nT_I, the immediate effects on inspiratory output (nT_I, inspiratory muscle activity and pressure output) will necessarily be attenuated. In the extreme, if triggering occurs at the very end of nT_I, changes in ventilator settings will have no immediate effect on any inspiratory variable. The opposite is true for immediate effects on expiratory events. When trigger delay is long, more of the inflation cycle occurs during nT_E. nT_E then becomes more sensitive to the duration of ventilator T_I and V_T. These observations probably explain, at least in part, the fact that immediate effects of ventilator settings on neural inspiratory events are weaker in mechanically ventilated patients than in alert normal subjects (e.g., compare [8] with [9]). In normal subjects, trigger delay is minimal (in view of absence of dynamic hyperinflation) and nT_I is generally longer than in ventilator dependent patients. A large fraction of nT_I occurs after triggering and is subject to the immediate effects of ventilator settings.

Subsequent Responses

A large number of studies have demonstrated an inverse relation between steady state respiratory output and level of support. This holds true regardless of mode of ventilation (VCV, PSV, proportional assist ventilation [PAV]), and whether output is expressed as pressure or electrical activity (e.g., [23, 27, 31, 34]).

Steady state responses to a change in ventilator settings represent the summation of the immediate responses (due to reflexes and intrinsic properties), to the extent these persist in the long term, and the contribution of other mechanisms that evolve more slowly (e.g., chemical drive). When ventilator assist is increased (higher V_T in VCV, higher PSV or higher gain in PAV), ventilation will immediately increase, resulting in a reduction in PCO_2, and vice versa. This will cause appropriate, but more slowly evolving, changes in respiratory output (e.g., [31]. In the event of an increase in support, there will be a chemically mediated gradual decrease in inspiratory muscle activity and, depending on the range of PCO_2 where the change is happening, there may also be a reduction in neural respiratory rate (the response of RR to PCO_2 at constant V_T is highly non-linear, being very flat in the low PCO_2 range and progressively increasing as PCO_2 increases [35]. The contribution of the fast responses (reflexes and mechanical responses) need not remain constant beyond the first one or two breaths. Several factors may modify the expression of these fast responses with time:

1. Adaptation of neural reflexes: When changes in PCO_2 are in a range where PCO_2 does not affect respiratory output (e.g., in the hypocapnic range in alert subjects) the immediate changes in inspiratory and expiratory output produced by changes in ventilator settings are sustained in the long term [4, 5]. Thus, neural adaptation, *per se*, is not likely to attenuate the responses observed immediately following a change in settings as these changes are maintained.

2. Subsequent changes in ventilator output: In VCV, the initial change in V_T will, necessarily, not change beyond the first 1–2 breaths. In PSV, however, the initial increase in V_T associated with an increase in pressure will, with time, be attenuated as inspiratory output is chemically downregulated [31, 36, 37]. The steady state V_T may even return to the V_T preceding the change [31, 36, 37]. This would necessarily eliminate the contribution of the mechanical responses (via intrinsic properties of respiratory muscles) and attenuate or eliminate the inspiratory timing responses. By contrast, because with higher PSV and lower inspiratory output, inflation tends to extend further into mechanical expiration, particularly in patients with a long mechanical time constant [24, 25, 38], the effect of fast responses on nT_E may be enhanced. RR may thus decrease with time, not because of relief of respiratory distress (although this may be a factor if distress existed before), but because of further extension of inflation into nT_E. This point should be kept in mind when neural RR decreases as PSV increases.

The converse is also true; an increase in neural RR as PSV is reduced need not reflect respiratory distress but may simply be the consequence of better synchrony between end of inflation and end of nT_I [24].

3. Changes in trigger delay: The chemically induced reduction in inspiratory output may increase trigger delay [39, 40]. As indicated above, this will attenuate or eliminate the impact of fast responses on inspiratory output while increasing the extension of inflation into nT_E. The latter effect may, again, cause further respiratory slowing and contribute to the steady state reduction in RR. Conversely, a reduction in trigger delay, produced by chemically mediated increase in inspiratory output, will decrease the amount of time inflation continues into nT_E, resulting in a steady state increase in RR, independent of distress.

It is clear that the mechanisms of changes in respiratory output in the steady state, following a change in ventilator settings, are complex and likely to vary considerably depending on ventilator mode, response to PCO_2, gain of the fast mechanisms, changes in trigger delay, etc. Viale et al. [31] described the breath by breath changes in respiratory output following institution of PSV in ventilator dependent COPD patients. There were minimal immediate changes in inspiratory activity, with most of the downregulation occurring gradually over the subsequent several breaths. Although this study nicely illustrated the operation of slow mechanisms (e.g., changes in PCO_2), it does not necessarily reflect the relative contribution of fast and slow mechanisms under other conditions. Thus, the authors studied COPD patients in whom neural reflexes are attenuated (see above), and they used a PSV level that resulted in V_T returning to baseline level in the long term. A higher PSV level may have increased steady state V_T, producing different results. The extent of trigger delay was also not reported.

Possible role of neuromechanical inhibition in mediating the slow responses: So far, discussion of responses to a change in ventilator settings included fast neural and mechanical mechanisms, to account for immediate responses, while the slower responses were attributed to changes in chemical drive. Dempsey and colleagues proposed the existence of a slow evolving inhibitory neural mechanism that occurs during mechanical ventilation (For summary of manifestations and evidence see [41]). This mechanism, if operative, could account for part of the slow downregulation that follows an increase in level of assist, and vice versa. Most of the work on neuromechanical inhibition in humans has centered on the development of central apnea during controlled mechanical ventilation delivered via a facial interface. The mechanism of central apnea under these circumstances has been debated [42] but, in any case, this expression of neuromechanical inhibition (apnea) is not relevant to assisted ventilation. Increasing the level of assist during assisted ventilation never results in apnea unless PCO_2 is allowed to decrease. There are conflicting reports as to whether there is slow non-chemical partial downregulation during assisted ventilation. Georgopoulos et al. [43], compared Pdi and Pmus during rebreathing, with and without PAV assist, in awake normal subjects. They found no evidence of downregulation at the same PCO_2, even though ventilation was higher by 20 l/min, and V_T was greater by 0.7 l, during PAV. By contrast Fauroux et al. [44] found, also in awake subjects, that during isocapnic pressure support,

Pdi measured at 0.25 and 0.5 sec from inspiratory onset was 1.0 and 1.3 cmH$_2$O, respectively, lower than the same measurements at baseline (i.e., before pressure support). At the same points in time, however, volume was at least twice as high during PSV than at baseline. This easily accounts for the Pdi difference (on the basis of the force-length relation, see above). The authors also found that peak E$_{di}$ was approximately half the baseline value during iso-capnic PSV. However, nT$_I$ was reduced by approximately the same percent so that the reduction in peak Edi could well represent the operation of the fast neural reflexes acting on nT$_I$ (i.e., one does not have to postulate slowly evolving reflexes to explain these findings). Wilson et al. [45] and Scheid et al. [46] found a reduction in P0.1, at iso-PCO$_2$, with the use of VCV [45] or PSV [46]. Interpretation of changes in P0.1 under conditions where volume history during expiration (i.e., just prior to the P0.1 measurement) is different, is fraught with uncertainty. Particularly when expiratory resistance is high (e.g., nose plus ventilator circuitry ([45]), an increase in V$_T$ may result in expiratory flow not reaching zero prior to the onset of inspiratory effort. Under these conditions, the period during which P0.1 is measured is associated with decrescendo expiratory flow. This artificially reduces the value of P0.1. Thus, if expiratory flow at the onset of inspiratory effort is 0.1 l/sec, and expiratory resistance is 10 cmH$_2$O/l/sec, P0.1 is reduced by 1.0 cmH$_2$O (10 cmH$_2$O/sec) even if true muscle pressure is the same. Figure 1 in [45] shows clearly that Paw had not stabilized prior to inspiratory effort, an occurrence that, under the circumstances of mechanical ventilation, indicates that expiratory flow did not reach zero prior to onset of inspiratory effort. In addition to P0.1, Wilson et al. [45] found a 50% reduction in the area under the Edi tracing when V$_T$ was doubled at isocapnia. These authors, however, did not take into account the reduction in nT$_I$ expected to occur under the circumstances. Two other studies are cited by advocates of neuromechanical inhibition as evidence for neuromechanical inhibition during assisted ventilation, even though these studies were not designed to test this concept (i.e., no effort was made to maintain isocapnia). Morrel et al. [37] are cited [41] as showing reduction in E$_{di}$ during PSV in the absence of changes in PCO$_2$. In reality, end-tidal carbon dioxide pressure (P$_{ET}$CO$_2$) decreased by 2 mmHg, a change that is large enough to account for the downregulation [36, 47]. The change in P$_{ET}$CO$_2$ was not significant because the number of observations was very small. Bonmarchand et al. [48] are also cited as showing an increase in P0.1 and Edi, with no change in PCO$_2$, when the initial time constant of PSV was increased, again suggesting non-chemical inhibition. In reality, PCO$_2$ increased significantly. The increase in PCO$_2$ (1.6 mmHg on average) could easily account for a 1.4 cmH$_2$O increase in P0.1 and the 60% increase in Edi. Furthermore, it is quite possible that reducing initial flow during PSV increased nT$_I$ (see above) so that part of the increase in Edi was due to the fast acting timing responses described earlier. It is clear that the evidence for the operation of neuromechanical inhibition during assisted ventilation is tenuous at best.

Impact of downregulation on patient-ventilator interaction: Downregulation of inspiratory pressure may result in changes in patient-ventilator interaction and breathing pattern. The type of change depends on the mode of ventilation, the mechanical time constant of the respiratory system (resistance*compliance; RC), and trigger sensitivity.

With PSV, when RC is long, reduction of inspiratory Pmus causes ventilator T_I to become longer, extending more into nT_E [24, 25, 38, 40]. At times (very long RC), ventilator T_I may be extremely long [24] (Fig. 1A). This extension into nT_E promotes the occurrence of ineffective efforts because lung volume is high when the next effort occurs [24, 25, 40]. The occurrence of an ineffective effort makes it possible for lung volume to decrease so that the effort following the ineffective effort succeeds in triggering the ventilator. In the presence of long RC, V_T tends to increase as a function of ventilator T_I [25]. The consequence of these effects (increase in V_T because of more PSV and a longer ventilator T_I, and reduction in ventilator rate because of ineffective efforts) is that breathing pattern, as judged from ventilator output, becomes slower and deeper, even though patient's RR may have changed little (compare Fig. 1A and 1B). The pattern and frequency of ineffective efforts depends on the RC, and the magnitude of downregulation. In mild cases, an ineffective effort may occur every now and then. In more severe cases, 2:1 (patient rate/ventilator rate) or higher rhythms (up to 6:1, personal observations) may occur. The occurrence of intermittent ineffective efforts moderates the decrease in PCO_2 so that central apnea does not occur.

When, during PSV, RC is short, there is no possibility for ventilator cycle to extend into nT_E [25, 38]. Maximum V_T is reached within nT_I and the ventilator continues to be triggered, delivering the maximum V_T for the PSV level in effect, with every effort. If PSV is increased to a level where $V_T * RR$ (i.e., minute ventilation [V_E]) is sufficient to reduce PCO_2 below apneic threshold, central apnea develops and is maintained until PCO_2 rises again above the apneic threshold [36]. A number of breaths are then triggered, reducing PCO_2 below the apneic threshold, and the cycle repeats. Thus, recurrent central apneas are observed under these conditions. Recurrent central apneas during PSV almost invariably reflect overassist in a patient with short RC; only the extremely rare patient has central apneas because of central nervous system (CNS) disease. In the event ventilator trigger sensitivity is poor under the same scenario (downregulation during PSV with short RC), central apnea may be averted because triggering stops before inspiratory effort decreases substantially, arresting the decline in PCO_2. Under these conditions, instead of recurrent central apneas, the pattern consists of a number of triggered breaths alternating with a number of untriggered breaths. This pattern is again indicative of overassist in a patient with short RC, and a ventilator with poor trigger sensitivity.

The above changes in patient-ventilator interaction need not only occur when assist level is increased. Downregulation of inspiratory output for any reason (sleep, administration of a sedative, correction of metabolic acidosis) may result in the same changes at the same PSV level. Thus, a patient may switch from the pattern of Figure 1B to that of 1A, or may develop recurrent central apneas, upon falling asleep or upon receiving a sedative. Conversely, a slow deeper pattern (e.g., Fig. 1A) may become rapid and shallow upon awakening or with any intervention that increases ventilatory drive (nursing intervention, visitors, etc.) giving rise to the false interpretation of respiratory distress. Thus, paradoxically, during PSV, V_T may decrease as inspiratory output increases (compare Fig. 1A and 1B).

With VCV, downregulation of inspiratory output following an increase in assist does not alter V_T or ventilator T_I. There is, accordingly, no possibility of the extreme non-synchrony (e.g., 3:1 rhythm and higher) observed during PSV on account of the potential for very long ventilator T_I. Intermittent ineffective efforts may occur, however, if the higher V_T results in more dynamic hyperinflation, while efforts become weaker [40]. Central apneas may also occur. However, these abnormalities tend to be 'masked' during VCV because of the back-up ventilator rate. Thus, depending on the back-up rate, an ineffective effort may soon be followed by a ventilator-triggered effort. Likewise, if the back-up rate is not very different from the patient's rate, the development of central apnea will not be obvious. Ventilation continues via the back-up rate and the only evidence for central apnea would be the disappearance of trigger efforts. Depending on the relation between back-up rate and patient rate (when patient makes efforts), central apnea may be maintained indefinitely, or ventilator rate may alternate between the back up rate and patient rate as central apnea comes and goes.

Clinical Implications
1. In VCV, inspiratory flow is often increased at the same V_T in order to reduce inspiratory muscle pressure output; excessive pressure output during VCV is usually evident by scooping of Paw (failure of Paw to rise quickly early in inspiration [49]). Although this procedure will tend to reduce inspiratory muscle pressure by reducing nT_I, and via mechanical feedback (force-length relation), the reduction may be mitigated by the increase in RR (more efforts per minute) and, possibly, by a faster rate of rise in inspiratory activity. The impact of these two offsetting responses on the unloading produced by increasing flow is currently unknown.
2. In VCV, inspiratory flow is also often increased to reduce ventilator T_I in order to provide more time for expiration, thereby reducing dynamic hyperinflation. The well documented increase in RR in response to this tactic mitigates the expected increase in mechanical T_E. In fact, there may be no change, or even a decrease in mechanical T_E [7]. When inspiratory flow is increased for this purpose, it is prudent to confirm directly what happened to mechanical T_E (from the ventilator display) and not assume that the change was effective.
3. When it is desired to increase V_E in VCV the increase in V_T should be associated concurrently with an increase in flow so that ventilator T_I is the same or shorter [6]. Increasing V_T at same flow will reduce RR [5, 6], thereby mitigating the increase in ventilation.
4. Extension of inflation into nT_E tends to lengthen that phase, thereby mitigating the increase in dynamic hyperinflation that would otherwise result from reduction in mechanical T_E. Nonetheless, unlike the case in alert subjects [6, 10], in ventilator dependent patients this response is, on average, quite weak [11]. Furthermore, these patients do not recruit expiratory muscles to expedite flow in the abbreviated time available for expiration [11]. It follows that extension of ventilator T_I into neural expiration will result in more dynamic hyperinflation, particularly in patients with high expiratory airway or tubing resistance. The increase in dynamic hyperinflation, coupled with some respiratory slowing, will result in lower ventilation and higher PCO_2 than would, otherwise, be the case.

This is particularly so with PSV where dynamic hyperinflation tends to lower V_T at the same P_{aw} [11], and where the tendency for extension of ventilator T_I into nT_E is high in patients with high resistance [25,38]. Expiratory muscles may be recruited in the steady state, because of the increase in chemical drive, but this will be at the expense of more inspiratory effort. In patients with high resistance, every effort should be made to minimize the extension of ventilator T_I into neural T_E.

5. The high initial flow during PSV promotes earlier termination of T_I with the result that nT_I often terminates very soon after triggering (e.g., see Fig 1. in [26]). The occurrence of the inflation phase largely during nT_E promotes dynamic hyperinflation and longer trigger delays [39, 40]. The ventilator then essentially cycles out of phase with neural cycle, thereby defeating the purpose of assisted ventilation; inspiration is loaded through most of nT_I, as it occurs prior to triggering, and expiration is loaded in view of continued inflation during nT_E.

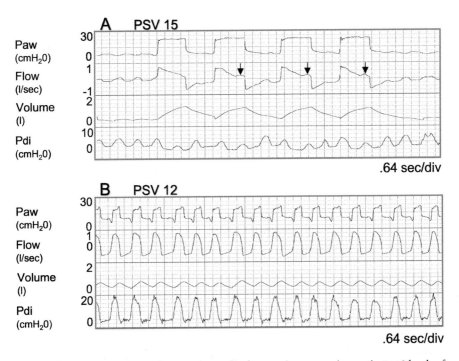

Fig. 1. Airway pressure, flow, volume and transdiaphragmatic pressure in a patient at 2 levels of pressure support. Note marked increase in ventilator rate as PSV decreased from 15 to 12 cmH2O. Patient rate, as judged from diaphragmatic pressure, did not increase. The increase in patient effort, resulting from lower assist, caused better synchrony between patient and ventilator; ventilator is now triggered with every effort as opposed to every 5th or sixth breath. In addition, the reduction in ventilator T_I, due to better synchrony, resulted in a much smaller V_T. The change in pattern from deep slow breathing to rapid shallow breathing, due to better synchrony, is often misinterpreted as respiratory distress. Arrows in panel A indicate new inspiratory efforts occurring during ventilator cycles triggered by earlier efforts.

.An increase in ventilator rate, even of a large magnitude, following a decrease in level of assist need not reflect distress. It is necessary first to establish that the increase in ventilator rate is not due to improved synchrony and reduction or loss of ineffective efforts (Fig.1). This can be done non-invasively by inspecting the Paw and flow tracings [24] for evidence of extra efforts that did not produce new ventilator cycles (these can occur during expiration [i.e., the traditional ineffective efforts] or during an inflation phase triggered by an earlier effort (Fig. 1A)). These extra efforts should be added to the ventilator rate to arrive at what actually happened to the patient's rate. Even if the patient's RR increased following a reduction in assist, it should not be presumed that the patient is developing distress, unless there are other manifestations of distress. Particularly with PSV, a reduction in assist, with a consequent increase in inspiratory effort, promotes better synchrony between end of ventilator cycle and end of nT_I. Extension of inflation into nT_E is reduced, resulting in reduction of nT_E (via built-in reflexes) and an increase in RR, independent of distress [24].

7. A spontaneous sudden increase in ventilator rate at the same PSV level need not reflect distress, particularly in the absence of other manifestations of distress. It could simply be the result of improved synchrony associated with a physiologic increase in inspiratory output related to awakening from sleep, subsidence of sedative effect, increase in metabolic rate due to movement, etc.

8. Recurrent central apneas almost invariably signify overassist in a patient with a short mechanical time constant (RC).

9. Recurrent central apneas and ineffective efforts are more likely to occur during sleep because of sleep related downregulation of respiratory output. Central apneas result in sleep fragmentation [50], and it is also quite possible that non-synchrony between patient and ventilator, of which ineffective efforts are only one expression (others being trigger delay and extension of inflation into nT_E), may disrupt sleep. Sleep fragmentation has several undesirable effects, including decrease in ventilatory response to hypercania and hypoxia [51], decreased respiratory muscle endurance [52] and increased metabolic rate [53], all factors that can adversely affect weaning. Furthermore, sleep deprivation decreases host immunity with predisposition for systemic infections [54, 55].

Variability in Ventilation and Breathing Pattern

Variability among Patients

Breathing patterns vary widely among normal subjects at rest, with V_T ranging from 5 to 17 ml/kg and RR ranging from 6 to 25 min^{-1} [56]. Until the advent of PAV [57] it was not possible to determine the breathing pattern desired by ventilator dependent patients since, with conventional modes, breathing pattern is to a considerable extent determined by ventilator settings. When patients are placed on PAV at a high level of assist (i.e., in the absence of distress), the breathing pattern is found to be as variable among patients as it is among normal subjects. Data on a limited number of patients have been published [24, 58]. In a much larger group (n=80, unpublished observations) the range of patient-selected V_T was 0.23–0.89 l

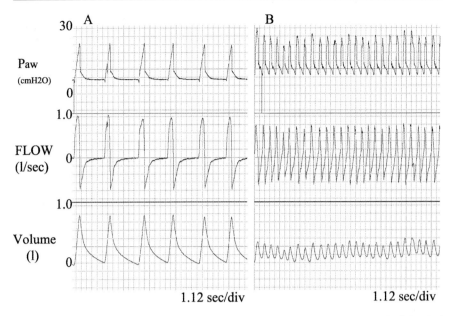

Fig. 2. Tracings illustrating greatly different breathing patterns in two patients on high level of PAV assist.

(0.50±0.18 l), corresponding to 4–15 ml/kg (7.0±2.5 ml/kg). Undistressed RR ranged from 8.4 to 43.3 min^{-1} (23.8±7.5 min^{-1}). In seven patients (9%) RR was >35. Mechanical T_I, which during PAV is similar to nTI [59], ranged 0.48 to 1.61 sec (0.96±0.24 sec). Undistressed f/V_T ratio ranged 10 to 171 (55±31). Eight patients (10%) had a ratio >110. Figure 2 shows two extremes of the range of breathing patterns observed. Undistressed V_E also varied widely (4.9 to 23.3, 11.2±3.6 l/min).

Clinical Implications
1. The clinician setting the ventilator does not know what V_T the patient wants. He/she will tend to use a standard formula (e.g., 10 ml/kg). Given the very wide range of desired V_T (4–15 ml/kg), the percentage of patients who would be satisfied with a given fixed formula is directly related to the V_T of the formula. If clinician-chosen V_T is 15 ml/kg, all patients will receive their desired V_T. However, since virtually all patients would be satisfied with a smaller V_T, with this high V_T prescription most patients will be subjected to unnecessary overdistension, with a consequent increase in risk of barotrauma. If the formula is 7 ml/kg, half the patients will get less than what they want and may become agitated. Of course, when a critically ill patient is agitated one does not know that this is because V_T is too small for the patient. The response would thus be to sedate the patient. The wide range of desired V_T, therefore, creates a no-win situation if one uses a fixed V_T prescription. There is either unnecessary overdistension or unnecessary sedation, depending on the V_T of the prescription.

2. Delivering a V_T that is higher than that desired by the patient does not automatically result in a proportionate reduction in RR [5, 6, 12]. Much depends on ventilator T_I (see above). However, even if ventilator T_I is long (>2.0 sec), the reduction in RR is not enough to offset the higher V_T, so that PCO_2 declines [5, 6]. It follows that providing a V_T that is higher than spontaneously chosen V_T will cause PCO_2 to be lower than it would be otherwise. In the long term this may reduce the PCO_2 set point. A decrease in PCO_2 set point translates into a greater ventilatory demand at the time of weaning and this may affect weanability. Furthermore, the downregulation of inspiratory output will promote non-synchrony or recurrent central apneas in PSV (see above). In VCV, back-up rate will maintain ventilation but, in doing so, it will maintain and aggravate the relative hypocapnia, favoring a greater reduction in PCO_2 set point in the long term.

3. The observation that a significant minority of patients (10%) choose a high RR and f/V_T ratio without distress calls for caution when interpreting high RR and f/V_T during a weaning trial. RR>35, or f/V_T > 100, need not, *per se*, reflect weaning failure. We have seen many cases in which weaning failure, diagnosed on the basis of rate or f/V_T criteria, turned out to be examples of spontaneously chosen breathing pattern; the same RR and f/V_T were maintained as PAV assist was increased from 0 to near 100%. Such patients were successfully extubated notwithstanding the 'unfavorable' breathing pattern during the weaning trial.

4. The wide range of adequate V_E in different patients (as illustrated by the spontaneously chosen V_E) illustrates the difficulty that would be encountered with closed-loop ventilation systems that aim to target a set V_E:

Variability with Time in the Same Patient

Unless comatose, mechanically ventilated patients are subject to many influences that normally affect ventilatory demand. Examples include sleep/wake transitions, motor activity, temperature changes, sedation, changes in pH, anxiety, etc. The extent to which these influence ventilatory demand over time in the typical ventilator dependent patient is unknown; with conventional ventilation (VCV, PSV), changes in V_T demand, or in patient RR, do not necessarily result in corresponding changes in ventilator output [1]. With PAV, however, it is possible to assess the changes in ventilatory demand over time. Figure 3 illustrates two examples in patients monitored for about 2 hours on PAV. These examples represent the extremes of responses observed in a limited sample of patients (n=20), randomly selected (for the sake of this review) from patients studied on PAV, and is not a comprehensive display of this type of variability. In each case the data represent one minute moving averages of V_E (to exclude breath by breath variability). In patient 1 (top panel) there were very frequent short term changes in V_E (1–3 minutes in duration) as well as slower changes; V_E decreased from a high value of approximately 12 l/min to 7.5 l/min in the span of an hour. There was a further reduction, with attenuation of the higher frequency fluctuations, as the patient went to sleep. Thus, in this patient, V_E changed by a factor of 2 in the span of 2 hrs. By contrast, in the other patient, both the higher frequency and slower changes were

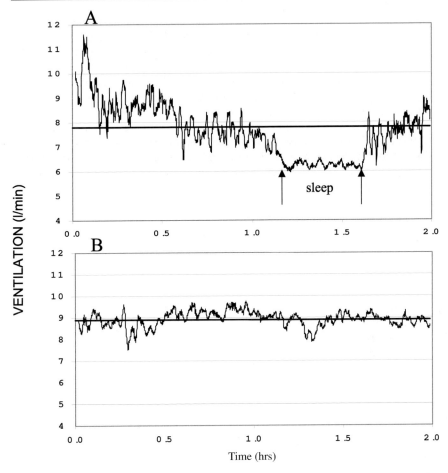

Fig. 3. 1 min moving average of ventilation in two patients followed on PAV for 2 hours. Note the substantial changes in ventilation with time in the top panel. Solid horizontal line is the overall average over the 2 hrs.

considerably attenuated. The example of Fig 3B is not shown to imply that some patients have inherently less variability than others. It is shown to reflect the minimum amount of variability observed in this sample. Clearly this patient could well have more variability under other circumstances.

The response of the ventilator to changes in demand (i.e., increase in inspiratory pressure output or patient RR) is very complex and depends on the mode used, specific settings in each mode and mechanical properties of the respiratory system. A review of this aspect is beyond the scope of this chapter (For review see [1]). It is sufficient here to point out that VCV does not permit any adjustment of V_T as demand increases. In PSV, although changes in inspiratory pressure can change V_T, the relation between change in effort and change in V_T is much attenuated [25,

34] because of the respiratory muscle weakness and abnormal mechanics that characterize ventilator dependent patients. Furthermore, peculiar situations may occur where an increase in effort, by improving synchrony, can result in a smaller V_T. The response of respiratory output to increasing demand, in the low to moderate drive range, is primarily through an increase in intensity of muscle activation per breath. Significant increases in RR occur only at high levels of respiratory drive. Ranieri et al. [60] contrasted the response to added deadspace in ventilator dependent patients while they were on PAV or PSV. On PAV the response was similar to that in normal subjects (principally an increase in V_T). In PSV, the response was primarily tachypneic and the sense of breathlessness was greater.

Clinical Implications
1. If ventilator settings are set for comfort during a period of high demand, the assist may become excessive when demand decreases, resulting in unnecessary overventilation, on average, as well as non-synchrony or central apneas.
2. If ventilator settings are set for comfort during a period of low demand, distress may develop when demand increases. The assist would then be increased but it would be unusual to decrease it again when demand decreases again. Thus, the net result of this variability is that, on average, assist and V_E will be higher than they would be if the assist changed with ventilatory demand. This may result in a lower than necessary average PCO_2 with the possibility of downregulation of PCO_2 set point.
3. Alternatively, frequent occurrence of episodes of tachypnea, related to physiologic changes in demand in the face of inability to alter ventilation appropriately, may lead to unnecessary investigations or excessive use of sedatives.

Breath by Breath Variability

Breath by breath variability in V_T, timing, flow rate and V_E is a prominent feature of breathing in healthy alert subjects [61, 62]. Its magnitude varies with level of vigilance, being less pronounced during sleep and minimal under anesthesia [63]. Breath by breath variability decreases in patients with weak muscles and abnormal mechanics [64, 65]. When the abnormal mechanics are offset by PAV, breath by breath variability becomes evident again. Typically, the coefficient of variation in ventilated patients on PAV is in the range of 10–40%, depending on their level of vigilance (personal observations). This is in the same range observed in normal subjects and indicates that the decrease in variability in patients with respiratory disease in not because they are unhealthy, per se, but is due to the effect of abnormal mechanics and weak muscles attenuating the ventilatory expression of breath by breath changes in inspiratory activity.

Clinical Implications
1. When, in a healthy subject, one measures average values of V_T, T_I and flow, then places the subject on VCV at the same settings as the average spontaneous values, the settings are not tolerated [12]. The subject requests more volume and flow. We believe that this is related to the fact that the fixed settings do not allow

a ventilatory expression of the spontaneous breath by breath changes in demand. Given that patients do display breath by breath changes in demand, it is possible that this phenomenon results in V_T and flow at which the patient feels comfortable being higher than the average values that would be tolerated if the patient were able to change V_T and flow at will. This needs to be confirmed, however.

2. There is considerable interest at present in the potential benefits to gas exchange of having breath by breath differences in V_T, and there is evidence to support this idea during controlled ventilation in animals [66, 67]. If these observations are confirmed in ventilator dependent patients on assisted ventilation, then current modes of assisted ventilation, which result in fairly monotonous V_T, may not be advantageous to gas exchange.

Conclusion

The study of control of breathing during mechanical ventilation is still in its infancy. Recent work in this area has shown that neural responses to different ventilator settings can alter the intended result of changes in ventilator settings and may lead to poor patient-ventilator interactions and central apneas. These changes in patient-ventilator interactions may, in turn, lead to diagnostic errors and delayed weaning. The documentation of a wide range in desired breathing patterns among different patients, of large changes in ventilatory demand from time to time in the same patient, and of substantial breath by breath variability in breathing demand, suggest that ventilatory modes that constrain ventilatory output within narrow limits may have adverse effects (over-ventilation, over-sedation or even worse gas exchange). Much additional work needs to be done to better define the implications of the knowledge gained in the past several years in this field.

References

1. Younes M, Georgopoulos D (1998) Control of breathing relevant to mechanical ventilation. In: Marini J, Slutsky A (Eds) Physiological Basis of Ventilatory Support. Vol 118, Lung Biology in Health and Disease. Marcel Dekker, New York Vol 118, pp: 1–74
2. Younes M, Riddle W (1981) A model for the relation between respiratory neural and mechanical outputs. I. Theory. J Appl Physiol 51:963–978
3. Corne S, Webster K, Younes M (2000) Effect of inspiratory flow rate on diaphragmatic motor output in normal subjects. J Appl Physiol 89:481–492
4. Puddy A, Younes M (1992) Effect of inspiratory flow rate on respiratory motor output in normal humans. Amer Rev Resp Dis 146:787–789
5. Tobert DG, Simon PM, Stroetz RW, Hubmayr RD (1997) The determinants of respiratory rate during mechanical ventilation. Am J Respir Crit Care Med 155:485–492
6. Laghi F, Karamchandani K, Tobin MJ (1999) Influence of ventilator settings in determining respiratory frequency during mechanical ventilation. Am J Respir Crit Care Med 160:1766–1770
7. Corne S, Gillespie D, Roberts D, Younes M (1997) Effect of inspiratory flow rate on respiratory rate in intubated ventilated patients. Am J Respir Crit Care Med 156:304–308

8. Kondili E, Prinianakis G, Anastasaki M, Georgopoulos D (2001) Acute effects of ventilator settings on respiratory motor output in patients with acute lung injury. Intensive Care Med 27:1147–1157
9. Fernandez F, Mendez M, Younes M (1999) Effect of ventilator flow-rate on respiratory timing in normal subjects. Am J Respir Crit Care Med 159:710–719
10. Laghi F, Segal J, Choe WK, Tobin MJ (2001) Effect of imposed inflation time on respiratory frequency and hyperinflation in patients with chronic obstructive pulmonary disease. Am J Respir Crit Care Med 163:1365–1370
11. Younes M, Kun J, Webster K, Roberts D (2002) Response of ventilator dependent patients to delayed opening of exhalation valve. Am J Respir Crit Care Med 166:21–30
12. Puddy A, Patrick W, Webster K, Younes M (1996) Control of breathing during volume-cycled ventilation in normal humans. J Appl Physiol 80:1749–1758
13. Younes M, Remmers J (1981) Control of tidal volume and respiratory frequency. In: Hornbein T (ed) Control of Breathing. Vol 17, Lung biology in Health and Disease. Marcel Dekker, New York, pp:617–667
14. von Euler C (1986) Brain stem mechanisms for generation and control of breathing pattern. In: Cherniack NS, Widdicombe JG (eds) Handbook of Physiology: The Respiratory System. Vol 2, Am Physiol Soc, Bethesda, pp:1–68
15. Sant'Ambrogio G (1982) Information arising from the tracheobronchial tree of mammals. Physiol Rev 62:531–569
16. Clark FJ, von Euler C (1972) On the regulation of depth and rate of breathing. J Physiol 222:267–295
17. Phillipson EA, Murphy E, Kozar LF (1976) Regulation of respiration in sleeping dog. J Appl Physiol 40:688–693
18. Younes M, Vaillancourt P, Milic-Emili J (1974) Interaction between chemical factors and duration of apnea following lung inflation. J Appl Physiol 36:190–201
19. Gautier H (1976) Pattern of breathing during hypoxia or hypercapnia of the awake or anesthetized cat. Respir Physiol 27:193–206
20. Georgopoulos D, Mitrouska I, Bshouty Z, Anthonisen NR, Younes M (1996) Effects of NREM sleep on the response of respiratory output to varying inspiratory flow. Am J Respir Crit Care Med 153:1624–1630
21. Iber C, Simon PM, Skatrud JB, Mahowald MW, Dempsey JA (1995) The Breuer-Hering reflex in humans: effects of pulmonary denervation and hypocapnia. Am J Respir Crit Care Med 152:217–224
22. Hamilton RD, Winning AJ, Horner RL, Guz A. The effect of lung inflation on breathing in man during wakefulness and sleep. Respir Physiol 73:145–154
23. Xirouhaki N, Kondili E, Mitrouska I, Siafakas N, Georgopoulos D (1999) Response of respiratory motor output to varying pressure in mechanically ventilated patients. Eur Respir J 14:508–516
24. Giannouli E, Webster K, Roberts D, Younes M (1999) Responses of ventilator dependent patients to different levels of pressure support and proportional assist. Am J Respir Crit Care Med 159:1716–1725
25. Younes M (1993) Patient-ventilator interaction with pressure-assisted modalities of ventilatory support. Semin Respir Med 14:299–322
26. Nava S, Bruschi C, Fracchia C, Braschi A, Rubini F (1997) Patient-ventilator interaction and inspiratory effort during pressure support ventilation in patients with different pathologies. Eur Respir J 10:177–183
27. Imsand C, Feihl F, Perret C, Fitting JW (1994) Regulation of inspiratory neuromuscular output during synchronized intermittent mechanical ventilation. Anesthesiology 80:13–22
28. Giuliani R, Mascia L, Recchia F, Caracciolo A, Fiore T, Ranieri VM (1995) Patient-ventilator interaction during synchronized intermittent mandatory ventilation. Effects of flow triggering. Am J Respir Crit Care Med 151:1–9

29. Polacheck J, Strong R, Arens J, Davies C, Metcalff I, Younes M (1980) Phasic vagal influence on inspiratory motor output in anesthetized man. J Appl Physiol 49:609–619

30. Tryfon S, Kontakiotis T, Mavrofridis E, Patakas D (2001) Hering-Breuer reflex in normal adults and in patients with chronic obstructive pulmonary disease and interstitial fibrosis. Respiration 68:140–144

31. Viale JP, Duperret S, Mahul P, et al (1998) Time course evolution of ventilatory responses to inspiratory unloading in patients. Am J Respir Crit Care Med 157:428–434

32. Jubran A, Van de Graaff WB, Tobin MJ (1995) Variability of patient-ventilator interaction with pressure support ventilation in patients with chronic obstructive pulmonary disease. Am J Respir Crit Care Med 152:129–136

33. Parthasarathy S, Jubran A, Tobin MJ (1998) Cycling of inspiratory and expiratory muscle groups with the ventilator in airflow limitation. Am J Respir Crit Care Med 158:1471–1478

34. Grasso S, Puntillo F, Mascia L, et al (2000) Compensation for increase in respiratory workload during mechanical ventilation. Pressure-support versus proportional-assist ventilation. Am J Respir Crit Care Med 161:819–826

35. Patrick W, Webster K, Puddy A, Sanii R, Younes M (1995) Respiratory response to CO_2 in the hypocapnic range in conscious humans. J Appl Physiol 79:2058–2068

36. Meza S, Mendez M, Ostrowski M, Younes M (1998) Susceptibility to periodic breathing with assisted ventilation during sleep in normal subject. J Appl Physiol 85:1929–1940

37. Morrell MJ, Shea SA, Adams L, Guz A (1993) Effects of inspiratory support upon breathing in humans during wakefulness and sleep. Respir Physiol 93:57–70

38. Yamada Y, Du HL (2000) Analysis of the mechanisms of expiratory asynchrony in pressure support ventilation: a mathematical approach. J Appl Physiol 88:2143–2150

39. Tobin MJ, Jubran A, Laghi F (2001) Patient-ventilator interaction. Am J Respir Crit Care Med 163:1059–1063

40. Leung P, Jubran A, Tobin MJ (1997) Comparison of assisted ventilator modes on triggering, patient effort, and dyspnea. Am J Respir Crit Care Med 155:1940–1948

41. Dempsey JA, Skatrud JB (2001) Apnea following mechanical ventilation may be caused by nonchemical neuromechanical influences. Am J Respir Crit Care Med 163:1297–1298

42. Younes M (2001) Apnea following mechanical ventilation cannot be due to neuromechanical influences. Am J Respir Crit Care Medicine 163: 1298–1301

43. Georgopoulos D, Mitrouska I, Webster K, Bshouty Z, Younes M (1997) Effects of inspiratory muscle unloading on the response of respiratory motor output to CO_2. Am J Respir Crit Care Med 155:2000–2009

44. Fauroux B, Isabey D, Desmarais G, Brochard L, Harf A, Lofaso F (1998) Nonchemical influence of inspiratory pressure support on inspiratory activity in humans. J Appl Physiol 85:2169–2175

45. Wilson CR, Satoh M, Skatrud JB, Dempsey JA (1999) Non-chemical inhibition of respiratory motor output during mechanical ventilation in sleeping humans. J Physiol 518:605–618

46. Scheid P, Lofaso F, Isabey D, Harf A (1994) Respiratory response to inhaled CO_2 during positive inspiratory pressure in humans. J Appl Physiol 77:876–882

47. Skatrud JB, Dempsey JA (1983) Interaction of sleep state and chemical stimuli in sustaining rhythmic ventilation. J Appl Physiol 55:813–822

48. Bonmarchand G, Chevron V, Chopin C, et al (1996) Increased initial flow rate reduces inspiratory work of breathing during pressure support ventilation in patients with exacerbation of chronic obstructive pulmonary disease. Intensive Care Med 22:1147–1154

49. Marini JJ, Smith TC, Lamb VJ (1988) External work output and force generation during synchronized intermittent mechanical ventilation. Effect of machine assistance on breathing effort. Am Rev Respir Dis 138:1169–1179

50. Parthasarathy S, Tobin MJ (2002) Effect of ventilator mode on sleep quality in critically ill patients. Am J Respir Crit Care Med 166:1423–1429

51. Schiffman PL, Trontell MC, Mazar MF, Edelman NH (1983) Sleep deprivation decreases ventilatory response to CO_2 but not load compensation. Chest 84:695–698

52. Chen H, Tang Y (1989) Sleep loss impairs inspiratory muscle endurance. Am Rev Respir Dis 140:907–909
53. Bonnet MH, Berry RB, Arand DL (1991) Metabolism during normal, fragmented, and recovery sleep. J Appl Physiol 71:1112–1118
54. Benca RM, Quintans J (1997) Sleep and host defences: a review. Sleep 20:1027–1037
55. Everson CA, Toth LA (2000) Systemic bacterial invasion induced by sleep deprivation. Am J Physiol 278: R905–R916
56. Jammes Y, Auran Y, Gouvermet J, Delpierre S, Grimaud C (1979) The ventilatory pattern of conscious man according to age and morphology. Bull Eur Physiopathol Respir 15:527–540
57. Younes M (1992) Proportional Assist Ventilation: A new approach to ventilatory support. Theory. Amer Rev Respir Dis 145:114–120
58. Marantz S, Patrick W, Webster K, Roberts D, Oppenheimer L, Younes M (1996) Response of ventilator dependent patients to different levels of proportional assist (PAV). J Appl Physiol 80:397–403
59. Appendini L, Purro A, Gudjonsdottir M, et al (1999) Physiologic response of ventilator-dependent patients with chronic obstructive pulmonary disease to proportional assist ventilation and continuous positive airway pressure. Am J Respir Crit Care Med 159:1510–1517
60. Ranieri VM, Giuliani R, Mascia L, et al (1996) Patient-ventilator interaction during acute hypercapnia: pressure-support vs. proportional-assist ventilation. J Appl Physiol 81:426–436
61. Davis JN, Stagg D (1975) Interrelationships of the volume and time components of individual breaths in resting man. J Physiol 245:481–498
62. Tobin MJ, Mador MJ, Guenther SM, Lodato RF, Sackner MA (1988) Variability of resting respiratory drive and timing in healthy subjects. J Appl Physiol 65:309–317
63. Read DJ, Freedman S, Kafer ER (1974) Pressures developed by loaded inspiratory muscles in conscious and anesthetized man. J Appl Physiol 37:207–218
64. Loveridge B, West P, Anthonisen NR, Kryger MH (1984) Breathing patterns in patients with chronic obstructive pulmonary disease. Am Rev Respir Dis 130:730–733
65. Brack T, Jubran A, Tobin MJ (2002) Dyspnea and decreased variability of breathing in patients with restrictive lung disease. Am J Respir Crit Care Med 165:1260–1264
66. Boker A, Graham MR, Walley KR, et al (2002) Improved arterial oxygenation with biologically variable or fractal ventilation using low tidal volumes in a porcine model of acute respiratory distress syndrome. Am J Respir Crit Care Med 165:456–462
67. Suki B, Alencar AM, Sujeer MK, et al (1998) Life-support system benefits from noise. Nature 393:127–128

Patient-ventilator Interactions

S. Parthasarathy and M. J. Tobin

Introduction

One of the main reasons for instituting mechanical ventilation is to decrease a patient's work of breathing [1]. To achieve this goal it is imperative that two pumps, the mechanical ventilator and the patient's respiratory muscles, interact in a smooth manner. To understand patient-ventilator interactions, it is necessary to evaluate the interplay between these two pumps at two different time frames: on a breath-to-breath basis, and within one breath. At the level of one breath, the interaction between a patient and a ventilator needs to focus on the following time points: the onset of ventilator triggering, the rest of inspiration after triggering, and the switch from inspiration to expiration.

Triggering and Inspiration

Ventilators provide positive-pressure assistance to a patient's inspiratory effort when the pressure in the ventilator circuit decreases by 1 to 2 cmH2O. The task of triggering the ventilator can require substantial effort [2]. Patients who struggle to reach the set sensitivity are unable to switch off their respiratory motor output immediately after successfully triggering the ventilator [3]. As a result, considerable effort can be expended during the period of mechanical inflation that follows the trigger phase, the so-called post-trigger phase. The increased effort in the post-trigger phase may arise because of an inadequate level of positive pressure in the inspiratory limb during the period immediately before and during the milliseconds after opening of the inspiratory valve [4]. In this situation, the increased effort during the post-trigger phase may offset the prime objective of the ventilator: to unload the respiratory muscles.

For a ventilator to function ideally, inspiratory assistance from the ventilator should coincide with the inspiratory effort of the patient. Most studies of patientventilator interaction have been based on indirect measurements, where the onset and offset of respiratory muscle activity have been estimated from recordings of airflow combined with airway, esophageal, or transdiaphragmatic pressures [2, 3, 5–7]. Parthasarathy and coworkers systematically evaluated the concordance between such indirect estimates and a more direct measurement of neural activity, namely the crural diaphragmatic electromyogram (EMG) [8]. Estimates of the duration of inspiration based on flow, esophageal pressure, and transdiaphragmatic pressures revealed substantial differences as compared with the duration of inspiration measured with the diaphragmatic EMG. The average differences ranged from 252 to 714 ms. The standard deviation of these differences ranged from 74 to 221 milliseconds. When inspiratory time measured on the recording of the diaphragmatic EMG was taken as the reference standard, the inspiratory time estimated from the transdiaphragmatic pressure (from the initial deflection of the signal until the signal returns to baseline) had a mean difference of 57% from the reference value and a scatter (± 2 SD) of 87% (Fig. 1). Given the magnitude of these discrepancies, conclusions about patient ventilator interactions based on indirect estimates of inspiratory time are susceptible to considerable error.

Apart from the research importance of the discrepancies between indirect estimates of a patient's inspiratory time and the true value of inspiratory time, the discrepancies can adversely affect the operation of the ventilator. Because the ventilator's algorithms are based on recordings of flow and airway pressure, errors in estimating the onset of inspiratory time may give rise to delay in triggering the ventilator, and errors in estimating the duration of inspiratory time that may cause mechanical inflation to persist into expiration (Figs. 2 and 3). A delay in opening of the inspiratory valve may arise from a decreased respiratory drive [6, 9] or increased intrinsic positive end-expiratory pressure (PEEPi) [8]. In five critically ill patients receiving mechanical ventilation, significant delays were noted between the onset of patient's inspiratory effort (measured by crural diaphragmatic electromyogram) and the onset of inspiratory flow [8] (Figs. 1 and 2). The delay between the onset of inspiratory effort and the time the ventilator was triggered was correlated with the level of PEEPi of the breaths (r = 0.59). This observation suggests that when elastic recoil pressure at the end of expiration is high, the subsequent inspiratory effort also needs to be proportionally increased if the ventilator is to be successfully triggered. A ventilator that is designed to sense the patient's effort at a neural level (diaphragmatic electromyogram) instead of sensing the final result of patient effort (changes in airway pressure or flow) should achieve better patient-ventilator synchrony [10]. The machine described by Sinderby and

--→

Fig. 1. Representative tracings of the raw crural diaphragmatic electromyogram (EMG), the processed diaphragmatic EMG achieved by removing EKG artifacts by computer, the moving average (MA) of the processed diaphragmatic EMG, esophageal pressure (Pes), and flow in a patient. The relationship between an indirect estimate of the onset of neural inspiratory time and its onset on the diaphragmatic EMG signal was assessed by calculation of the phase angle, expressed in degrees. In this example, the onset of inspiratory time is estimated as occurring earlier (negative phase angle of 15 degrees) by Pes-based measurements and later (positive phase angle of 110 degrees) by flow-based measurements. The duration of inspiratory time as estimated by Pes (hatched horizontal bar) is longer than the true inspiratory time measured by the diaphragmatic EMG (note that the hatched bar is wider than 0 to 360 degrees on the solid black bar of the reference measurement). The duration of inspiratory time as estimated by flow-based measurements is shorter (clear horizontal bar) than the true inspiratory time measured by diaphragmatic EMG (note that the open white bar is narrower than 0 to 360 degrees on the solid black bar of the reference measurement). Modified from [8] with permission

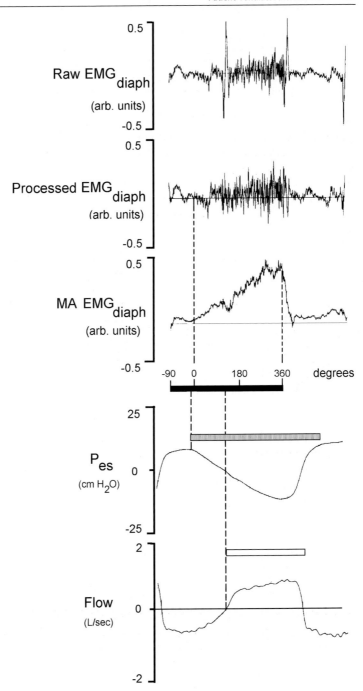

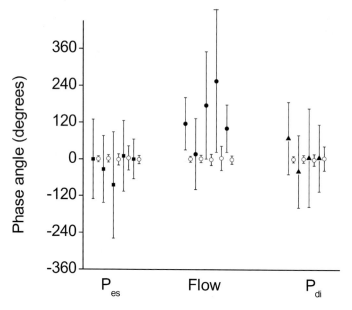

Fig. 2. The phase angle between the indirect estimate of the onset of neural inspiratory time and its reference measurement in each patient during mechanical ventilation; estimates from the esophageal pressure (Pes) tracings are shown as closed squares, estimates from flow tracings are shown as closed circles, and estimates from transdiaphragmatic pressure (Pdi) tracings are shown as closed triangles. The closed symbols represents the mean difference (bias) in phase angle; the open symbols to the right of each closed symbol represents the mean difference between the two measurements noted during the reproducibility testing of the reference measurement. The error bars represent ± 2 SD (twice the precision). A positive value in the phase angle indicates a delay in onset of inspiratory time for the flow-based measurements. Modified from [8] with permission

coworkers shows promise in that regard. This machine has yet to undergo rigorous evaluation, especially within the ICU.

Some patients have a high elastic load, secondary to hyperinflation, and a low respiratory drive. As a result, inspiratory effort will be insufficient to successfully trigger the ventilator [6]. The increased use of bedside displays of pressure and flow tracing has led to a growing awareness of the frequency with which patients fail to trigger a ventilator [8–12]. When receiving high levels of pressure support or assist-control ventilation, a quarter to a third of a patient's inspiratory efforts may fail to trigger the machine [9]. The number of ineffective triggering attempts increases in direct proportion to the level of ventilator assistance [9]. Some authors have recommended reducing the level of pressure support as a means of decreasing the number of ineffective triggering attempts [13]. While this approach should decrease the number of failed triggering attempts, it is likely to be accompanied by a decrease in ventilator assistance. At present, there are no rules of how best to achieve a good balance.

In a study of factors contributing to ineffective triggering, a decrease in the magnitude of inspiratory effort at a given level of assistance was not the cause of

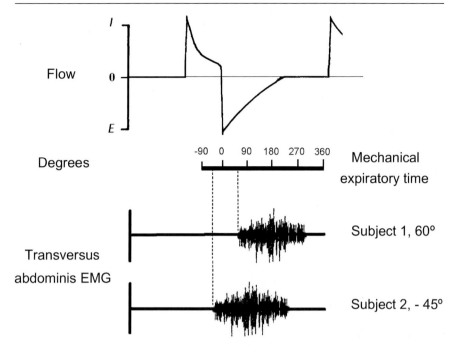

Fig. 3. The relationship of neural expiratory time to mechanical expiratory time was assessed by measuring the phase angle, expressed in degrees. If neural activity began simultaneously with the machine, the phase angle was zero. If neural activity began after the offset of mechanical inflation, the phase angle was positive (60 degrees for Subject 1). If neural activity began before the machine, the phase angle was negative (–45 degrees for Subject 2). Modified from [12] with permission

ineffective triggering. Indeed, effort was 38% higher during non-triggering attempts than during the triggering phase of attempts that successfully opened the inspiratory valve [9]. Significant differences, however, were noted in the characteristics of the breaths before the triggering and non-triggering attempts. Breaths before non-triggering attempts had a higher tidal volume (V_T) than did the breaths before triggering attempts, 486 ± 19 and 444 ± 16 ml, respectively, and a shorter expiratory time, 1.02 ± 0.04 and 1.24 ± 0.03 seconds, respectively. An abbreviated expiratory time does not allow the lung to return to its relaxation volume, leading to an increase in elastic recoil pressure. Indeed, PEEPi was higher at the onset of non-triggering attempts than at the onset of triggering attempts: 4.22 ± 0.26 versus 3.25 ± 0.23 cmH$_2$O. Thus, non-triggering results from premature inspiratory efforts that are not sufficient to overcome the increased elastic recoil associated with dynamic hyperinflation [9].

An elevated PEEP$_i$ may result from an increase in elastic recoil pressure or expiratory muscle activity. The relative contributions of these two factors to ineffective triggering were investigated in healthy subjects receiving pressure support and in whom airflow limitation was induced with a Starling resistor [12]. PEEPi was more than 30% higher at the onset of nontriggering attempts than before triggering attempts similar to the situation in critically ill patients [9]. The magnitude of expiratory effort, quantified as the expiratory increase in gastric pressure, did not differ before triggering and non-triggering attempts. In contrast, elastic recoil, estimated as gross PEEPi minus the increase in gastric pressure, was higher before non-triggering attempts than before triggering attempts: for example, 14.1 and 4.9 cmH$_2$O, respectively, at pressure support of 20 cmH$_2$O. That non-triggering was caused by the elastic recoil fraction of PEEPi, not that resulting from expiratory effort, suggests that external PEEP might be clinically useful in reducing ineffective triggering.

Inspiration-expiration Switching

Although the magnitude of expiratory effort does not appear to influence the success of triggering attempts, the time that expiratory efforts commence in relation to the cycling of the ventilator is an important factor. Parthasarathy and coworkers [12] quantified the relationship between the onset of expiratory muscle activity, measured with a wire electrode in the subject's transversus abdominis, and the termination of mechanical inflation by the ventilator (Fig. 3). When mechanical inflation extends into the early part of the patient's (neural) expiration, resulting in a negative phase angle, the time available for unopposed exhalation is shortened. The inadequate time for exhalation leads to hyperinflation with an associated increase in elastic recoil. As a result, patients need to generate greater inspiratory effort to successfully trigger the ventilator. In this way, the time that a patient commences an expiratory effort (in relation to cycling-off of mechanical inflation) partly determines the success of the ensuing inspiratory effort in triggering the ventilator. Younes and coworkers [14] studied 50 patients ventilated in the proportional-assist mode. Exhalation was delayed intermittently by briefly delaying the opening of the exhalation valve. In response to a delay in the opening of the expiratory valve, all but 5 of 50 patients developed an increase in the duration of neural expiratory time. The increase in duration of neural expiratory time, however, did not entirely offset the delay in expiration. Consequently, dynamic hyperinflation worsened. In a computer-simulated model, Du et al. found that the introduction of delays in the onset of expiration resulted in equivalent increases in dynamic hyperinflation [15].

A patient's neural inspiratory time can also be longer than the inflation time of the machine. If the machine delivers the set V_T before the end of a patient's neural inspiratory time, ventilator assistance will cease while the patient continues to make an inspiratory effort – with double triggering (two ventilator breaths for a single effort) a likely consequence [16]. Algorithms that achieve better coordination between the end of mechanical inflation and the onset of a patient's expiration should lessen this form of patient-ventilator asynchrony, although such algorithms have yet to be rigorously evaluated in patients [17].

The algorithm for 'cycling-off' of mechanical inflation during pressure support varies among brands, but most manufacturers employ some fall in inspiratory flow [13]. Problems arise with the algorithms in patients with chronic obstructive pulmonary disease (COPD), because increases in resistance and compliance produce a slow time-constant of the respiratory system. The longer time needed for flow to fall to the threshold value can cause mechanical inflation to persist into neural expiration. In 12 patients with COPD receiving pressure support of 20 cmH2O, five recruited their expiratory muscles while the machine was still inflating the thorax [18]. As anticipated, the patients who recruited their expiratory muscles during mechanical inflation had a greater time constant than did the patients who did not exhibit expiratory muscle activity.

Setting of Inspiratory Flow And V$_T$

When a patient is first connected to a ventilator, inspiratory flow is set at some default value, such as 60 l/min. Many critically ill patients have an elevated respiratory drive and the initial setting of flow may be insufficient to meet flow demands. As a result, patients will struggle against their own respiratory impedance and that of the ventilator, with consequent increase in the work of breathing. To minimize this likelihood, clinicians commonly employ a much higher flow, e.g., 80 to 100 l/min. Recent studies, however, suggest that a high flow setting may be counterproductive in this situation.

In healthy subjects, Puddy and Younes [19] found that an increase in inspiratory flow from 30 to 90 l/min caused respiratory frequency to increase from 8.8 to 14.1 breaths/min. The increase in frequency was nearly complete within the first two breaths and did not change thereafter despite the development of respiratory alkalosis. In addition to the effect of delivered flow on frequency, investigators have shown that frequency is influenced by delivered V$_T$ – an effect seen under isocapnic conditions, hypocapnic conditions, and during wakefulness and sleep [6, 19].

When studying the effects of a change in a ventilator's flow or V$_T$, the results may be influenced unwittingly by simultaneous changes in ventilator inspiratory time. When inspiratory flow is increased and V$_T$ kept constant, ventilator inspiratory time must decrease. When V$_T$ is increased and inspiratory flow kept constant, ventilator inspiratory time must increase. Laghi and coworkers [20] undertook a series of experiments in healthy volunteers to identify the influence of flow, V$_T$ and ventilator inspiratory time by varying one while keeping the others constant. For inspiratory flows of 30, 60, and 90 l/min, the respective frequencies were 12.9, 15.5, and 18.2 breaths/min. Because V$_T$ was kept constant, an increase in flow was accompanied by a proportional decrease in ventilator inspiratory time. The increase in frequency was proportional to the decrease in ventilator inspiratory time (r = – 0.69). When flow and V$_T$ were held constant and ventilator inspiratory pauses of as much as 2 sec were imposed, frequency again changed as a function of ventilator inspiratory time (r = – 0.86). When flow was increased from 30 to 60 l/minute and V$_T$ adjusted to maintain a constant ventilator inspiratory time, frequency decreased from 17.9 to 16.0 breaths/min. This series of observations shows that imposed inspiratory time can determine frequency independently of delivered inspiratory flow and V$_T$ [20]. The findings have clinical implications. Clinicians often increase V$_T$ to lower carbon dioxide tension. An increase in V$_T$ without change in inspiratory flow, however, must be accompanied by a longer inspiratory time, which is likely to decrease frequency. The consequent change in minute ventilation and carbon dioxide will fall short of that intended.

Shortening the time of inflation during mechanical ventilation has been convincingly shown to cause tachypnea in healthy subjects. The response in patients with COPD might be different because of time-constant inhomogeneities in their lungs. To investigate this issue, Laghi and colleagues [21] studied 10 patients with COPD during assist-control ventilation. Decreasing the time of mechanical inflation, achieved through an increase in inspiratory flow from 30 to 90 l/min, caused a 29% increase in respiratory frequency, a 10% increase in expiratory time, and a 9% decrease in PEEPi. Decreasing the time of mechanical inflation, achieved through shortening of an applied inspiratory pause from 2 to 0 sec, caused a 40% increase in frequency, a 30% increase in expiratory time, and a 14% decrease in PEEPi. In both experiments, decreases in the time of mechanical inflation caused a decrease in inspiratory effort. The authors conclude that strategies that shorten the time of mechanical inflation cause tachypnea in patients with COPD, but that PEEPi does not increase because the time for exhalation is also prolonged.

Clinicians usually wish to deliver relatively low V_T in patients with acute respiratory distress syndrome (ARDS). In 10 patients with ARDS, de Durante and coworkers [22] determined whether the increase in respiratory rate that accompanies the use of a low V_T would result in PEEPi. When the patients were ventilated with a V_T of 12 ml/kg, respiratory rate was 14 breaths per minute, PEEPi was 1.4 cmH_2O, and total PEEP (including an external PEEP of 10.3 cmH_2O) was 11.7 cmH_2O. When the patients were ventilated with a V_T of 6 ml per kg, respiratory rate was 34 breaths per minute, PEEPi was 5.8 cmH_2O, and total PEEP was 16.3 cmH_2O. Thus, a high respiratory rate that accompanies use of a low V_T in patients with ARDS can produce PEEPi, and potentially result in levels of total PEEP that are greater than those intended.

Breath-by-breath Differences

Breath-by-breath changes in patient-ventilator interaction could arise because of ventilator-related factors (mode of ventilation) [9], patient-related factors (intrinsic breath-by-breath variability) [23], or a combination of both [24]. Intermittent mandatory ventilation (IMV) was the first mode designed to provide graded levels of assistance. By design, this mode attempts to support some breaths (mandatory) while providing no support to intervening (spontaneous, non-mandatory) breaths [2]. Many years elapsed after the introduction of IMV before it was recognized that patients have difficulty in adapting to the intermittent nature of the assistance [25].

In patients receiving IMV because of an acute exacerbation of COPD, Imsand and colleagues noted that at greater than 60% of machine assistance, the work of breathing was only modestly reduced [26]. The degree of inspiratory muscle rest achieved by IMV was not directly proportional to the level of machine assistance. The study suggested that the inspiratory motor output is not regulated breath-by-breath but rather is constant for a given level of machine assistance. Hence when the mandatory breaths did not render a sufficient level of ventilatory assistance, an increased respiratory drive resulted, and this persisted at a greater than desired level during both the mandatory and non-mandatory breaths [26].

A higher than desired level of respiratory drive due to the lack of support during the non-mandatory, or spontaneous breaths, can be decreased by the addition of pressure support to IMV [9]. Pressure support of 10 cmH2O when added to IMV decreased patient effort during the mandatory ventilator breaths, and the decrease in patient effort was related to the decrease in respiratory drive during the intervening breaths (r = 0.67) [9]. In other words, the reduction in drive during the intervening breaths achieved by adding pressure support was carried over to the mandatory breaths, facilitating greater unloading. Combining IMV and pressure support provides a sometimes useful means of achieving a high level of assistance; the combination has a clinical advantage when it is difficult to achieve a high inspiratory flow in the assist-control mode, as with the Siemens 900C ventilator (Siemens Corporation, New York, NY). Pressure support and IMV are commonly combined in a given patient. In an international survey of mechanical ventilation [27], this combination tied with assist-control ventilation as the most commonly used mode of ventilation in North America (34% for each).

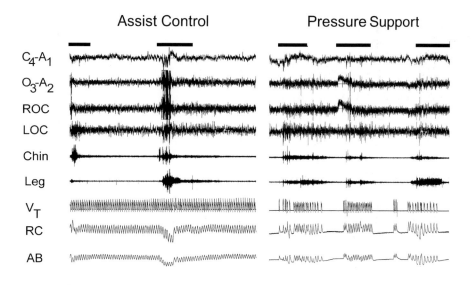

Fig. 4. Polysomnographic tracings during assist-control ventilation and pressure support in a representative patient. Electroencephalogram (C4-A1, O3-A2), electrooculogram (ROC, LOC), electromyograms (Chin and Leg), integrated tidal volume (VT), rib-cage (RC), and abdominal (AB) excursions on respiratory inductive plethysmography are shown. Arousals and awakenings, indicated by horizontal bars, were more numerous during pressure support than during assist-control ventilation. Modified from [24] with permission

In the international survey, pressure support was used as the sole mode of ventilation in up to 15% (range, 5 to 34%) of ventilated patients and in 36% (range, 21 to 45%) of patients being weaned. Pressure support, which is devoid of the back-up respiratory rate, may allow central apneas to occur in healthy subjects [28]. Such central apneas may cause arousals from sleep. Accordingly, Parthasarathy and Tobin [24] studied whether critically ill patients developed central apneas and consequent arousals from sleep during pressure support. Eleven critically ill patients were randomized to both assist-control ventilation and pressure support. Sleep fragmentation, measured as the sum of arousals plus awakenings, was greater during pressure support than during assist-control ventilation: 79 versus 54 events per hour. Six of the 11 patients developed central apneas during pressure support but not during assist-control ventilation by virtue of the backup rate (Fig.4). Heart failure was more common in the six patients who developed apneas than in the five patients without apneas: 83 versus 20%. The authors concluded that critically ill patients experience greater fragmentation of sleep during pressure support than

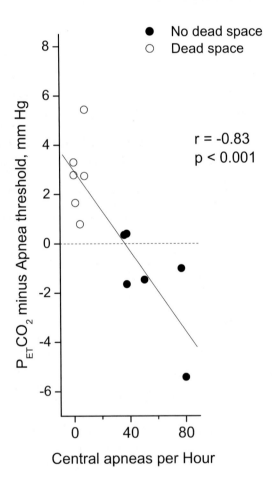

Fig. 5. The difference between average end-tidal CO_2 and the apnea threshold is plotted against the number of central apneas per hour in six patients. Closed symbols represent pressure support alone. Open symbols represent pressure support with added deadspace. The average end-tidal CO_2, measured during both sleep and wakefulness, strongly correlated with the mean number of central apneas ($r = -0.83$, $p < 0.001$). Modified from [24] with permission

during assist-control ventilation because of the development of central apneas, and that this effect is especially prominent in patients with heart failure.

The coefficient of variation of the level of end-tidal CO_2 was greater during pressure support than during assist-control ventilation: 8.7 ± 1.4 versus $4.7 \pm 0.7\%$. Among the patients with central apneas, adding dead space increased end-tidal PCO_2 by 4.3 mmHg. This intervention caused a decrease in the coefficient of variation of end-tidal CO_2, and a decrease in the sum of arousals plus awakenings (from 83 to 44 events per hour). The number of central apneas was most closely related to the difference between end-tidal CO_2 (during a mixture of wakefulness and sleep) and the apnea threshold point ($r = -0.83$; Fig. 5).

Significant differences in breathing pattern were noted between sleep and wakefulness during both pressure support and assist-control ventilation. In patients receiving pressure support, respiratory rate was 32.6% lower and end-tidal CO_2 was 11.0% higher during sleep than during wakefulness. In patients receiving assist-control ventilation, respiratory rate was 14.9% lower and end-tidal CO_2 was 4.6% higher during sleep than during wakefulness. The differences in the breathing pattern between wakefulness and sleep were greater for pressure support than for assist-control ventilation. In clinical practice, the level of pressure support is adjusted in accordance with a patient's respiratory rate, which provides reasonable guidance as to a patient's inspiratory effort [18]. Because respiratory rate is lower during sleep as compared with wakefulness, if a physician adjusts pressure support according to a patient's sleeping respiratory rate, patient effort will likely increase on awakening.

Ventilator settings are commonly adjusted in accordance with arterial blood gas measurements. With pressure support, end-tidal CO_2 was up to 7 mmHg higher during sleep as compared with wakefulness. The coefficient of variation for end-tidal CO_2 during pressure support was 8.1% (range, 1.5 to 10.3%). Differences of this magnitude between sleep and wakefulness, arising from variations in CO_2, may cause physicians to change ventilator settings when a change is not necessary. Consequently, under-ventilation or over-ventilation may result [16]. Studies of patient-ventilator interaction should therefore control for the state of the patient: wakefulness or sleep.

Abnormal breathing patterns, such as Cheyne-Stokes respiration or central apneas, may lead to sleep fragmentation in critically-ill ventilated patients. In ambulatory patients, sleep disruptions may result in activation of the sympathetic nervous system, which, in turn, can decrease myocardial contractility and increase cardiac arrhythmias [29]. Deliberate variations in breathing pattern, without the introduction of apneas, however, may improve oxygenation [30, 31]. In guinea pigs with endotoxin-induced lung injury, Arold and coworkers [32] determined whether an imposed variability in V_T is beneficial. Tidal volumes were varied randomly by 10, 20, 40, and 60% of the average value (rate was adjusted to achieve a constant minute ventilation). Compared with conventional ventilation, an increase in the variability of V_T to 40% of the average value produced a decrease in lung elastance of 14% and an increase in PO_2 from 42 to 54 mmHg; an increase in the variability of V_T to 60% of the average value produced a 29% decrease in elastance and no further improvement in PO_2. A 20% increase in the variability of V_T was not beneficial. The authors conclude that deliberate attempts to vary delivered V_T produce improvements in lung mechanics and oxygenation in mechanically ventilated animals with acute lung injury, and that the benefit depends on the degree of imposed variability.

Conclusion

Unsatisfactory patient-ventilator interaction is associated with delays in inspiration, delays in exhalation, non-triggering of the ventilator, wasted muscle effort [8, 9, 12], and inadequate respiratory muscle rest [1]. In undertaking studies of patient-ventilator interactions, careful attention needs to be given to the accuracy and reliability of measures of inspiratory time and expiratory time. In addition, the patient's sleep-wakefulness state needs to be carefully characterized.

References

1. Tobin MJ (2001) Advances in mechanical ventilation. N Engl J Med 344:1986–1996
2. Sassoon CSH, Gruer SE (1995) Characteristic of the ventilator pressure- and flow-trigger variables. Intensive Care Med 21:159–168
3. Marini JJ, Capps JS, Culver BH (1985) The inspiratory work of breathing during assisted mechanical ventilation. Chest 87:612–618
4. Aslanian P, El Atrous S, Isabey D et al (1998) Effects of flow triggering on breathing effort during partial ventilatory support. Am J Respir Crit Care Med 157:135–143
5. Lessard MR, Lofaso F, Brochard L (1995) Expiratory muscle activity increases intrinsic positive end-expiratory pressure independently of dynamic hyperinflation in mechanically ventilated patients. Am J Respir Crit Care Med 151:562–569
6. Tobert DG, Simon PM, Stroetz RW, Hubmayr RD (1997) The determinants of respiratory rate during mechanical ventilation. Am J Respir Crit Care Med 155:485–492
7. Jubran A, Tobin MJ (1997) Pathophysiologic basis of acute respiratory distress in patients who fail a trial of weaning from mechanical ventilation. Am J Respir Crit Care Med 155:906–915
8. Parthasarathy S, Jubran A, Tobin MJ (2000) Assessment of neural inspiratory time in ventilator-supported patients. Am J Respir Crit Care Med 160:546–552
9. Leung P, Jubran A, Tobin MJ (1997) Comparison of assisted ventilator modes on triggering, patients' effort, and dyspnea. Am J Respir Crit Care Med 155:1940–1948
10. Sinderby C, Navalesi P, Beck J et al (1999) Neural control of mechanical ventilation in respiratory failure. Nature Med 5:1433–1436
11. Giannouli E, Webster K, Roberts D, Younes M (1999) Response of ventilator-dependent patients to different levels of pressure support and proportional assist. Am J Respir Crit Care Med 159:1716–1725
12. Parthasarathy S, Jubran A, Tobin MJ (1998) Cycling of inspiratory and expiratory muscle groups with the ventilator in airflow limitation. Am J Respir Crit Care Med 158:1471–1478
13. Brochard L (1994) Pressure support ventilation. In: Tobin MJ (ed) Principles and Practice of Mechanical Ventilation. McGraw-Hill, New York, pp: 239–257
14. Younes M, Kun J, Webster K, Roberts D (2002) Response of ventilator-dependent patients to delayed opening of exhalation valve. Am J Respir Crit Care Med 166:21–30
15. Du H, Ohtsuji M, Shigeta M et al (2002) Expiratory asynchrony in proportional assist ventilation. Am J Respir Crit Care Med 157:135–143
16. Younes M (1995) Interactions between patients and ventilators. In: Roussos C (ed) The Thorax, 2nd edn. Marcel Dekker, New York, pp 2367–2420

17. Yamada Y, Du H (2000) Analysis of the mechanisms of expiratory asynchrony in pressure upport ventilation: a mathematical approach. J Appl Physiol 88:2143–2150
18. Jubran A, Van de Graaff WB, Tobin MJ (1995) Variability of patient-ventilator interaction with pressure-support ventilation in patients with COPD. Am J Respir Crit Care Med 152:129–136
19. Puddy A, Younes M (1992) Effect of inspiratory flow rate on respiratory output in normal subjects. Am Rev Respir Dis 146:787–789
20. Laghi F, Karamchandani K, Tobin MJ (1999) Influence of ventilator settings in determining respiratory frequency during mechanical ventilation. Am J Respir Crit Care Med 160: 1766–1770
21. Laghi F, Segal J, Choe W, Tobin MJ (2001) Effect of imposed inflation time on respiratory frequency and hyperinflation in patients with chronic obstructive pulmonary disease. Am J Respir Crit Care Med 163:1365–1370.
22. de Durante G, del Turco M, Rustichini L et al (2002) ARDSNet lower tidal volume ventilatory strategy may generate intrinsic positive end-expiratory pressure in patients with acute respiratory distress syndrome. Am J Respir Crit Care Med 165:1271–1274
23. Tobin MJ, Yang KL, Jubran A, Lodato RF (1995) Interrelationship of breath components in neighboring breaths of normal eupneic subjects. Am J Respir Crit Care Med 152:1967–1976
24. Parthasarathy S, Tobin MJ (2002) Effect of ventilator mode on sleep quality in critically ill patients. Am J Respir Crit Care Med. 166:1423–1429
25. Marini JJ, Smith TC, Lamb VJ (1988) External work output and force generation during synchronized intermittent mechanical ventilation: effect of machine assistance on breathing effort. Am Rev Respir Dis 138:1169–1179
26. Imsand C, Feihl F, Perret C, Fitting JW (1994) Regulation of inspiratory neuromuscular output during synchronized intermittent mechanical ventilation. Anesthesiology 80:13–22
27. Esteban A, Anzueto A, Alia I et al (2000) How is mechanical ventilation employed in the intensive care unit? An international utilization review. Am J Respir Crit Care Med 161: 1450–1458
28. Meza S, Mendez M, Ostrowski M, Younes M (1998) Susceptibility to periodic breathing with assisted ventilation during sleep in normal subjects. J Appl Physiol 85:1929–40
29. Meredith IT, Broughton A, Jennings GL, Esler MD (1991) Evidence of a selective increase in cardiac sympathetic activity in patients with sustained ventricular arrhythmias. N Engl J Med 325:618–24
30. Mutch WAC, Harms S, Graham MR, Kowalski SE, Girling LG, Lefevre GR (2000) Biologically variable or naturally noisy mechanical ventilation recruits atelectatic lung. Am J Respir Crit Care Med 162:319–323
31. Boker A, Graham MR, Walley KR et al (2002) Improved arterial oxygenation with biologically variable or fractal ventilation using low tidal volumes in a porcine model of acute respiratory distress syndrome. Am J Respir Crit Care Med 165:456–462
32. Arold A, Mora R, Lutchen KR, Ingenito EP, Suki B (2002) Variable tidal volume ventilation improves lung mechanics and gas exchange in a rodent model of acute lung injury. Am J Respir Crit Care Med 165:366–371

Physiological Rationale for Ventilation of Patients with Obstructive Diseases

J. Mancebo

Introduction

Chronic obstructive pulmonary disease (COPD) is a disorder characterized by a slowly progressive airflow obstruction, and the main pathophysiological finding is expiratory airflow limitation [1]. The slow expiratory airflow rates are mainly caused by peripheral airway narrowing, and functional residual capacity (FRC, resting lung volume) is dynamically determined [1, 2]. Indeed, expiration is interrupted by the subsequent inspiration before the respiratory system has enough time to reach its resting volume. This is termed dynamic hyperinflation. The loss of lung recoil which occurs in the most severe cases, enhances the degree of dynamic hyperinflation. In addition, small airway collapse during tidal expiration exacerbates hyperinflation. When lungs deflate in COPD patients, dynamic airway compression occurs, and this additionally limits expiratory flow [3]. In severe COPD patients, the loss of elastic recoil favors airways collapse at low lung volumes. At low lung volumes, maximal expiratory flows are independent of expiratory muscle effort and only depend on passive elastic recoil. Consequently, when COPD patients contract their expiratory muscles and pleural pressure increases, this compresses the airways and limits, even more, the expiratory flow [3].

The presence of dynamic hyperinflation implies that alveolar pressure at end-expiration is higher than airway pressure at mouth opening (the so called intrinsic-positive and-expiratory pressure [PEEPi], or auto-PEEP). These abnormalities require increased pleural pressure swings to overcome the increased mechanical loads: resistive, due to airway narrowing, and elastic, due to dynamic hyperinflation [1]. Furthermore, the altered respiratory system mechanics, in particular the hyperinflation, decreases the resting length of inspiratory muscles (mainly the diaphragm) thus reducing their ability to lower intrapleural pressure [3]. Such a disadvantageous diaphragmatic configuration implies that for a given drive, the pressure generating capacity decreases, or the diaphragm will necessitate more inspiratory drive to generate a given pressure [4].

Mechanical derangements are associated with abnormalities in intrapulmonary gas exchange, mainly due to severe ventilation to perfusion mismatching. As a result, arterial blood gases show hypoxemia and hypercapnia [5]. Finally, in order to compensate the expiratory flow limitation and to maintain the minute ventilation adapted to the metabolic needs, the patients with COPD increase their mean inspiratory flow and lung volume. Such a compensatory strategy is characterized by a rapid and shallow breathing pattern [3].

Acute Respiratory Failure in Patients With COPD

During an acute exacerbation of COPD, patients usually show profound alterations in gas exchange (hypoxemia and hypercapnia), and when oxygen is administered to relieve the low arterial PO_2, hypercapnia worsens. This is mainly due to an increase in ventilation/perfusion heterogeneity with an increased dead space to tidal volume (V_T) ratio, and to a decrease in minute ventilation because of the removal of the hypoxic stimulus [3]. As a consequence, there is a further reduction in arterial pH. Inspiratory work of breathing further augments due to increases in both airway resistance (because of bronchoconstriction, inflammation, secretions, etc.) and dynamic hyperinflation (not only because of an increase in respiratory rate, but also because of increased minute ventilation for instance due to fever, which is frequent during the acute exacerbations). These factors, together with a rapid and shallow breathing pattern, lead to a vicious circle, consisting of progressive hypercapnia (because the dead space to V_T ratio increases), acidosis, increase in respiratory rate (and further increase in dynamic hyperinflation) and additional increases in work of breathing.

In this scenario, before a respiratory or cardiac arrest ensues, mechanical ventilation is envisaged in order to improve gas exchange, provide rest to the respiratory muscles and, allow time to recover from the initial insult leading to the acute exacerbation. Mechanical ventilation can be provided via invasive (intubation of the trachea) or non-invasive means (via an appropriate interface, usually a mask). The fundamental importance of non-invasive ventilation (NIV) in this clinical setting is covered in another chapter of this book. Nevertheless, despite the major benefits attributable to NIV, there is still a fraction of patients who will need intubation and mechanical ventilation.

Once intubation and mechanical ventilation is first instituted, patients are usually kept under controlled modes. This allows for muscle rest and gas exchange improvement. When spontaneous inspiratory activity resumes, assisted ventilatory modes are commonly employed. Once the patient is stabilized, discontinuation of mechanical ventilation is envisaged. These three phases will be commented on below.

Controlled Mechanical Ventilation

Immediately after sedation and intubation of the trachea, great care has to be taken when adjusting the ventilatory parameters. Sedation may *per se* diminish arterial blood pressure. However, a rapid respiratory rate, either delivered manually via an Ambu-bag or with a mechanical ventilator, may also cause severe hypotension due to the increase in intrathoracic pressure associated with auto-PEEP [6]. This happens because, in the presence of highly compliant lungs, a high fraction of increased alveolar pressure is transmitted to intrathoracic vessels, thus decreasing venous return and ventricular preload. In this setting, a brief discontinuation of ventilation restores blood pressure.

When patients are first connected to the ventilator, usually in volume controlled ventilation, a moderate inspired oxygen concentration (FiO_2, usually 0.4) is sufficient to reverse hypoxemia since intrapulmonary shunting of blood plays virtually no role in explaining the low PaO_2. In COPD patients, hypoxemia (arterial oxygen saturation below 90%) refractory to oxygen supplementation should prompt a search for associated disturbances. Prevention of hyperventilation is important not only to avoid further hyperinflation, but also to avoid respiratory alkalosis which may lead to seizures and cardiac dysfunction. Since COPD patients with hypercapnia retain sufficient bicarbonate to normalize arterial pH, even at $PaCO_2$ of 60 to 70 mmHg, minute ventilation should be adjusted to keep a normal pH and not to normalize the $PaCO_2$. This is commonly achieved with V_T about 8 ml/kg and respiratory rates about 15 per minute.

In these patients, it is crucial to analyze the time course of the passive expiratory airflow curve (Fig. 1). A slow expiratory airflow persisting until onset of next inspiration, is a hallmark of dynamic hyperinflation [2, 7–11]. Importantly, a number of simple calculations may help in properly adjusting the ventilatory settings. First, an end-expiratory occlusion (up to three seconds) will allow equilibration of alveolar pressure and pressure at the airway opening in most instances. When dynamic hyperinflation exists, the airway pressure will increase above the PEEP level (if any) set in the ventilator. The difference between static airway pressure at the end of the expiratory occlusion and the external PEEP fixed in the ventilator is the static auto-PEEP. The sum of external PEEP plus the auto-PEEP is the total PEEP. With the patient ventilated in a volume controlled mode and constant inspiratory flow, a subsequent end-inspiratory occlusion will allow to measure the passive elastic recoil pressure of the respiratory system (the static airway pressure at the end of the inspiratory occlusion, or Pplat). The peak inspiratory airway pressure (Ppeak) is that measured at the end of V_T delivery. With these parameters, and during constant flow inflation, resistance and compliance of the respiratory system can be easily calculated.

Resistance is the quotient between Ppeak minus Pplat divided by inspiratory flow. Compliance is the quotient between V_T divided by Pplat minus total PEEP. The product of resistance times compliance is the time constant of the respiratory system and determines the rate of passive lung emptying. Assuming a linear compliance and resistance, the time course of volume changes follows an exponential equation. Such an equation predicts that three time constants are needed to passively decrease volume to 5% of its initial value [8, 12]. In other words, assuming a COPD patient with a respiratory system resistance of 20 $cmH_2O/l/s$ and a respiratory system compliance of 0.05 l/cmH_2O, a duration of expiration of 3 second (3 x 20 x 0.05) will be needed to passively exhale 95% of the inspired V_T. This could be achieved with a respiratory rate of 15 breaths/min and an inspiratory to expiratory ratio of 1/3. The same rate but a shorter inspiratory to expiratory ratio (for instance 1/2), would be insufficient to provide complete emptying since expiratory time is 2.66 seconds. A respiratory rate of 20 breaths/min could never achieve this objective, since total breath duration is three seconds.

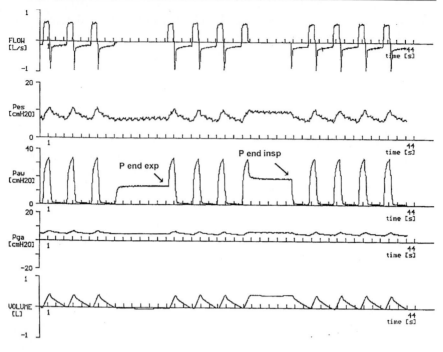

Fig. 1. From top to bottom tracings of airflow (flow), esophageal pressure (Pes), airway pressure (Paw), gastric pressure (Pga) and tidal volume (volume). Each mark on the time axis denotes one second. These tracings were obtained in a completely relaxed, passively ventilated COPD patient. Expiratory flow is interrupted by the beginning of each machine delivered breath. A prolonged end-expiratory occlusion allows to recognize the presence of a static auto-PEEP (Pend exp) of about 14 cmH2O. A prolonged end-inspiratory occlusion allows to measure the static recoil pressure of the respiratory system (P end insp). These values, together with peak Paw, airflow and tidal volume, allow to calculate resistance, compliance, and the respiratory system time constant.

Setting the ventilator rate and the inspiratory to expiratory ratio according to such simple measurements, will minimize the degree of dynamic hyperinflation and its hemodynamic and mechanical untoward effects. If expiratory time is insufficient to allow for passive emptying, this will generate further hyperinflation and a higher end-inspiratory elastic recoil pressure. This, in turn, will generate a new steady state when the increase in lung volume and recoil pressure result in a mean maximal expiratory flow equal to that determined by the ventilator settings. Actually, mean expiratory flow (tidal volume/expiratory time [V_T/T_E]) is the principal ventilator setting influencing the degree of dynamic hyperinflation [8, 13]. In other words, if a COPD patient has a V_T/T_E of 0.2 l/s, he/she cannot accommodate an imposed ventilatory V_T/T_E of 0.5 l/s without increasing end-expiratory lung volume. Of course, the use of bronchodilators, low resistance ventilator tubings and valves, and large bore endotracheal tubes, will minimize the degree of dynamic hyperinflation.

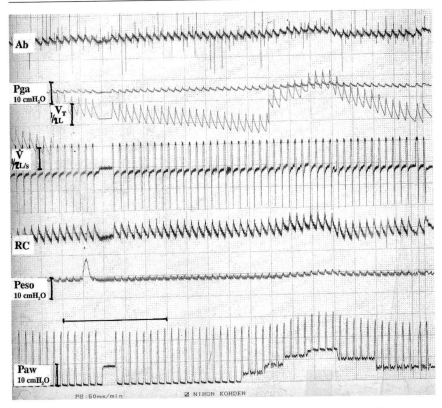

Fig. 2. From top to bottom tracings of abdominal volume displacement (Ab) assessed by inductive plethysmography, gastric pressure (Pga), tidal volume (V_T), airflow (V), thoracic volume displacement (RC), esophageal pressure (Peso) and airway pressure (Paw). Horizontal bar on the time axis denotes one minute. These tracings were obtained in a completely relaxed, passively ventilated COPD patient. End expiratory occlusion showed an static auto-PEEP of 8 cmH$_2$O (left). Note that progressive addition of external PEEP up to 7 cmH$_2$O did not change Paw or RC signals. When PEEP levels higher than auto-PEEP values were added (right), a clear increase in Paw and an upward shift in the RC were seen, suggesting a further augmentation in lung volume.

In passively ventilated patients, an alternative way to estimate the amount of auto-PEEP induced by dynamic airway collapse, is by adding at progressive steps small amounts of external PEEP. External PEEP will not increase Ppeak or Pplat until reaching the level of auto-PEEP. In other words if auto-PEEP is, say 8 cmH$_2$0, adding external PEEP up to 8 cmH$_2$O will not much change end-inspiratory pressures (Fig. 2). Clinical data obtained in COPD patients under controlled mechanical ventilation, indicate that adding extrinsic PEEP, up to 85% of auto-PEEP, does not worsen neither hemodynamics, gas exchange, or respiratory system mechanics [14, 15]. In one of these studies, however, it was pointed out that the effects of external PEEP on individual patients was largely unpredictable, in part because of non-linear pressure-volume relationships [15].

Ventilator Settings

Tuxen and Lane [13] studied the effects of ventilatory pattern on the degree of hyperinflation, airway pressures and hemodynamics in patients with severe airflow obstruction. These authors observed that end-inspiratory lung volume was increased by dynamic hyperinflation as much as 3.6 ± 0.4 l above the apneic FRC depending on ventilator settings. When V_T was increased and/or when expiratory time was decreased either by an increase in rate (and hence minute ventilation) or by a decrease in inspiratory flow (at constant minute ventilation), dynamic hyperinflation worsened. Pulmonary hyperinflation was associated with increased alveolar, central venous and, esophageal pressures as well as with systemic hypotension.

These authors demonstrated that, at constant minute ventilation, mechanically ventilated airflow obstructed patients exhibited the lowest degree of dynamic hyperinflation when ventilation was performed at high inspiratory airflows and long expiratory time [13]. Above all, imposed mean expiratory flow was the main determinant of hyperinflation. In a related study, Connors and coworkers [16] observed that higher airflow rates improved gas exchange in patients mechanically ventilated due to COPD, presumably because of decreased dynamic hyperinflation. Georgopoulos et al. [17] studied a group of passively ventilated COPD patients at constant respiratory rate and V_T. The authors also documented that shortening expiratory time (by decreasing inspiratory flow or by adding an end-inspiratory pause) had a major influence on respiratory system mechanics, gas exchange and hemodynamics. These findings were explained by significant increases in auto-PEEP and trapped gas volume above the passive FRC when expiratory time was shortened.

At the present time, and according to the physiological data available, a general recommendation can be made when initiating volume controlled mechanical ventilation in COPD patients: set a moderate FiO_2, usually 0.4 suffices to improve hypoxemia. Arterial oxygen saturation about 90% is acceptable in these individuals. Initiate ventilation with a respiratory rate of 15/min, V_T about 8 ml/kg and constant inspiratory flow 60-90 l/min. Inspiratory to expiratory ratio should be set at 1/3 or shorter (1/4, 1/5). Readjust these parameters once basic respiratory variables (resistance and compliance) have been measured. Provide enough ventilation to keep a normal pH, not a normal $PaCO_2$.

External PEEP can be added to counterbalance auto-PEEP due to expiratory flow limitation. However, when patients are passively ventilated, the total impedance of the respiratory system, including the elastic extraload due to auto-PEEP, is overcome by the ventilator. In passively ventilated subjects under volume controlled mechanical ventilation, the ventilator will generate more or less airway pressure depending on the pressure needed to overcome total elastance and the pressure needed to overcome total resistance. An important notion is that external PEEP is needed to counterbalance auto-PEEP when patients have spontaneous inspiratory efforts. In this scenario, external PEEP will counterbalance the elastic mechanical load induced by auto-PEEP, thus decreasing inspiratory muscle effort [18]. It has to be taken into account that external PEEP does nothing with regards the degree of dynamic hyperinflation, either in passively ventilated patients or in patients with spontaneous inspiratory efforts. The amount of dynamic hyperinflation is the same, regardless of the external PEEP levels. Adjust the trigger at maximal sensitivity and check there is no auto-triggering. Although trigger variable is useless in passively ventilated patients, a proper trigger adjustment will insure that patients are not burdened when spontaneous inspiratory activity resumes. The same holds true for external PEEP.

Assisted Mechanical Ventilation

In every assisted mode, the ventilator responds in front of a patient's inspiratory effort. With respect to pressure and flow triggering systems, modern mechanical ventilators offer a high performance of both systems. Although the differences between these two systems are small in terms of added work of breathing, flow triggering seems to be slightly superior to pressure triggering [19].

When COPD patients under volume controlled mechanical ventilation resume spontaneous inspiratory activity, and thus trigger the mechanical breaths, the expiratory time is no longer constant. This implies that expired (not inspired) V_T might change on a cycle per cycle basis and modify the degree of dynamic hyperinflation. This may alter patient-ventilator synchrony and cause subsequent wasted inspiratory efforts. Such a phenomenon happens because the pressure generated by the inspiratory muscles is not sufficient to overcome the extraload imposed by auto-PEEP and the trigger sensitivity of the ventilator [20]. The presence of wasted inspiratory efforts is influenced by the level of mechanical assist and is observed in both, volume and pressure assisted modes. As far as the level of ventilator assist increases (in terms of volume or pressure delivered at each triggered breath), the number of wasted inspiratory efforts increases. This, however, is accompanied by a decrease in the sensation of dyspnea and a decrease in inspiratory effort. When the level of assist is diminished, there are less wasted inspiratory efforts but the inspiratory effort and the sensation of dyspnea both augment [21]. It follows that a balance needs to be achieved when delivering assisted ventilation. A high level of assistance, although associated with feeble inspiratory efforts and maximal unloading, will induce patient-ventilator dysynchrony. A low level of assistance, although associated with minor patient-ventilator dysynchrony, will be accompanied by a vigorous inspiratory muscle effort.

Assisted ventilation can be delivered via volume controlled breaths or pressure limited breaths (usually pressure support ventilation, PSV). Both modes can provide appropriate respiratory muscle unloading, provided that flow rate is adequately set during volume controlled breaths [22]. An interesting point is the effect of imposed inspiratory flow when volume assist-controlled ventilation is used. A number of authors have shown that increases in inspiratory flow are associated with an increase in respiratory rate. In COPD patients this is an important issue. Laghi and coworkers [23] recently showed that in non-intubated COPD subjects, when inspiratory time was decreased by shortening the inspiratory pause, the respiratory frequency and time for exhalation both significantly increased. This significantly decreased auto-PEEP. Also, when inspiratory time was decreased by increasing flow (from 30 to 90 l/min), this significantly increased rate and time to exhale. Again, auto-PEEP significantly diminished. Authors hypothesized that overdistension of fast-time constant lung units during early inflation increased time for expiration (probably because a vagal discharge). Additionally, the higher inspiratory flow rates also decreased respiratory drive and inspiratory effort.

With pressure support, the inspiratory flow rate depends on the amount of delivered pressure, the mechanical properties of the respiratory system and the inspiratory muscle effort [24]. Cycling-off is flow dependent in pressure support ventilation, and varies according to the machine. Some ventilators cycle-off at 25% of peak inspiratory flow, others cycle-off at low levels of flow (for instance 5% of peak inspiratory flow), others allow free manipulation of cycling-off. Also, pressurization ramp differs among ventilators, and some machines allow for caregiver setting of this variable. Both, cycling-off and pressurization ramp may profoundly influence patient-ventilator interactions. Generally speaking, the less steep pressure ramps increase patient work of breathing [25], whereas cycling-off at very low flow levels may profoundly influence breathing pattern, in particular when patients have a long respiratory system time constant [26]. Pressure support levels are adjusted, at the bedside, to the lowest level providing comfortable breathing. Data derived from clinical research suggest that the most appropriate pressure support level is that giving as a result a patient respiratory rate of 25–30 breaths/min [27]. This goal is commonly achieved with 15 to 20 cmH_2O of pressure support, but large inter-individual variations exist.

In COPD patients under assisted mechanical ventilation, the presence of auto-PEEP increases the work of spontaneous breathing [18]. When patients start inspiration during spontaneous breathing, they must first generate a sufficiently high negative pressure to counterbalance auto-PEEP before inspiratory airflow begins. This extraload is the product of V_T times the auto-PEEP level, and represents a non-negligible amount of total inspiratory effort [27–31]. In COPD patients on assisted ventilatory modes, the application of external PEEP to compensate for auto-PEEP due to flow limitation, decreases the inspiratory effort to initiate an assisted breath and has a major impact on the total breathing workload [18, 28, 31]. The effects of external PEEP will also depend upon the severity and homogeneity of the obstructive process, the minute ventilation requirement, the activity of expiratory muscles, and the existence of dynamic airway collapse [32]. Figures 3 and 4 show the effects of adding external PEEP in a patient with dynamic hyperinflation and ventilated with pressure support.

During assisted breathing, however, auto-PEEP measurement is cumbersome and invasive. Accurate measurements need placement of esophageal and gastric balloons. Usually, auto-PEEP is estimated from simultaneous recordings of esophageal pressure and airflow, from the change in esophageal pressure preceding the start of inspiratory flow. Unfortunately, this is true only when expiratory muscles are relaxed. When expiratory muscle recruitment exists, as frequently happens in COPD patients [33, 34], then a correction needs to be made to take into account the amount of abdominal pressure (gastric pressure) transmitted to the thorax [35]. Although auto-PEEP usually implies dynamic hyperinflation, the two are not synonymous. Lung volume can be normal in the setting of persistent flow at the end of exhalation when recruitment of the expiratory muscles is huge. As a consequence, alveolar pressure will be positive, and the gradient of alveolar to central airway pressure will produce an auto-PEEP effect.

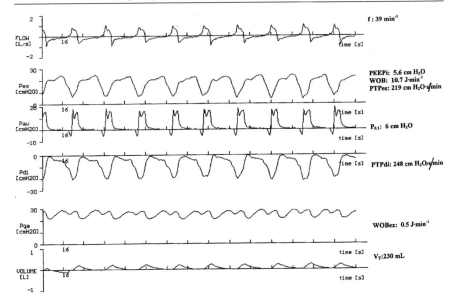

Fig. 3. From top to bottom tracings of airflow (flow), esophageal pressure (Pes), airway pressure (Paw), transdiaphragmatic pressure (Pdi), gastric pressure (Pga) and tidal volume (volume). Each mark on the time axis denotes one second. These tracings were obtained in a COPD patient during weaning from mechanical ventilation while ventilated with 15 cmH$_2$O pressure support ventilation (PSV) and zero end-expiratory pressure (ZEEP). Legends at the right show some physiological measurements. Note the high inspiratory drive as assessed by the airway occlusion pressure (P$_{0.1}$) during the triggering phase, and the recruitment of expiratory muscles. WOB: work of breathing.

During PSV, the airway occlusion pressure (P0.1), measured from the airway pressure during the phase of ventilator triggering, has been proposed to assess the effects of external PEEP in patients with auto-PEEP [36]. In a study carried out in COPD patients under mechanical ventilation, significant correlations were found between changes in P0.1 versus the changes in work of breathing when external PEEP was changed from zero to five and ten cmH$_2$O, indicating that P0.1 and work of breathing changed in the same direction. A decrease in P0.1 with PEEP indicated a decrease in auto-PEEP with a specificity of 71% and a sensitivity of 88%, and a decrease in work of breathing with a specificity of 86% and a sensitivity of 91% [36].

The Asthmatic Patient

Acute changes in lung mechanics experienced by patients with severe bronchospasm due to asthma attacks are similar to those observed in COPD during acute exacerbations. However, the pathophysiology of asthma may differ substantially from that of COPD. Increased airway collapsibility due to destruction of the lung parenchyma and loss of lung elastic recoil is a main feature of COPD patients. In asthma, the increases in bronchomotor tone, and inflammatory infiltration may

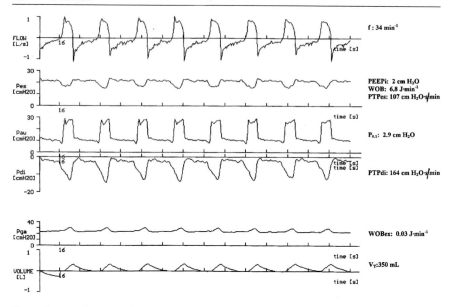

Fig. 4. Same patient as in figure 3, ventilated with the same pressure support ventilation (PSV) level but adding 10 cmH2O external PEEP. The inspiratory drive and respiratory muscle effort markedly decreased.

stiffen the airway walls and decrease collapsibility, despite considerable reduction in airway caliber [1, 37]. Additionally, in asthmatic patients, a decrease in lung compliance due to hyperinflation and widespread airway closure has been described, and in these circumstances end-inspiratory plateau pressure may be a better marker of hyperinflation than PEEPi [38]. Moreover, contrary to what occurs in COPD, these factors are usually generalized and reversible with pharmacologic treatment in the case of severe asthma [37].

Current data [37, 39–42] indicate that the ventilatory strategy in acute asthma should favor relatively small V_T and higher inspiratory airflow to preserve expiratory time, in order to minimize hyperinflation, barotrauma and hypotension. This objective could be achieved with inspiratory flows of 80 to 100 l/min (and high peak airway pressure), V_T below 10 ml/kg and alveolar plateau pressures not higher than 25–30 cmH2O [37]. The respiratory rate should be adjusted at relatively low frequencies (about 10 cycles/min), so as to minimize hyperinflation as much as possible and maintain arterial pH in an acceptable range (pH > 7.20).

An important aspect related to mechanical ventilation in asthma is to avoid complications rather than to achieve normocapnia. The low respiratory rates together with small V_T can lead to hypoventilation and severe hypercapnia. Darioli and Perret [40], used controlled hypoventilation in status asthmaticus in a series of 40 patients, and $PaCO_2$ values as high as 90 mmHg were tolerated for more than 24 hours. Complications were a transient hypotension in 40% of patients and barotrauma was observed in only three patients. In a large study by Williams and coworkers [43], it was observed that the risk of hypotension and barotrauma were best predicted by the end-inspiratory lung volume. Indeed, 65% of patients with end-inspiratory lung volume 1.4 l above FRC, had severe complications. Ventilatory adjustments should be ideally based on the level of dynamic hyperinflation, not on $PaCO_2$, so as to maintain the level of dynamic hyperinflation below a safe limit. This corresponds to an end-inspiratory lung volume (above FRC) below 20 ml/kg [44].

Current data in the literature suggest that the risks of increased end-inspiratory airway pressure (reflecting the amount of trapped gas volume above FRC), are much larger than those of permissive hypercapnia. Despite the fact that permissive hypercapnia is contraindicated in the presence of raised intracranial pressure and may cause adverse effects in patients with some forms of cardiovascular disease and patients with preexisting epilepsy, it is probably the safest approach to ventilate patients exhibiting acute severe asthma [39, 42, 45].

Discontinuation of Mechanical Ventilation

Weaning or liberation from mechanical ventilation in COPD patients, as in any other condition, begins when the precipitating cause of the acute respiratory failure is partially or totally reversed. The aim of this process is to hasten the withdrawal of the ventilator and ultimately proceed with extubation of the trachea. In clinical practice, the possible liberation from mechanical ventilation should be evaluated at least daily [46]. Once the patient is considered able to breathe without mechanical assistance, a spontaneous breathing trial can be carried out using a T-tube or low pressure support levels (about 7 cmH_2O) for between 30 and 120 minutes [47, 48]. This process, although successful in the vast majority (about 70%) of intubated mechanically ventilated patients, is particularly difficult when COPD is present [49–51]. Probably, equally successful discontinuation of mechanical ventilation can be achieved with volume assist-controlled mechanical ventilation and daily trials of spontaneous breathing, or with PSV with reductions between 2 and 4 cm H_2O in inspiratory pressure, as frequently as tolerated [49, 52].

In COPD patients, the most frequent cause of failure during a spontaneous breathing trial, is respiratory pump failure [3, 30, 51, 53, 54]. Other causes, however, need to be ruled out. Respiratory muscle dysfunction because of weakness, atrophy because of excessive rest, or drug-induced myopathy (corticosteroids and neuromuscular blocking agents) may further aggravate the respiratory pump performance in COPD patients [55]. Additionally, gas exchange abnormalities, psychological dependence on the ventilator and, particularly, congestive heart failure [56] may explain weaning failure.

Moreover, the weaning phase is a 'stress' test for these patients, and this may be a relevant issue not only because of its respiratory effects but also because of its cardiovascular effects [57–60]. Thus, if the hemodynamic function is not well preserved, weaning can fail. Recent studies [59, 60] have shown that, in COPD patients, the degree of dynamic hyperinflation is a constraint on V_T expansion during exercise. In these patients, inspiratory capacity is reduced because of dynamic hyperinflation. The reduction in inspiratory capacity as exercise progresses (because further hyperinflation due to increases in end-expiratory lung volume), implies that V_T is closer to total lung capacity (near the flat upper part of the pressure-volume relationship). These abnormalities contribute to exercise intolerance, dyspnea, and marked CO_2 retention [59, 60]. Interestingly, patients with an emphysematous profile had faster rates of dynamic hyperinflation and greater constraints on V_T during exercise [59]. These data, together with the hemodynamic profile of emphysematous patients, makes it possible that weaning outcomes are heavily influenced by cardiovascular status. Indeed, Scharf and coworkers [61] studied a group of 120 non-intubated patients with severe emphysema in whom right-heart catheterization was performed. Patients with previously diagnosed pulmonary vascular disease, ischemic heart disease or congestive heart failure were excluded. The main findings of this study included a high prevalence of elevated pulmonary artery pressure and wedge pressure. Mean cardiac index, at rest, was in the low normal range. The authors concluded that although resting cardiovascular function was well preserved, it may become impaired with exercise [61].

Although suggested for long time [3], few studies have documented clear-cut ventricular failure during discontinuation of mechanical ventilation. Lemaire et al. [62] described the hemodynamic response during weaning in fifteen COPD patients. They observed an increase in the pulmonary artery occlusion pressure during the shift from assist-control mechanical ventilation to spontaneous breathing. Authors concluded that the left ventricular dysfunction made the weaning process even more difficult in COPD patients. Richard et al. [63] also showed a decrease in left ventricular ejection fraction in COPD subjects without coronary artery disease during the weaning phase, and hypothesized that heart dysfunction was secondary to an increase in left ventricular afterload. Jubran et al. [64] studied the hemodynamic changes during weaning in a series of patients, most of them having COPD. One group of patients failed to be weaned, while the other group was successfully weaned. During full mechanical ventilatory support, physiological variables were similar between the two groups. When a spontaneous breathing trial was initiated, successfully weaned patients showed an increase in both cardiac output and oxygen transport in comparison with the values recorded during mechanical ventilation. These phenomena were not observed in unsuccessfully weaned patients. Moreover, in this latter group a decrease in both mixed venous oxygen saturation and oxygen transport, were documented. Furthermore, an increase in arterial blood pressure was observed in these patients. So, if congestive heart failure leading to acute cardiogenic pulmonary edema develops, this will generate additional hypoxemia and will further increase the mechanical load of the respiratory system [7], thus jeopardizing weaning from mechanical ventilation.

Frequent clinical manifestations of decompensated cardiovascular disease during weaning are dyspnea, anxiety, tachypnea, tachycardia, wheezing, hypoxemia and hypercapnia. These are common in COPD patients as well. As these signs and symptoms are not specific, they are difficult to differentiate from respiratory pump failure alone. Proper differential diagnosis may require invasive tests.

Conclusion

Proper implementation of invasive mechanical ventilation in COPD patients is not easy and requires appropriate knowledge of respiratory and cardiovascular system physiology. Although invasive mechanical ventilation is lifesaving, once these patients are intubated and mechanically ventilated, they are prone to develop substantial morbidity and mortality, not only because of severe respiratory derangement but because of frequently associated comorbidities. Ideally, the duration of mechanical ventilation should be as short as possible. This is feasible provided drug therapy is adequately administered, the ventilatory strategies and discontinuation of mechanical ventilation are optimized, and complications are diagnosed and treated early.

References

1. Pride NB, Macklem PT (1986) Lung mechanics in disease. In: Handbook of Physiology, Section 3, vol. III : The Respiratory System. Mechanics of Breathing, part 2. American Physiological Society, Bethesda, pp:659–692
2. Kimball WR, Leith DE, Robins AG (1982) Dynamic hyperinflation and ventilator dependence in chronic obstructive pulmonary disease. Am Rev Respir Dis 126:991–995
3. Derenne J, Fleury B, Pariente R (1988) Acute respiratory failure of chronic obstructive pulmonary disease. Am Rev Respir Dis 138:1006–1033
4. Aubier M, Murciano D, Fournier M, Milic Emili J, Pariente R, Derenne JP (1980) Central respiratory drive in acute respiratory failure patients with chronic obstructive pulmonary disease. Am Rev Respir Dis 1980:191–199
5. Roca J, Rodriguez-Roisin R (1998) Distributions of alveolar ventilation and pulmonary blood flow. In: Physiological Basis of Ventilatory Support. Marini JJ, Slutsky AS (eds) Marcel-Dekker, New York, pp:311–344
6. Pepe PE, Marini JJ (1982) Occult positive end-expiratory pressure in mechanically ventilated patients with airflow obstruction.The auto-PEEP effect. Am Rev Respir Dis 216:166–169
7. Broseghini C, Brandolese R, Poggi R, et al (1988) Respiratory mechanics during the first day of mechanical ventilation in patients with pulmonary edema and chronic airway obstruction. Am Rev Respir Dis 138:355–361
8. Hubmayr RD (1994) Setting the ventilator. In: Tobin MJ (ed) Principles and Practice of Mechanical Ventilation. McGraw-Hill, New York, pp:191–206
9. Rossi A, Gottfried SB, Higgs BD, Zocchi L, Grassino A, Milic-Emili J (1985) Respiratory mechanics in mechanically ventilated patients with respiratory failure. J Appl Physiol 58:1849–1858
10. Rossi A, Polese G, Brandi G (1991) Dynamic hyperinflation. In: Marini JJ, Roussos Ch (eds) Ventilatory Failure. Update in Intensive Care and Emergency Medicine, vol 15. Springer-Verlag, Berlin, pp:199–218
11. Rossi A, Polese G, Brandi G, Conti G (1995) Intrinsic positive end-expiratory pressure (PEEPi). Intensive Care Med 21:522–536
12. Hubmayr RD, Abel MD, Rehder K (1990) Physiologic approach to mechanical ventilation. Crit Care Med 18:103–113
13. Tuxen D, Lane S (1987) The effects of ventilatory pattern on hyperinflation, airway pressures, and circulation in mechanical ventilation of patients with severe airflow obstruction. Am Rev Respir Dis 136:872–879

14. Ranieri MV, Giuliani R, Cinnella G, et al (1993) Physiologic effects of positive end-expiratory pressure in patients with chronic obstructive pulmonary disease during acute ventilatory failure and controlled mechanical ventilation. Am Rev Respir Dis 147:5–13
15. Georgopoulos D, Giannouli E, Patakas D (1993) Effects of extrinsic positive end-expiratory pressure on mechanically ventilated patients with chronic obstructive pulmonary disease and dynamic hyperinflation. Intensive Care Med 19:197–203
16. Connors AF, McCaffree DR, Gray BA (1981) Effect of inspiratory flow rate on gas exchange during mechanical ventilation. Am Rev Respir Dis 124:533–537
17. Georgopoulos D, Mitrouska I, Markopoulou K, Patakas D, Anthonisen NR (1995) Effects of breathing patterns on mechanically ventilated patients with chronic obstructive pulmonary disease and dynamic hyperinflation. Intensive Care Med 21:880–886
18. Smith TC, Marini JJ (1988) Impact of PEEP on lung mechanics and work of breathing in severe airflow obstruction. J Appl Physiol 65:1488–1499
19. Aslanian P, Brochard L (1998) Partial ventilatory support. In: Marini JJ, Slutsky AS (eds) Physiological Basis of Ventilatory Support. Marcel-Dekker, New York, pp:817–846
20. Patessio A, Purro A, Appendini L, et al (1994) Patient-ventilator mismatching during pressure support ventilation in patients with intrinsic PEEP. Am J Respir Crit Care Med 151:562–569
21. Leung P, Jubran A, Tobin M (1997) Comparison of assisted ventilator modes on triggering, patient effort and dyspnea. Am J Respir Crit Care Med 155:1940–1948
22. Cinnella G, Conti G, Lofaso F, et al (1996) Effects of assisted ventilation on the work of breathing: volume-controlled versus pressure-controlled ventilation. Am J Respir Crit Care Med 153:1025–1033
23. Laghi F, Segal J, Choe WK, Tobin MJ (2001) Effect of imposed inflation time on respiratory frequency and hyperinflation in patients with chronic obstructive pulmonary disease. Am J Respir Crit Care Med 163:1365–1370
24. Brochard L (1994) Pressure support ventilation. In: Tobin MJ (ed) Principles and Practice of Mechanical Ventilation. Mc Graw-Hill, New York, pp:239–257
25. Chiumello D, Pelosi P, Croci M, Bigatello LM, Gattinoni L (2001) The effects of pressurization rate on breathing pattern, work of breathing, gas exchange and patient comfort in pressure support ventilation. Eur Respir J 18:107–114
26. Yamada Y, Du HL (2000) Analysis of the mechanisms of expiratory asynchrony in pressure support ventilation: a mathematical approach. J Appl Physiol 88: 2143–2150
27. Jubran A, Van de Graaff WB, Tobin MJ (1995) Variability of patient-ventilator interaction with pressure support ventilation in patients with chronic obstructive pulmonary disease. Am J Respir Crit Care Med 152:129–136
28. Purro A, Appendini L, Patessio A, et al (1998) Static intrinsic PEEP in COPD patients during spontaneous breathing. Am J Respir Crit Care Med 157:1044–1050
29. Petrof BJ, Legaré M, Goldberg P, Milic-Emili J, Gottfried SB (1990) Continuous positive airway pressure reduces work of breathing and dyspnea during weaning from mechanical ventilation in severe chronic obstructive pulmonary disease (COPD). Am Rev Respir Dis 141: 281–289
30. Fleury B, Murciano D, Talamo C, Aubier M, Pariente R, Milic Emili J (1985) Work of breathing in patients with chronic obstructive pulmonary disease in acute respiratory failure. Am Rev Respir Dis 131:822–827
31. Appendini L, Purro A, Patessio A, et al (1996) Partitioning of inspiratory muscle workload and pressure assistance in ventilator-dependant COPD patients. Am J Respir Crit Care Med 154: 1301–1309
32. Tuxen DV (1989) Detrimental effects of positive end-expiratory pressure during controlled mechanical ventilation of patients with severe airflow obstruction. Am Rev Respir Dis 140:5–9
33. Ninane V, Rypens F, Yernault JC, De Troyer A (1992) Abdominal muscle use during breathing in patients with chronic airflow obstruction. Am Rev Respir Dis 146:16–21
34. Ninane V, Yernault JC, De Troyer A (1993) Intrinsic PEEP in patients with chronic obstructive pulmonary disease. Role of expiratory muscles. Am Rev Respir Dis 148:1037–1042

35. Lessard MR, Lofaso F, Brochard L (1995) Expiratory muscle activity increases intrinsic positive end-expiratory pressure independently of dynamic hyperinflation in mechanically ventilated patients. Am J Respir Crit Care Med 151:562–569
36. Mancebo J, Albaladejo P, Touchard D, et al (2000) Airway occlusion pressure to titrate positive end-expiratory pressure in patients with dynamic hyperinflation. Anesthesiology 93:81–90
37. Corbridge TC, Hall JB (1995) The assessment and management of adults with status asthmaticus. Am J Respir Crit Care Med 151:1296–1316
38. Leatherman JW, Ravenscraft SA (1996) Low measured auto-positive end-expiratory pressure during mechanical ventilation of patients with severe asthma: Hidden auto-positive end-expiratory pressure. Crit Care Med 24:541–546
39. Leatherman JW (1998) Mechanical ventilation in severe asthma. In: Marini JJ, Slutsky AS (eds) Physiological Basis of Ventilatory Support. Marcel-Dekker, New York, pp:1155–1185
40. Darioli R, Perret C (1984) Mechanical controlled hypoventilation in status asthmaticus. Am Rev Respir Dis 129:385–387
41. Manthous CA (1995) Management of severe exacerbations of asthma. Am J Med 151:298–308
42. Tuxen DV (1994) Permissive hypercapnia. In: Tobin MJ (ed) Principles and Practice of Mechanical Ventilation. Mc Graw-Hill, New York, pp:371–392
43. Williams TJ, Tuxen DV, Scheinkestel CD, Czarny D, Bowes G (1992) Risk factors for morbidity in mechanically ventilated patients with acute severe asthma. Am Rev Respir Dis 146:607–615
44. Tuxen DV, Williams TJ, Scheinkestel CD, Czarny D, Bowes G (1992) Use of measurement of pulmonary hyperinflation to control the level of mechanical ventilation in patients with acute severe asthma. Am Rev Respir Dis 146:1136–1142
45. Feihl F, Perret C (1994) Permissive hypercapnia. How permissive should we be? Am J Respir Crit Care Med 150:1722–1737
46. Ely EW, Baker AM, Dunagan DP, et al (1996) Effect on the duration of mechanical ventilation of identifying patients capable of breathing spontaneously. N Engl J Med 335:1864–1869
47. Esteban A, Alia I, Gordo F, et al (1997) Extubation outcome after spontaneous breathing trials with T-tube or pressure support ventilation. Am J Respir Crit Care Med 156:459–465
48. Esteban A, Alia I, Tobin MJ, et al (1999) Effect of spontaneous breathing trial duration on outcome of attempts to discontinue mechanical ventilation. Spanish Lung Failure Collaborative Group. Am J Respir Crit Care Med 159:512–518
49. Brochard L, Rauss A, Benito S, et al (1994) Comparison of three methods of gradual withdrawal from ventilatory support during weaning from mechanical ventilation. Am J Respir Crit Care Med 150: 896–903
50. Vallverdú I, Calaf N, Subirana M, Net A, Benito S, Mancebo J (1998) Clinical characteristics, respiratory functional parameters and outcome of a 2-hour T-piece trial in patients weaning from mechanical ventilation. Am J Respir Crit Care Med 158:1855–1862
51. Jubran A, Tobin MJ (1997) Pathophysiologic basis of acute respiratory distress in patients who fail a trial of weaning from mechanical ventilation. Am J Respir Crit Care Med 155:906–915
52. Esteban A, Frutos F, Tobin MJ, et al (1995) A comparison of four methods of weaning patients from mechanical ventilation. N Engl J Med 332:345–350
53. Tobin MJ, Perez W, Guenther SM, et al (1986) The pattern of breathing during successful and unsuccessful trials of weaning from mechanical ventilation. Am Rev Respir Dis 134:1111–1118
54. Vassilakopoulos T, Zakynthinos S, Roussos C (1998) The tension-time index and the frequency/tidal volume ratio are the major pathophysiologic determinants of weaning failure and success. Am J Respir Crit Care Med 158:378–385
55. Mancebo J (1996) Weaning from mechanical ventilation. Eur Respir J 9:1923–1931
56. Jubran A (2002) Weaning-induced cardiac failure. In: Mancebo J, Net A, Brochard L (eds) Mechanical Ventilation and Weaning. Update in Intensive Care and Emergency Medicine, Vol. 36, Springer-Verlag, Berlin, pp:184–192
57. Chatila W, Ani S, Guaglianone D, Jacob B, Amoateng-Adjepong Y, Manthous CA (1996) Cardiac ischemia during weaning from mechanical ventilation. Chest 109:1577–1583

58. Jones NL, Killian KJ (2000) Exercise limitation in health and disease. N Engl J Med 343:632–641
59. O'Donnell DE, Revill SM, Webb KA (2001) Dynamic hyperinflation and exercise intolerance in chronic obstructive pulmonary disease. Am J Respir Crit Care Med 164:770–777
60. O'Donnell DE, D'Arsigny C, Fitzpatrick M, Webb KA (2002) Exercise hypercapnia in advanced chronic obstructive pulmonary disease: The role of lung hyperinflation. Am J Respir Crit Care Med 166:663–668
61. Scharf SM, Iqbal M, Keller C, Criner G, Lee S, Fessler HE (2002) Hemodynamic characterization of patients with severe emphysema. Am J Respir Crit Care Med 166:314–322
62. Lemaire F, Teboul JL, Cinotti L, et al (1988) Acute left ventricular dysfunction during unsuccessful weaning from mechanical ventilation. Anesthesiology 69:171–179
63. Richard C, Teboul JL, Archambaud F, Hebert JL, Michaut P, Auzepy P (1994) Left ventricular function during weaning of patients with chronic obstructive pulmonary disease. Intensive Care Med 20:181–186
64. Jubran A, Mathru M, Dries D, Tobin MJ (1998) Continuous recordings of mixed venous oxygen saturation during weaning from mechanical ventilation and the ramifications thereof. Am J Respir Crit Care Med 158:1763–1769

Role of the Clinician in Adjusting Ventilator Parameters During Assisted Ventilation

L. Brochard

Introduction

This chapter addresses the role of assessing patient-ventilator synchrony at the bedside and optimizing ventilatory settings during assisted ventilation. The hypothesis is that it is better for the patient to have a ventilator working in synchrony with the patients own inspiratory and expiratory rhythm. Although this is likely to be true in general, in some circumstances it probably does not matter so much. To what extent the clinician has to repeatedly make optimal adjustments of ventilatory settings is sometimes difficult to determine. It is important, however, to realize that improper adjustments can generate major dysynchrony, make the patient uncomfortable, and/or unnecessarily increase the work of breathing. This is also probably a major reason for administration or increase in sedation. Whether automated systems making these adjustments based on reasonable physiological grounds will benefit both the patient and the clinician is also an interesting and important question for the future of intensive care medicine [1, 2].

Mechanisms explaining patient-ventilator dysynchrony are explored with greater details in another chapter. Whereas the interaction between the patient and the ventilator has often been described as a fight, this chapter will also suggest that a similar fight may exist between the clinician and the ventilator.

Because mechanical ventilation is delivered on a 24-hour basis, inadequate adjustment leading to excessive work of breathing may potentially have important consequences on global metabolism, regional blood flow redistribution and respiratory muscle performance. However, at the opposite end, excessive unloading of the respiratory muscles inducing disuse atrophy may rapidly change muscle fiber components and profoundly reduce respiratory muscle force and endurance.

Controlled Mechanical Ventilation

When the ventilator assumes the entire work of breathing, and the patient's respiratory muscles are inactive, a risk exists that inactivity of the diaphragm leads to disuse atrophy of the respiratory muscles. In animal studies, passive ventilation has been shown to induce detrimental effects on diaphragm muscle function [3–6]. In sedated and paralyzed baboons, transdiaphragmatic pressure and endurance decreased significantly after eleven days of controlled mechanical ventilation [3].

In anesthetized rats, two days of controlled mechanical ventilation reduced dia-phragm muscle force-generating capacity by 42% compared with control animals breathing spontaneously [4]. A recent study demonstrated also that the reduction in diaphragm force-generating capacity with controlled mechanical ventilation was time dependent and that the injury to the muscles accounted for the reduction in diaphragm muscle force [5]. How much these experimental data apply to patients and whether experimental data are able to reproducing the clinical situation of patient-triggered ventilation is difficult to determine. The available data, however, constitute an important incentive for the clinician to avoid or minimize fully controlled mechanical ventilation.

Despite the fact that the supposed role of controlled ventilation (as set on the ventilator) is to take over all the work of breathing, it is important to realize that the patient can still produce active work during controlled mechanical ventilation, provided that no pharmacological paralysis is used [7]. Depressing the respiratory drive with sedation usually turns down the active work of breathing, but persistence of major metabolic abnormalities and of lung injury constitute important stimuli for the respiratory centers. Applied minute ventilation, through settings of tidal volume (V_T) and respiratory rate, is a major determinant of the respiratory drive and of the adaptation of the patient to the ventilatory conditions [7, 8]; indirectly, it will determine the amount of sedation that the clinician judges necessary to keep the patient comfortable. Proper adjustment of the sedation level to minimize its side effects has important clinical consequences, especially on the duration of mechanical ventilation [9]. Whether some ventilatory modes allowing spontaneous breathing superimposed on standard ventilatory settings facilitate the use of lower levels of sedation, has already been suggested, but will need to be tested in further studies [10].

Triggering the Ventilator Inspiration

Auto-triggering

One risk of the modern, highly sensitive, triggering systems is auto-triggering (Fig. 1). Transmission of cardiac oscillations in terms of flow or pressure can be sufficient to trigger the ventilator, and can result in dangerous hyperventilation in a sedated or even paralyzed patient [11]. Through a better control of expiration, inspiratory triggers have been made more and more sensitive to minimize the extra-work due to the triggering mechanisms. Among the new sensitive systems, whether some systems are less prone than others to self-triggering has not been well addressed yet, though could have important clinical consequences [12]. Clinicians should seek for self-triggering especially in case of hyperventilation. Oscillation of resident water in the ventilator circuit can also be responsible for self-triggering.

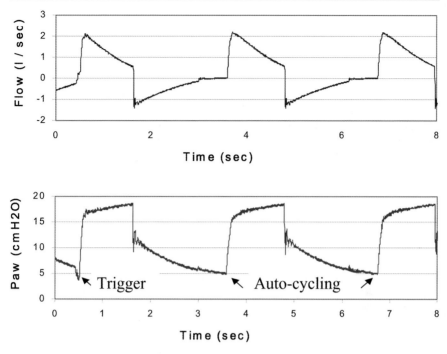

Fig. 1. Auto-cycling occurs when non respiratory airflow or pressure oscillations or leaks mimic an inspiratory effort. These tracings show airway pressure (Paw) and flow; the first cycle is triggered by the patient, as evidenced by a negative airway deflection, whereas the two following cycles do not show any evidence of patient activity (auto-cycling).

Pressure Versus Flow Triggering

Flow triggering systems have theoretical advantages over the classical pressure-triggering systems in that they never let the patient breathe against a closed circuit. Most bench and clinical evaluations have found some advantages to the newer flow-triggering systems [13–15]. Aslanian et al. found, however, that this advantage was clinically detectable only with pressure support ventilation and not with assist-control [15]. There were two main reasons. First, the advantage of one system over the other was small and the expected benefit in terms of work of breathing was less than 10% of the total patient work. Second, an inadequate setting of the peak-flow during assist-control ventilation had much more weight than the trigger effect, and masked any advantage of one system over the other. Lastly, results of experimental and clinical studies generally indicate that manufacturers have brought major improvements to the triggering systems of newer-generation ventilators [16]. The last generation of ventilators has improved the pressure-trigger systems, which now offer very similar performance to the flow-trigger systems in terms of time delay and imposed work of breathing.

Positive End-expiratory Pressure and Dynamic Hyperinflation

Patients with acute exacerbation of chronic obstructive pulmonary disease (COPD) who require intubation and mechanical ventilation frequently exhibit dynamic hyperinflation responsible for an auto or intrinsic positive end-expiratory pressure (PEEPi). Because the problem of intrinsic or (auto-) PEEP concerns the onset of inspiration, clinicians often ask whether increasing the sensitivity of the inspiratory trigger would reduce the work of breathing induced by hyperinflation [17]. The triggering systems are based on the detection of a small pressure drop relative to baseline (pressure-triggering system) or on the presence of a small inspiratory flow (flow-triggering systems). Unfortunately, increasing the trigger sensitivity has no, or only a marginal, effect on the consequences of hyperinflation. The reason for this lack of effect relates to the need for the inspiratory trigger to sense changes in airway pressure or in inspiratory flow, whereas PEEPi is a phenomenon which takes place during expiration before the triggering system can be activated.

Addition of external PEEP is one of the main ventilator adjustments that can counteract some of the effects of dynamic hyperinflation [18–21]. The presence of PEEPi implies that alveolar pressure at end expiration is higher than airway opening pressure, thus creating a problem for triggering the ventilator. The three main reasons explaining the generation of PEEPi and dynamic hyperinflation are:

1. the expiratory time between two spontaneous, patient-triggered or mandatory breaths is too short to allow complete lung emptying with regards to the time constant of the respiratory system, i.e., the product of compliance times resistance (including the endotracheal tube and the expiratory circuit of the ventilator).
2. Expiratory dynamic flow limitation caused by small airway collapse is a frequent further cause of air trapping and dynamic hyperinflation with PEEPi, especially but not exclusively in patients with chronic lung disease.
3. Activation of the expiratory muscles until the end of expiration with concomitant relaxation at the onset of the next inspiratory effort [22–24].

This latter phenomenon increases PEEPi but does not result in dynamic hyperinflation. In addition, measurements of PEEPi supposed to reflect hyperinflation, would markedly overestimate hyperinflation in case of expiratory muscle recruitment [24].

Adding external PEEP in mechanically ventilated COPD patients with dynamic hyperinflation has the ability to decrease the elastic workload that inspiratory muscles must overcome before triggering the ventilator. The addition of external PEEP in patients with PEEPi and flow limitation usually decreases the inspiratory effort done to initiate an assisted breath. This effect is variable from one patient to another, and the addition of external PEEP can also increase the degree of pulmonary hyperinflation. In addition, although external PEEP reduces work of breathing, it does not minimize hyperinflation. The level of dynamic hyperinflation is not modified by external PEEP, unless this PEEP is set higher than the minimal level of regional PEEPi, increasing hyperinflation. This can aggravate the working conditions of the respiratory muscles by placing them at a mechanical disadvantage and result in significant hemodynamic compromise by decreasing venous return and increasing right ventricular outflow resistance [21, 25]. Accordingly, a method to titrate external PEEP would be desirable to allow an optimal setting of mechanical ventilation in patients with dynamic hyperinflation. Titration of external PEEP to approximately 80% of the average static PEEPi limits the risk of overinflation and hemodynamic effects, and brings benefits in terms of reduction in patient effort [25]. Unfortunately, and to a large extent because of the frequent activity of the expiratory muscles, optimal measurement of PEEPi is made very difficult at the bedside [24].

Mancebo et al. suggested that measurement of occlusion pressure (P0.1), during the assisted breaths of mechanical ventilation could help to estimate the effects of external PEEP to reduce the inspiratory work of breathing [20]. P0.1 is the pressure generated at the airway opening in the first 100 ms of an occluded inspiration. It has the great advantage that it can be estimated from the airway pressure (Paw) tracing during the effort to trigger the ventilator. Using a large number of breaths for this calculation, the authors found that this measurement well paralleled the changes in work of breathing.

Triggering the Ventilator Expiration

The end of the patient's inspiratory time is difficult to determine for the ventilator and the time at which the ventilator terminates inspiration and opens the exhalation valve defines the beginning of the expiration process, for the ventilator, but also for the patient [26, 27]. Regarding the criteria used for terminating the breath, i.e., the cycling criteria, little effort has been provided towards a specific recognition of the end of a patient's effort. During assist-control ventilation, the breath is terminated on a time criterion independent of patient effort. The ventilator primarily controls the flow, and the insufflation time depends on the peak flow setting and V_T set on the ventilator by the clinician. The total inspiratory time can be prolonged by the addition of a pause or a plateau at end-insufflation. During pressure support ventilation (PSV), termination of the breath may be closer to a patient's neural signal than using a preset inspiratory time. The decelerating flow signal is used to determine the time at which the ventilator switches to expiration. Because the inspiratory flow should be influenced by the patient's effort at any time of the breath, this criterion is influenced by a signal directly coming from the patient. Unfortunately, this off-switch criterion is influenced by complex interference [28, 29]; the time constant of the respiratory system can vary the time at which the flow peaks, and, therefore, the time at which the flow threshold can be reached. For instance, in a patient with high respiratory resistance, the flow can become almost flat and a small percentage of the peak-flow will occur very late; the value of flow used as a threshold criterion can also make a large difference, especially in case of prolonged insufflation time. This latter parameter can now be adjusted on some ventilators, and the clinician must be aware of the possibility to generate or avoid dysynchrony at the end of the breath. The level of pressure applied at the opening of the respiratory system also influences the peak flow and the time of this peak; lastly, the remaining inspiratory effort at the end of the breath will also influence this criterion [30]. Many examples of dysynchrony occurring at the end

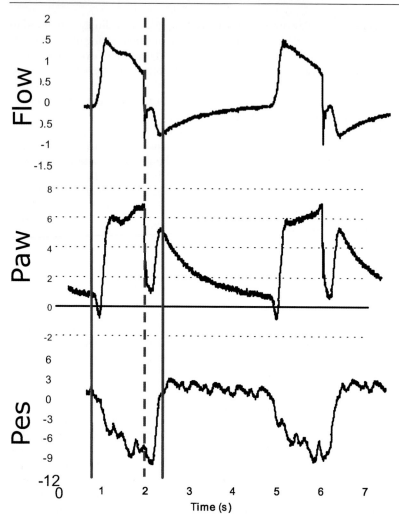

Fig. 2 Example of dysynchrony due to an insufflation time shorter than the inspiratory effort. Tracings of airway pressure (Paw), flow and esophageal pressure (Pes) are shown. The inspiratory effort is prolonged beyond the end of the inspiration (dashed line) and creates a sudden drop of airway pressure at the onset of expiration, followed by a normal expiration.

of the breath have been described, especially for high levels of PSV and in patients with high respiratory resistance (Fig. 2). This factor is also crucial in case of leaks, such as during non invasive ventilation (NIV).

In addition, delayed expiration, as frequently observed with inadequate settings during assisted ventilation, may influence the level of dynamic hyperinflation and worsen PEEPi [26, 27].

Tidal Volume, Peak-Flow, and Inspiratory Time

Adjusting the inspiratory time to match a patient's neural inspiratory time is potentially very important and is only automated, at least partially, with proportional assist ventilation. For the clinician, the first approach is to understand that the settings of volume, flow and inspiratory time are linked in a way that depends on the specific type of ventilator used. In particular, some ventilators propose to adjust the inspiration to expiration ratio in addition to the peak-flow setting. This is done with the purpose of calculating a plateau time or of recalculating an ideal inspiratory time during synchronized-intermittent mandatory ventilation (SIMV). Clinicians should be aware that they thus need to differentiate the insufflation time and the inspiratory time.

Since the seminal studies of Marini et al. [31, 32], of Ward et al. [7] and later of Cinnella et al. [8], the influence of the peak-flow setting on the patient's work of breathing has clearly been demonstrated as well as the importance of a proper adjustment for the clinician. In this regard, pressure-assisted modes deliver higher peak-flows than volume-controlled modes for a similar mean inspiratory flow and V_T. They may, therefore, be easier to adapt to patient comfort. For this reason, new ventilators have new servo controlled modes, where pressure-control or pressure-support is the way to deliver the breath but which are also volume-targeted. The intent is to offer the clinician both the safety of a pre-set volume and the comfort provided by a pressure-supported mode. Unfortunately, they bring more confusion than real benefits [33]. In case of increased ventilatory demand, they will react as an inversely proportional mode of assisted ventilation.

Once it was shown that high inspiratory flows were necessary, it was subsequently shown that this had an influence on a patient's respiratory frequency [34, 35]. Laghi et al. elegantly showed that this was primarily due to modifications of inspiratory time [36]. When patients look uncomfortable during assisted ventilation, flow is commonly increased to achieve a better match with patient demand. This results in a decrease in ventilator inflation time and, may thus allow more time for exhalation. Because tachypnea can also ensue, whether the time for exhalation is really prolonged and hyperinflation decreased is doubtful. The consequences of increasing frequency on hyperinflation, therefore, remain to be studied. In patients with moderate to severe COPD non-invasively ventilated, and using V_T sufficient to ensure comfort, Laghi et al. found that alterations in imposed ventilator inflation time produced increases in frequency but also decreases in PEEPi and inspiratory effort, whether these changes in inspiratory time were achieved by increasing delivered inspiratory flow or by decreasing ventilator inspiratory pause [36]. The data by Laghi et al. show that a decrease in ventilator inflation time does indeed allow more time for exhalation despite the development of tachypnea. Higher inspiratory flow also decreases respiratory drive and effort, which can help to improve patientventilator interaction.

Pressure-support Ventilation

The debate about the best level of pressure support to set has been compared to a classic in critical care medicine, that on the best PEEP [37]. An individual adjustment of the pressure support is indeed important in order to maintain enough inspiratory muscle activity while avoiding risk of respiratory muscle fatigue. Some have advocated the need for simple, clinically applicable techniques for measuring the inspiratory effort at the bedside in mechanically ventilated patients [38, 39]. The P0.1 has been used as a surrogate for patient work of breathing and has been shown to parallel changes in effort during changes in pressure support level [38]. Foti et al. showed that the difference between airway pressure at the end of inspiration and the elastic recoil pressure of the respiratory system obtained with an end-inspiratory pause was a good estimate of the pressure developed by the inspiratory muscles at end inspiration [30]. This measurement can be performed by simply activating the inspiratory hold button on the ventilator, and can simply be taken from the analog airway pressure display. In a group of non-obstructed patients with acute respiratory failure, this index was also a good reflection of the overall patient effort [30]. This method is best suited for research purposes, however, and there is no universally accepted method to titrate PSV. Clinical examination, especially regarding the use of accessory muscles of inspiration, and measurements of respiratory frequency are probably the more appropriate methods [40, 41]. The optimal level of respiratory frequency may be difficult to determine individually, although a threshold around 30 breaths per minute is probably acceptable for many patients, as shown by measurements of respiratory efforts [40, 41] and as used in automated algorithms to drive a ventilator [1, 2]. Clinicians should be aware, however, that the frequency displayed by the ventilator may differ from the real frequency of the patient in case of missing efforts [42]. This is especially true when high levels of pressure support are used in patients with COPD, and should be suspected by visual inspection of the flow-time curve.

Non-invasive Ventilation and Leaks

Although NIV is generally perceived as more comfortable for patients than invasive mechanical ventilation, mask (or interface) intolerance remains a major cause of NIV failure [43]. Failure rates range from below 10% to over 40%, despite the best efforts of skilled caregiver staff. Thus, improvements in mask design that enhance comfort and reduce complication rates are needed, with the presumption that they will lead to improved tolerance and reduced NIV failure rates [44]. Leaks create major dysynchrony that the clinician needs to recognize. In case of leaks, attempts to minimize the leaks must be performed and should include readjustment of the mask and decrease of the delivered pressures [45]. Once leaks persist, minimizing their consequences on patient-ventilator interaction becomes important. During PSV, adjustment of the cycling-off criterion or addition of an inspiratory time limit will help in avoiding prolonging the ventilator's inspiration long after the end of the patient's neural inspiratory time [46]. These useful settings are, however, sometimes difficult to access on the ventilator panel. In other cases, they are not provided, or can only be obtained indirectly.

References

1. Dojat M, Harf A, Touchard D, Laforest M, Lemaire F, Brochard L (1996) Evaluation of a knowledge-based system providing ventilatory management and decision for extubation. Am J Respir Crit Care Med 153:997–1004
2. Dojat M, Harf A, Touchard D, Lemaire F, Brochard L (2000) Clinical evaluation of a computer-controlled pressure support mode. Am J Respir Crit Care Med 161:1161–1166
3. Anzueto A, Peters JI, Tobin MJ, et al (1997) Effects of prolonged controlled mechanical ventilation on diaphragmatic function in healthy adult baboons. Crit Care Med 25:1187–1190
4. Le Bourdelles G, Viires N, Boczkowski J, Seta N, Pavlovic D, Aubier M (1994) Effects of mechanical ventilation on diaphragmatic contractile properties in rats. Am J Respir Crit Care Med 149:1539–1544
5. Sassoon CS, Caiozzo VJ, Manka A, Sieck GC (2002) Altered diaphragm contractile properties with controlled mechanical ventilation. J Appl Physiol 92:2585–2595
6. Sassoon CS (2002) Ventilator-associated diaphragmatic dysfunction. Am J Respir Crit Care Med 166:1017–1018
7. Ward ME, Corbeil C, Gibbons W, Newman S, Macklem PT (1988) Optimization of respiratory muscle relaxation during mechanical ventilation. Anesthesiology 69:29–35
8. Cinnella G, Conti G, Lofaso F, et al (1996) Effects of assisted ventilation on the work of breathing : volume-controlled versus pressure-controlled ventilation. Am J Respir Crit Care Med 153:1025–1033
9. Kress JP, Pohlman AS, O'Connor MF, Hall JB (2000) Daily interruption of sedative infusions in critically ill patients undergoing mechanical ventilation. N Engl J Med 342:1471–1477
10. Putensen C, Zech S, Wrigge H, et al (2001) Long-term effects of spontaneous breathing during ventilatory support in patients with acute lung injury. Am J Respir Crit Care Med 164:43–49
11. Imanaka H, Nishimura M, Takeuchi M, Kimball WR, Yahagi N, Kumon K (2000) Autotriggering caused by cardiogenic oscillation during flow-triggered mechanical ventilation. Crit Care Med 28:402–407
12. Prinianakis G, Kondili E, Georgopoulos D (2003) Effects of the flow waveform method of triggering and cycling on patient-ventilator interaction during pressure support. Intensive Care Med (in press)
13. Sassoon CS (1992) Mechanical ventilator design and function: the trigger variable. Respir Care 37:1056–1069
14. Stell IM, Paul G, Lee KC, Ponte J, Moxham J (2001) Noninvasive ventilator triggering in chronic obstructive pulmonary disease. A test lung comparison. Am J Respir Crit Care Med 164: 2092–2097
15. Aslanian P, El Atrous S, Isabey D, et al (1998) Effects of flow triggering on breathing effort during partial ventilatory support. Am J Respir Crit Care Med 157:135–143
16. Richard JC, Carlucci A, Breton L, et al (2002) Bench testing of pressure support ventilation with three different generations of ventilators. Intensive Care Med 28:1049–1057
17. Brochard L (2002) Intrinsic (or auto-) positive end-expiratory pressure during spontaneous or assisted ventilation. Intensive Care Med 28:1552–1554
18. Gottfried SB (1991) The role of PEEP in the mechanically ventilated COPD patient. In: Marini JJ, Roussos C (eds) Ventilatory Failure: Update in Intensive Care and Emergency Medicine. Springer-Verlag, Heidelberg, pp:392–418
19. Smith TC, Marini JJ (1988) Impact of PEEP on lung mechanics and work of breathing in severe airflow obstruction. J Appl Physiol 65:1488–1499

20. Mancebo J, Albaladejo P, Touchard D, et al (2000) Airway occlusion pressure to titrate positive end-expiratory pressure in patients with dynamic hyperinflation. Anesthesiology 93:81–90
21. O'Donoghue FJ, Catcheside PG, Jordan AS, Bersten AD, McEvoy RD (2002) Effect of CPAP on intrinsic PEEP, inspiratory effort, and lung volume in severe stable COPD. Thorax 57:533–539
22. Ninane V, Yernault JC, De Troyer A (1993) Intrinsic PEEP in patients with chronic obstructive pulmonary disease. Am Rev Respir Dis 148:1037–1042
23. Ninane V, Rypens F, Yernault JC, De Troyer A (1992) Abdominal muscle use during breathing in patients with chronic airflow obstruction. Am Rev Respir Dis 146:16–21
24. Lessard MR, Lofaso F, Brochard L (1995) Expiratory muscle activity increases intrinsic positive end-expiratory pressure independently of dynamic hyperinflation in mechanically ventilated patients. Am J Respir Crit Care Med 151:562–569
25. Ranieri MV, Giuliani R, Cinnella G, et al (1993) Physiologic effects of positive end-expiratory pressure in patients with chronic obstructive pulmonary disease during acute ventilatory failure and controlled mechanical ventilation. Am Rev Respir Dis 147:5–13
26. Brochard L (2002) When ventilator and patient's end of inspiration don't coincide: what's the matter? Am J Respir Crit Care Med 166:2–3
27. Younes M, Kun J, Webster K, Roberts D (2002) Response of ventilator-dependent patients to delayed opening of exhalation valve. Am J Respir Crit Care Med 166:21–30
28. Yamada Y, Du HL (2000) Analysis of the mechanisms of expiratory asynchrony in pressure support ventilation: a mathematical approach. J Appl Physiol 88:2143–2150
29. Hotchkiss JRJ, Adams AB, Stone MK, Dries DJ, Marini JJ, Crooke PS (2002) Oscillations and noise: inherent instability of pressure support ventilation? Am J Respir Crit Care Med 165:47–53
30. Foti G, Cereda M, Banfi G, Pelosi P, Fumagalli R, Pesenti A (1997) End-inspiratory airway occlusion: a method to assess the pressure developed by inspiratory muscles in patients with acute lung injury undergoing pressure support. Am J Respir Crit Care Med 156:1210–1216
31. Marini JJ, Rodriguez RM, Lamb V (1986) The inspiratory workload of patient-initiated mechanical ventilation. Am Rev Respir Dis 134:902–909
32. Marini JJ, Smith TC, Lamb VT (1988) External work output and force generation during synchronized intermittent mechanical ventilation. Am Rev Respir Dis 138:1169–1179
33. Sottiaux TM (2001) Patient-ventilator interactions during volume-support ventilation: asynchrony and tidal volume instability—a report of three cases. Respir Care 46:255–262
34. Puddy A, Patrick W, Webster K, Younes M (1996) Respiratory control during volume-cycled ventilation in normal humans. J Appl Physiol 80:1749–1758
35. Fernandez R, Mendez M, Younes M (1999) Effect of ventilator flow rate on respiratory timing in normal humans. Am J Respir Crit Care Med 159:710–719
36. Laghi F, Karamchandani K, Tobin MJ (1999) Influence of ventilator settings in determining respiratory frequency during mechanical ventilation. Am J Respir Crit Care Med 160:1766–1770
37. Rossi A, Appendini L (1995) Wasted efforts and dysynchrony: is the patient-ventilator battle back? Intensive Care Med 21:867–870
38. Alberti A, Gallo F, Fongaro A, Valenti S, Rossi A (1995) P0.1 is a useful parameter in setting the level of pressure support ventilation. Intensive Care Med 21:547–553
39. Conti G, Cinnella G, Barboni E, Lemaire F, Harf A, Brochard L (1996) Estimation of occlusion pressure during assisted ventilation in patients with intrinsic PEEP. Am J Respir Crit Care Med 154:907–912
40. Brochard L, Harf A, Lorino H, Lemaire F (1989) Inspiratory pressure support prevents diaphragmatic fatigue during weaning from mechanical ventilation. Am Rev Respir Dis 139:513–521
41. Jubran A, Van de Graaff WB, Tobin MJ (1995) Variability of patient-ventilator interaction with pressure support ventilation in patients with chronic obstructive pulmonary disease. Am J Respir Crit Care Med 152:129–136

42. Leung P, Jubran A, Tobin MJ (1997) Comparison of assisted ventilator modes on triggering, patient effort, and dyspnea. Am J Respir Crit Care Med 155:1940–1948
43. Carlucci A, Richard J-C, Wysocki M, Lepage E, Brochard L, and the SRLF collaborative group on mechanical ventilation (2001) Noninvasive versus conventional mechanical ventilation. An epidemiological survey. Am J Respir Crit Care Med 163:874–880
44. Hill NS (2002) Saving face: better interfaces for noninvasive ventilation. Intensive Care Med 28:227–229
45. Lellouche F, Maggiore SM, Deye N, et al (2002) Effect of the humidification device on the work of breathing during noninvasive ventilation. Intensive Care Med 28:1582–1589
46. Calderini E, Confalonieri M, Puccio PG, Francavilla N, Stella L, Gregoretti C (1999) Patient-ventilator asynchrony during noninvasive ventilation: the role of expiratory trigger. Intensive Care Med 25:662–667

Neurally-adjusted Ventilatory Assist

C. Sinderby, J. Spahija, and J. Beck

Introduction

In today's commercially available mechanical ventilators, the systems for controlling the assist are almost exclusively based on pneumatic technologies, responding to changes in airway pressure, flow, and/or volume in the respiratory circuit. The use of pneumatic technologies to control delivery of ventilatory assist has, however, been reported to have limitations [1] and there have been suggestions that the use of control signals obtained closer to the respiratory centers, may improve the control of ventilatory assist [2].

Neurally adjusted ventilatory assist (NAVA) uses diaphragm electrical activity, measured via an esophageal probe or modified nasogastric tube, to control the assist delivered by the ventilator [3]. With NAVA, the pressure delivered by the ventilator is a function of the neural output to the diaphragm (diaphragm electrical activity) [3].

Figure 1 shows a schematic description of the set-up used for NAVA. The electrical activity of the diaphragm is obtained with an array of electrodes placed in the esophagus at the level of the diaphragm. The signals are amplified and acquired into an on-line processing unit. To optimize signal to noise ratio of the diaphragm electrical activity, the position of the diaphragm with respect to the electrode array is determined [4] and signals are processed with the double subtraction technique [5]. The processed signal is then amplified and outputted to a servo-ventilator, which then delivers assist in proportion to the diaphragm electrical activity [3].

Since NAVA is based on the neural output to the diaphragm, it is not limited by the same factors as conventional systems using airway pressure, flow, and/or volume. The main factors of interest can be summarized as below (in no particular order):

- Airway resistance
- Respiratory system elastance
- Inspiratory muscle function
- Intrinsic positive end-expiratory pressure (PEEPi)
- Air leaks in the system

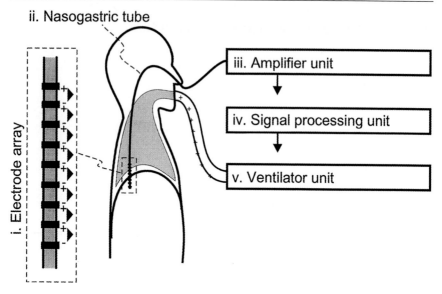

ii. Nasogastric tube

iii. Amplifier unit

iv. Signal processing unit

v. Ventilator unit

i. Electrode array

Fig. 1. Description of the setup used for NAVA. Electrode array arrangement (i), attached to a nasogastric tube (ii) normally used for feeding or other purposes. The electrode array is positioned in the esophagus at the level of and perpendicular to the crural diaphragm such that the active muscle creates an electrically active region around the electrode. Signals from each electrode pair on the array are differentially amplified (iii) and digitized into a personal computer, and filtered (iv) to minimize the influence of cardiac electric activity, electrode motion artifacts, and common noise, as well as other sources of electrical interference. The processed signal's intensity value is displayed for monitoring purposes or fed to the ventilator (v) to control the timing and/or levels of the ventilatory assist. From [3] with permission

Airway Resistance

Resistance of the respiratory airways signifies the amount of pressure required to generate a given airway flow. Airway resistance varies within and between inspiration and expiration and changes with lung disease and lung volume. In practical terms, an increased resistance means that an increased pressure is needed to generate the same flow, and hence increased airway resistance will demand more respiratory muscle activation, i.e., increased diaphragm electrical activation, to increase pressure. If an increase in resistance is not accompanied by a sufficient increase in inspiratory muscle activity and pressure generation, inspiratory flow will decrease. This suggests that, if flow is to be defended, increased inspiratory resistance must result in an increased neural drive to breathe. Thus one can anticipate that the larger the inspiratory resistance, the larger the increase in neural inspiratory drive, if the original breathing pattern is to be maintained.

Figure 2 shows a healthy subject breathing at rest on NAVA (left panels), and the response to increased inspiratory and expiratory resistance (middle panels). As depicted in the two uppermost panels, inspiratory volume and flow profiles are similar between periods where the subject is breathing with and without an inspi-

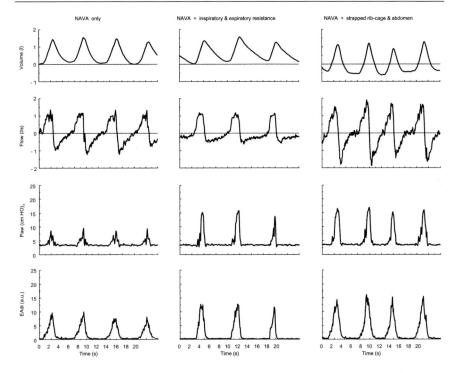

Fig. 2. Influence of increased resistive and elastic loads in a healthy subject breathing with neurally adjusted ventilatory assist (NAVA). From top to bottom, panels show: volume, flow, airway pressure (Paw), and diaphragm electrical activity (EAdi). *Left panels:* unrestricted breathing with NAVA. *Middle panels:* same subject breathing on NAVA through an inspiratory/expiratory airflow resistance (inserted between ventilator circuit and mouthpiece). *Right panels:* the same subject breathing on NAVA when having ribcage and abdomen strapped with elastic bandage. The gain level for NAVA is the same during all conditions.

ratory resistive load. The addition of flow resistance increased the diaphragm electrical activity, which in turn increased the applied pressure to the airways (Paw) such that flow and volume could remain relatively unaltered. Consequently, without a need for quantifying the actual resistive load, the required assist is automatically delivered with NAVA. If the increased load is large and continuous, the gain factor for NAVA, which may be too low to fully compensate for the increased load, may need to be increased.

Respiratory System Elastance

Elastance of the respiratory system denotes the pressure required to produce a given change in lung volume. Similar to airway resistance, respiratory system elastance varies between inspiration and expiration and changes with chest wall/lung disease and elastic recoil increases with increased lung volumes. To maintain breathing with a given tidal volume (V_T) and at the same end-expiratory lung volume in the presence of an increased elastic load, it is necessary to increase pressure generation and activation of the inspiratory muscles.

Figure 2 depicts a healthy subject breathing at rest on NAVA (left panels), and the response to an increased inspiratory elastic load (right panels). As illustrated in the two uppermost panels, inspiratory volume profiles are similar between periods where the subject is breathing with and without elastic load, whereas inspiratory flow is slightly increased. As a consequence of the added elastic load, diaphragm electrical activity increased, which caused the applied Paw to be increased by NAVA, such that more assist was delivered in the presence of the inspiratory elastic load.

Similar to resistive loading, the required assist is automatically delivered with NAVA, without a need for quantifying the actual elastic load. Extra-pulmonary elastic and resistive loads (e.g., visco-elastic properties of the abdomen) will also be included in this neural control loop [6]. Again, in the case that the increased load is large and continuous, there may be a need to adjust the gain settings of NAVA.

Inspiratory Muscle Function

Inspiratory muscle function depends on the neuro-mechanical coupling, the latter characterized by the force that a muscle can generate for a given (maximal or submaximal) neural activation. Any factor that alters the contractile properties of the muscle, e.g., altered lung volume influences the inspiratory muscle activation [7]. For example, if breathing occurs at an increased end-expiratory lung volume and/or with increased V_T, activation must be increased in order to maintain the same pressure output. Although this, in part, is due to increased respiratory system elastic recoil, more importantly it is due to impaired muscle function secondary to, e.g., an impaired length-tension relationship [8]. Adding to the complexity, it should be noted that resistance is expected to decrease at elevated lung volumes, which may partially compensate for the demand of increased pressure and activation, caused by the weakness and the increased elastance.

Figure 3 shows how a healthy subject breathing at rest on NAVA (left panels) responds to an increased end-expiratory lung volume (right panels). As depicted in the uppermost panels, the inspiratory volumes and flow profiles are similar between periods where the subject is breathing with and without an increase in end-expiratory lung volume. In response to hyperinflation, there was an increase in diaphragm electrical activity, which increased the Paw delivered by NAVA, while ventilation, esophageal pressure (Pes), gastric pressure (Pga), and transdiaphragmatic pressure (Pdi) remained relatively unchanged. This shows that NAVA, via intrinsic feedback loops, can automatically adjust ventilatory assist, whereas, with conventional ventilation, one would need to quantify the changes in elastance and resistance, as well as the weakness, in order to manually adjust the level of assist that is necessary to maintain the same breathing pattern.

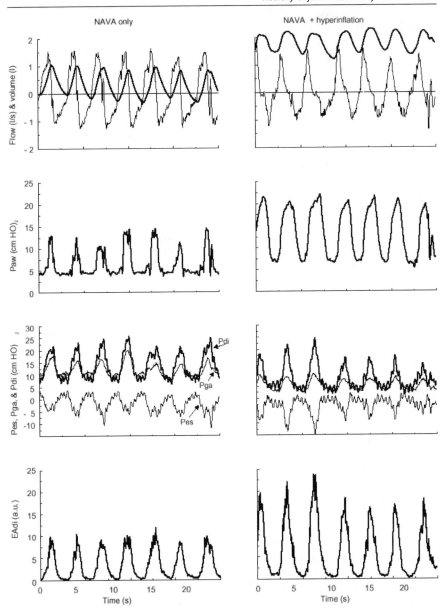

Fig. 3. Effect of increased end-expiratory lung volume (EELV) in a healthy subject breathing with neurally adjusted ventilatory assist (NAVA). Left panels show tidal breathing with NAVA and right panels show the same subject breathing on NAVA when hyperinflated (achieved by actively trying to increase EELV by maintaining slight diaphragm activity during expiration and by applying external PEEP). The gain level for NAVA is the same during both conditions. From top to bottom, panels show: volume (thick line), flow (thin line), airway pressure (Paw), esophageal, gastric and transdiaphragmatic (Pes, Pga, Pdi) pressures, and diaphragm electrical activity (EAdi).

Intrinsic PEEP

PEEPi occurs when the expiratory time is shorter than the time needed to deflate the lung/chest wall to an elastic equilibrium point [9, 10]. Consequently, the onset of airway pressure, flow and volume (detected at the airway opening), will not occur until inspiratory (pleural) pressure generation exceeds the PEEPi level, causing a delay relative to the neural onset of inspiration. PEEPi can be caused by both altered patient respiratory mechanics and inappropriate ventilator settings [10, 11].

With respect to triggering mechanical ventilation with a pneumatic trigger (flow, pressure or volume), PEEPi acts as a threshold load forcing an increase of the total activation and mechanical effort necessary to trigger the assist [12], which delays the onset of inspiratory deflections in airway pressure, flow, and volume relative to the neural onset of inspiration.

To overcome the problems associated with PEEPi, an external positive pressure can be applied (extrinsic PEEP) in order to counterbalance PEEPi [13, 14]. However, PEEPi varies on a breath-by-breath basis, and titration of extrinsic PEEP is clinically difficult and unreliable in spontaneously breathing subjects [15–17]. Furthermore, excessively applied extrinsic PEEP will produce hyperinflation [18].

In the presence of PEEPi, NAVA can initiate assist without delay, independent of whether extrinsic PEEP is applied or not [3].

Air Leaks in the System

Leaks in the respiratory circuit are a problem for pneumatically-controlled ventilator systems. In the presence of leaks, pneumatic triggering may cause either false triggering or no triggering depending on the trigger algorithm used [1, 19]. Cycling-off of ventilatory assist may frequently malfunction during leaks and control of assist delivery becomes inaccurate [19]. With proportional assist ventilation (PAV), which uses flow and volume in combination with measured constants for elastance and resistance (according to the equation of motion), a leak in the respiratory circuit (unless corrected in the formula) will by definition cause the assist to be un-proportional to the predicted muscle pressure generation (Pmus).

NAVA delivers ventilatory assist according to a function continuously calculated from the measured diaphragm electrical activity, where the mechanical ventilator's servo system is continuously adjusting the level of assist, depending on the magnitude of diaphragm electrical activity [3]. The limiting factor for leak compensation is, therefore, the pressure generating capacity of the ventilator. Due to the independence of diaphragm electrical activity from airway pressure, flow and volume, triggering and cycling off with NAVA is not affected by leaks [20].

Issues Pertaining to the Application of NAVA

Similar to all other modes of mechanical ventilation, NAVA uses an upper safety pressure limit, such that, in case of an artifact of disproportionate amplitude, the patient is protected. Potentially, all patient groups could benefit from the use of

NAVA as long as the respiratory center, phrenic nerve, neuromuscular junction, and diaphragm fibers are functional and there is no contraindication or limitation to insertion of an esophageal probe or a nasogastric tube.

Measurements of diaphragm electrical activity, an electrical signal in the microvolt range, in an electrically noisy environment such as the intensive care unit (ICU), with the electrode located in the electrically active esophagus (peristalsis) and next to the heart, is a challenge. An understanding of the behavior of esophageal recordings of the diaphragm electrical signal relative to those of non-diaphragmatic origin is a pre-requisite. Electrode configuration/design and signal processing algorithms, such as the double subtraction technique [5], have made it possible to improve signal to noise ratio to levels suitable for neural control of mechanical ventilation and to account for changes in muscle to electrode distance and electrode filtering [4, 5, 21, 22]. Implementation of custom-designed filters helps to reduce disturbances, and algorithms capable of sensing disturbances are used for their detection and elimination through replacement [5, 23, 24]. The above, in combination with carefully selected hardware components, (i.e., low noise amplifiers), makes it possible to accurately measure the diaphragm electrical activity in the esophagus with an electrode array.

A frequently recurring criticism of the measurement of diaphragm electrical activity with esophageal electrodes during spontaneous breathing is that the signal strength is affected by changes in muscle length and/or lung volume. This critique is based on studies of evoked diaphragm compound muscle action potentials [25] or outdated methodology that does not control for interelectrode distance [26]. Using appropriate methodology, diaphragm electrical activity obtained during spontaneous breathing is not artifactually influenced by changes in muscle length, chest wall configuration and/or lung volume [7, 27].

Measurements of diaphragm electrical activity with an esophageal electrode represent signals obtained from a limited region of the activated crural portion of the diaphragm, and therefore the method could be criticized as not being representative of the whole diaphragm. Studies in healthy subjects [27], patients with chronic obstructive pulmonary disease (COPD) [28], and patients with acute respiratory failure [29], however, show that esophageal recordings of diaphragm electrical activity correspond well to both costal diaphragm electrical activity and to estimates representing global diaphragm activation. This is further supported by animal studies [30, 31]. Given that diaphragm electrical activity increases with respiratory impairment [28, 32], one could assume that as the respiratory muscles are activated closer to their maximum, there are fewer `degrees of freedom' with which the crural and costal portions can vary their activation patterns with respect to each other.

Future Potentials of NAVA

By overcoming the problems associated with the current technology for ventilator triggering, NAVA should improve patient-ventilator interaction and patient comfort during assisted mechanical ventilation, regardless of patient-ventilator interface and presence of leaks. Since the diaphragm electrical activity increases with the extent of respiratory dysfunction [28, 32], the use of NAVA over current technology should be particularly apparent in patients with the most severe respiratory dysfunction. This would be especially true for pre-term neonates who have high breathing frequencies and very small V_T [33], and who use uncuffed small bore endotracheal tubes (which result in high system impedance, air leaks and difficulty in reliably measuring flow and volume).

A major cause of ventilator induced lung injury (VILI) is regional over-distension of alveoli and airways, caused by excessive lung stretch (volutrauma), which in association with partial lung collapse (atelectrauma) can cause extensive damage to the lungs and initiate inflammatory processes leading to chronic lung injury [34, 35]. Consequently, a preferred strategy for mechanical ventilation is to keep the airways from collapsing and avoid excessive lung volumes. In adult patients, this is usually performed in the context of limiting V_T and limiting plateau pressures. This approach has been successful [36], but the values chosen for V_T and plateau pressure are somewhat arbitrary. One novel approach is to have the patient's own 'defense mechanisms' limit the degree of lung distension by providing V_T and lung stretch as 'dictated' by the patient by applying NAVA. In this way, the patient's own afferent feedback system would act to limit the degree of lung distension, without the need for arbitrary V_T and pressures [37].

Conclusion

NAVA is a new mode of mechanical ventilation that responds to central respiratory demand, via intrinsic neural, chemical, and mechanical feedback loops, such that if there is a change in metabolism, load, muscle function, stress (physical or psychological), or presence of leaks, the assist will always act to compensate.

By improving patient-ventilator interaction, during both invasive and non-invasive ventilation, NAVA has the potential to reduce ventilator-related complications, reduce the incidence of lung injury, facilitate weaning from mechanical ventilation, and decrease the duration of stay in the ICU and overall hospitalization.

References

1. Hill L (2001) Flow triggering, pressure triggering, and autotriggering during mechanical ventilation. Crit Care Med 28:579–581
2. Sassoon CSH, Foster GT (2001) Patient-ventilator asynchrony. Curr Opin Crit Care. 7:28–33
3. Sinderby C, Navalesi P, Beck J, et al (1999) Neural control of mechanical ventilation in respiratory failure. Nature Med 5:1433–1436
4. Beck J, Sinderby C, Lindström L, Grassino A. (1996) Influence of bipolar esophageal electrode positioning on measurements of human crural diaphragm EMG. J Appl Physiol 81:1434–1449
5. Sinderby C, Beck J, Lindström L, Grassino A (1997) Enhancement of signal quality in esophageal recordings of diaphragm EMG. J Appl Physiol 82:1370–1377
6. Sinderby C, Ingvarsson P, Sullivan L, Wickström I, Lindström L (1992) The role of the diaphragm in trunk extension in tetraplegia. Paraplegia 30:389–395
7. Beck J, Sinderby C, Lindström L, Grassino A (1998) Effects of lung volume on diaphragm EMG signal strength during voluntary contractions. J Appl Physiol 85:1123–1134

8. Gauthier AP, Verbanck V, Estenne M, Segebarth C, Macklem PT, Paiva M (1994) Three-dimensional reconstruction of the in vivo diaphragm shape at different lung volumes. J Appl Physiol 76: 495–506

9. Rossi A, Polese G, Brandi G, Conti G (1995) The intrinsic positive end expiratory pressure (PEEPi): physiology, implications, measurement, and treatment. Intensive Care Med 21:522–536

10. Ranieri VM, Grasso S, Fiore T, Giuliani R (1996) Auto positive end expiratory pressure and dynamic hyperinflation. Clin Chest Med 17:379–394

11. Pepe PE, Marini JJ (1982) Occult positive end-expiratory pressure in mechanically ventilated patients with airflow obstruction. Am Rev Respir Dis 126:166–170

12. Aslanian P, Atrous S, Isabey D, et al (1998) Effects of flow triggering on breathing effort during partial ventilatory assist. Am J Respir Crit Care Med 157:135–143

13. Petrof B, Legare M, Goldberg P, Milic-Emili J, Gottfried SB (1990) Continuous positive airway pressure reduces work of breathing and dyspnea during weaning from mechanical ventilation in severe chronic obstructive pulmonary disease. Am Rev Respir Dis 141:281–288

14. Appendini L, Patessio A, Zanaboni S, et al (1994) Physiologic effects of positive end-expiratory and mask pressure support during exacerbations of chronic obstructive pulmonary disease. Am J Respir Crit Care Med 149:1069–1076

15. Ninane V, Yernault JC, De Troyer A (1993) Intrinsic PEEP with chronic obstructive pulmonary disease. Role of expiratory muscles. Am Rev Respir Dis 148:1037–1042

16. Lessard MR, Lofaso F, Brochard L (1995) Expiratory muscle activity increases intrinsic positive end-expiratory pressure independently of dynamic hyperinflation in mechanically ventilated patients. Am J Respir Crit Care Med 151:562–569

17. Maltais F, Reissmann H, Navalesi P, et al (1994) Comparison of static and dynamic measurements of intrinsic PEEP in mechanically ventilated patients. Am J Respir Crit Care Med 150:1318–1324

18. Ranieri VM, Giuliani R, Cinnella G, et al (1993) Physiologic effects of positive end-expiratory pressure in patients with chronic obstructive pulmonary disease during acute ventilatory failure and controlled mechanical ventilation. Am Rev Respir Dis 147:5–13

19. Calderini E, Confalonieri M, Puccio PG, Francavilla N, Stella L, Gregoretti C (1999) Patient-ventilator asynchrony during non-invasive ventilation: the role of the expiratory trigger. Intensive Care Med 25:662–667

20. Beck J, Gottfried S, Spahija J, Comtois N, Sinderby C (2001) Influence of respiratory system leaks on neurally adjusted Ventilatory assist (NAVA). Am J Respir Crit Care Med 163:A132 (abst)

21. Sinderby CA, Comtois AS, Thomson RG, Grassino AE (1996) Influence of the bipolar electrode transfer function on the electromyogram power spectrum. Muscle Nerve 19:290–301

22. Sinderby C, Friberg S, Comtois N, Grassino A (1996) Chest wall muscle cross-talk in the canine costal diaphragm electromyogram. J Appl Physiol 81:2312–2327

23. Sinderby C, Lindstrom L, Grassino AE (1995) Automatic assessment of electromyogram quality. J Appl Physiol 79:1803–1815

24. Aldrich T, Sinderby C, McKenzie D, Estenne M, Gandevia S (2002) ATS/ERS Statement on Respiratory Muscle Testing: Part 3. Electrophysiologic techniques for the assessment of respiratory muscle function. Am J Respir Crit Care Med 166:518–624

25. Gandevia SC, McKenzie DK (1986) Human diaphragmatic EMG: changes with lung volume and posture during supramaximal phrenic stimulation. J Appl Physiol 60:1420–1428

26. Brancatisano A, Kelly SM, Tully A, Loring SH, Engel LA (1989) Postural changes in spontaneous and evoked regional diaphragmatic activity in dogs. J Appl Physiol 66:1699–1705

27. Sinderby C, Lindström L, Comtois N, Grassino AE (1996) Effects of diaphragm shortening on the mean action potential conduction velocity. J Physiol (Lond) 490:207–214

28. Sinderby C, Beck J, Weinberg J, Spahija J, Grassino A (1998) Voluntary activation of the human diaphragm in health and disease. J Appl Physiol 85:2146–2158

29. Beck J, Gottfried SB, Navalesi P, et al (2001) Electrical activity of the diaphragm during pressure support ventilation in acute respiratory failure. Am J Respir Crit Care Med 164:419–424
30. Lourenco RV, Cherniack NS, Malm JR, Fishman AP (1966) Nervous output from the respiratory centers during obstructed breathing. J Appl Physiol 21:527–533
31. Aubier M, Trippenbach T, Roussos C (1981) Respiratory muscle fatigue during cardiogenic shock. J Appl Physiol 51:499–508
32. De Troyer A, Leeper JB, McKenzie DK, Gandevia SC (1997) Neural drive to the diaphragm in patients with severe COPD. Am J Respir Crit Care Med 155:1335–1340
33. Durang M, Rigatto H (1981) Tidal volume and respiratory frequency with bronchopulmonary dysplasia (BPD). Early Hum Dev 5:55–62
34. Clark RH, Gerstmann DR, Jobe AH, Moffit ST, Slutsky AS, Yoder BA (2001) Lung injury in neonates: Causes, strategies for prevention, and long-term consequences. J Pediatr 139:478–486
35. Tremblay LN, Slutsky AS (1998) Ventilator induced lung injury: from barotrauma to biotrauma. Proc Assoc Am Physicians 110:482–488
36. ARDS Network (2000) Ventilation with lower tidal volumes as compared with traditional tidal volumes for acute lung injury and the acute respiratory distress syndrome. N Engl J Med 18:1301–1308
37. Beck J, Spahija J, DeMarchie M, Comtois N, Sinderby C (2002) Unloading during neurally adjusted ventilatory assist (NAVA). Eur Respir J 20:637s (abst)

Liberating Patients from Mechanical Ventilation: What Have We Learned About Protocolizing Care?

J. W.W. Thomason and E. W. Ely

Introduction

In this chapter, we will discuss the cornerstones of liberating patients from mechanical ventilation, with special attention to protocols and recent advances over
the past 5 years. We will also review the historical sequence of landmark trials in
weaning (Table 1), suggest future trends in research, and try to dispel some key
myths regarding weaning [1]. Because of the continued, pervasive use of the term
`weaning' in modern critical care literature, we must first define this term. While
historically used to imply a deliberate process of *slowly* withdrawing ventilatory
support, we will use the term 'weaning' to imply the safe yet *rapid* removal from
mechanical ventilation as early as possible after identifying that the patient is able
to breathe spontaneously. In accordance with this definition, and for ease of
reading, we will use 'weaning' interchangeably with 'liberating from mechanical
ventilation'. Another point of emphasis is that weaning should be regarded as an
interdisciplinary process reliant upon physicians, nurses, respiratory therapists (or
their counterparts outside of the United States), pharmacists, and other members
of the intensive care unit (ICU) team of healthcare professionals.

The Agency for Healthcare Research and Quality (AHCPR), the American
College of Chest Physicians (ACCP), and the American Association of Respiratory
Care recently published clinical practice guidelines which represent a fresh look at
the state-of-the-art in this field [2]. This report was listed in Krieger's 2002 "top ten
list in mechanical ventilation" [3], and along with Tobin's recent update on advances in mechanical ventilation [4], should be considered mandatory reading for
all intensivists and pulmonologists.

To efficiently review and expand upon the AHCPR guidelines, this chapter is
structured to address several commonly encountered questions regarding weaning:
1. What is the role of 'weaning parameters'?
2. What is a 'spontaneous breathing trial' and how is one performed?
3. What were the pivotal investigations that led to modern day weaning protocols?
4. What data support 'real life' implementation of weaning protocols?
5. What advice can increase the success of implementation?
6. Is there a relationship between weaning success and sedation practices?

What is the Role of 'Weaning Parameters'?

Over 66 independent predictors of success for weaning have been identified over the past 30 years. These early studies stimulated numerous hypothesis-driven randomized controlled trials (RCTs), many of which have formed the backbone of the modern evidence based weaning approach (Table 1). In general, physicians do not discontinue mechanical ventilation efficiently, which results in a 'weaning time' of about two thirds of the total ventilator time [5, 6]. Our predictions of whether patients can have mechanical ventilation successfully discontinued are often inaccurate, with positive and negative predictive values of only 50 and 67%, respectively [7]. As well, half of patients who extubate themselves prematurely do not require reintubation within 24 hours [8–11].

Table 1. Key trials and evidence-based reviews of weaning from mechanical ventilation[*]

Building Blocks	Author [ref]	Year	Main findings/comments
I	Yang & Tobin [15]	1991	f/V_T (rapid shallow breathing index)
II	Brochard et al. [18]	1994	SBT and PSV weaning found to be better
	Esteban et al. [19]	1995	than IMV weaning – no 'control' arm
III	Ely et al. [20]	1996	Protocols with 'team approach' and SBTs
	Kollef et al. [22]	1997	were superior to physician-directed
	Marelich et al. [24]	2000	
Refining Years			
IV	Vallverdu et al. [62]	1998	SBTs equally effective at 30 minutes
	Esteban et al. [37]	1999	versus 120 minutes with PSV of up
	Perren et al. [38]	2002	to 7 cm, 1/3rd of failures occur after 30 min
V	Ely et al. [13]	1999	SBTs may be safely performed in patients
	Khamiees et al. [12]	2001	who are hemodynamically stable and have
	Epstein et al.	2003	modest oxygen requirements (?regardless
	(unpublished data)		of any specific f/V_T value)
VI	Kollef et al. [53]	1998	Nurse driven sedation protocols, bolus
	Brook et al. [57]	1999	dosing of sedatives, and the daily cessation
	Kress et al. [52]	2000	of sedatives can each shorten a patient's
			length of stay on the ventilator
Clinical Practice Guidelines			
VIII	MacIntyre et al. [2]	2001	Evidenced-based guidelines for ventilator
	Jacobi et al. [51]	2002	weaning and sedation in ICU

[*] This table provides a historical overview of selected trials of liberating patients from mechanical ventilation that serve as the foundation for the recommendations in this chapter. V_T: tidal volume; SBT: spontaneous breathin trial; PSV: pressure support ventilation; IMV: intermittent mandatory ventilation

One of the most commonly employed weaning parameters, the ratio of respiratory frequency (f) to tidal volume (V_T), has recently been re-evaluated [12]. Epstein and colleagues (unpublished data presented at the American Thoracic Society Meeting in May, 2001) prospectively studied the utility of the f/V_T as a screening tool for 304 adult patients among three separate ICUs. The patients were randomized to two parallel groups, each of whom had an f/V_T measured daily using a Wright's spirometer while on zero pressure support. Group 1 consisted of 151 patients who were allowed to progress to a spontaneous breathing trial (SBT) after a liberal daily screen (including a $PaO_2/FiO_2 \geq 150$, positive end-expiratory pressure [PEEP] ≤ 5 cmH2O, hemodynamic stability on minimal vasopressors, arousable to command, and requiring endotracheal tube suctioning $\leq$ every 2 hours) regardless of the result of their f/V_T. In contrast, the 153 patients randomized to group 2 were not allowed to undergo an SBT unless they passed the daily screening criteria *and* their recorded f/V_T was 105. Although the two groups were demographically equal, Epstein found no difference in time on the ventilator, extubation failure, need for a tracheotomy, mortality, or length of stay in the ICU (Table 2). These data suggest that it is safe to allow a patient to undergo an SBT, despite the f/V_T. It is supportive of recent data from Khamiees et al. [12], who similarly found no difference between successful versus unsuccessful extubations based upon the f/V_T used as a weaning parameter. In addition, of the 1,167 total patients studied by Ely et al. [13], 1 of 4 patients who were successfully extubated never passed daily screen criteria which included an f/V_T.

Table 2. Incorporation of rapid shallow breathing index and outcomes in mechanical ventilation

	f/V_T not included in weaning decision n = 151	f/V_T included in weaning decision n = 153	P value
Mechanical ventilation days*	6 (3, 10)	6 (3, 11)	0.77
Hospital days*	19 (13, 35)	19 (10, 37)	0.62
ICU days*	9 (6, 17)	9 (5, 15)	0.64
Reintubation n. (%)[+]	28 (18)	23 (15)	0.40
Mortality n. (%)	40 (26)	34 (22)	0.38
Tracheotomy n. (%)	10 (7)	6 (4)	0.30
Unplanned extubation n. (%)	14 (9)	9 (6)	0.25

* values are expressed as median ($\pm$ interquartile range)
[+]defined as the need for reintubation within 72 hours after planned extubation
Note: Comparison of the outcome between parallel study groups for Epstein et al. [13]. Group 1 consisted of 151 patients who were allowed to progress to a spontaneous breathing trial (SBT) after a liberal daily screen (including a $PaO_2/FiO_2 \geq 150$, PEEP ≤ 5 cmH2O, hemodynamic stability on minimal vasopressors, arousable to command, and requiring endotracheal tube suctioning no more than every 2 hours) regardless of the result of their f/V_T. Group 2 consisted of 153 patients who were not allowed to undergo an SBT unless they passed the daily screening criteria *and* their recorded f/V_T was ≤ 105.

Table 3. Criteria to qualify for spontaneous breathing trial (SBT)

Patients receiving mechanical ventilation for respiratory failure should undergo a formal assessment of discontinuation potential if the following criteria are satisfied:

- Evidence for some reversal of the underlying cause of respiratory failure;
- Adequate oxygenation (i.e.; PaO_2/FiO_2 ratio >150 to 200; requiring positive end-expiratory pressure [PEEP] $\leq$ 5 to 8 cmH$_2$O; FiO$_2$ 0.4 to 0.5); and pH (e.g., $\geq$ 7.25);
- Hemodynamic stability, as defined by the absence of active myocardial ischemia and the absence of clinically significant hypotension (i.e.; a condition requiring no vasopressor therapy or therapy with only low-dose vasopressors such as dopamine or dobutamine, < 5 µg/kg/min), and
- The capability to initiate an inspiratory effort.

Note: The decision to use these criteria must be individualized. Some patients not satisfying all of the above criteria (e.g., patients with chronic hypoxemia values below the thresholds cited) may be ready for attempts at discontinuation of mechanical ventilation [2]. On the other hand, there are times in which a patient will meet these criteria and the clinician will appropriately elect to continue without an SBT. These criteria are guidelines only and should not be considered as absolutes.

Those who are advocates of weaning parameters attempt to identify patients who have a high likelihood of 'fatigue' soon after extubation. Laghi et al. [14] recently tried to clarify the role of 'low-frequency fatigue' as it may relate to diaphragm weakness and weaning failure. This entity is also known as long-lasting fatigue, which is a result of muscle injury and may last for days. Twitch transdiaphragmatic pressures were carefully recorded on 11 weaning failure patients and 8 weaning success patients both before and after SBTs. Despite greater mechanical load and diaphragmatic effort experienced in the weaning failure group, no evidence of low-frequency fatigue was found. This small study lays the foundation for advancing our understanding of the diaphragm and its role in the physiology of weaning failure.

In considering the recent body of literature reviewed above, weaning parameters, may best be regarded as 'common-sense' safety criteria that should be applied individually prior to initiating a patient's SBT. Table 3 lists the range of such criteria recommended by the AHCPR [2]. As detailed in this report, any single weaning parameter used in isolation serves poorly and can only be used as an adjunct to clinical experience. Indeed, the likelihood ratios (the expression of the odds that a given test result will be present in a patient with a given condition) for all of these parameters are less than 3, implying only moderate shifts in post-test probability after their use (Table 4).

Therefore, weaning parameters should be inclusive, rather than exclusive, and patients should be allowed to progress to spontaneous breathing at the earliest possible time point. As well, when parameters are used as a screening process prior to a more definitive SBT, they should be performed with a high degree of standardization. This may be possible if one person performs all of the measures [15]. Unfortunately, this degree of accuracy is a major obstacle in current daily practice. In an interesting investigation to determine the actual methods used by registered

Table 4. Predictive values for individual weaning parameters[*]

Predictor	Likelihood ratio	Sensitivity (%)	Specificity (%)
Minute ventilation (10-12 liters)	1.2	50	40
Respiratory rate	1.6	97	31
Tidal volume (325 ml)	1.5	76	36
f/V_T (100 breaths/minute/liter)	2.8	84	42
Negative inspiratory force (-25 to 30cmH$_2$O)	1.5	60	47
Daily screen	2.7	88	67

[*]AHCPR pooled results for weaning parameters [2].

respiratory therapists to obtain weaning parameters, Hoo et al. [16] distributed a questionnaire to local registered respiratory therapists. Among 102 registered respiratory therapists serving nine different hospitals, wide variations regarding both weaning parameter definitions and how to obtain them were revealed. Specifically, there was no consensus on the mode of ventilation used during the process, the time before recording the parameters, or even how to record a parameter such as respiratory rate (e.g., ventilator display vs watching the patient). Furthermore, there was wide variation between registered respiratory therapists at the same institution.

What were the Pivotal Investigations that led to Modern Day Weaning Protocols?

In an early investigation of weaning parameters [17], it was noted that this clinical decision is often arbitrary, "based on judgment and experience". Despite numerous efforts to determine the best method of weaning patients from mechanical ventilation, it was not until 1994 that any RCT showed one method (pressure support ventilation, or PSV) to be superior to others [18]. The following year, however, another well performed RCT showed seemingly conflicting results, with SBTs leading to earlier extubation among mechanically ventilated patients [19]. Although these investigations reached contradictory conclusions, these trials showed that:
1. weaning strategies influence the duration of mechanical ventilation
2. the specific criteria used to initiate changes in ventilatory support influence outcome
3. the most ineffective approach was intermittent mandatory ventilation (IMV), a previously widely-used strategy.

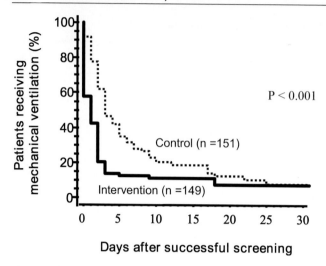

Fig.1. Kaplan Meier curve showing effect of therapist and nurse-driven protocol on duration of mechanical ventilation as compared to non-protocolized approach using attending physicians as key decision makers. Despite higher severity of illness in the intervention group, those patients were off of mechanical ventilation an average of 2 days earlier as compared to the control group. From [20] with permission

In the first prospective study to incorporate a 'control', non-protocolized arm versus a registered respiratory therapist driven protocol we enrolled 300 mechanically ventilated medical and nonsurgical cardiac patients into a RCT in which the treatment group was weaned using a two-step process of screening by registered respiratory therapists followed by daily SBTs for patients who 'passed' the screen [20]. The outcomes of the investigation included removal from mechanical ventilation two days earlier in the protocol-directed group despite a higher severity of illness (Fig. 1), 50% fewer complications, and a reduction in the cost of ICU stay by $5,000 per patient. Subsequent implementation of this protocol in 530 patients at another large medical center was associated with a similar reintubation rate (6%) and no increased risk of mortality [21].

Simultaneous to our study, Kollef and colleagues [22] were conducting another RCT (n=357) of protocol-directed versus physician-directed weaning in four ICUs (two medical and two surgical). This investigation incorporated three separate weaning protocols because of difficulty in achieving consensus among different units, underscoring the practical challenges facing implementation of protocols. The protocol-directed group incorporated an amalgam of SBTs, PSV, and synchronized IMV (SIMV) protocols, and demonstrated an earlier initiation of weaning efforts and a median duration of mechanical ventilation of 35 hours versus 44 hours in the physician-directed group.

Two other RCTs have compared protocol-based weans to conventional weans. One very small trial (15 patients) compared a computer-directed wean to a physician-directed wean and found trends in favor of the computer-directed wean in both non-extubation and reintubation rates [23]. In a more recent investigation that included 335 patients (~50% surgical, predominantly trauma), Marelich and colleagues [24] showed that the use of a weaning protocol incorporating multiple daily SBT assessments shortened the median duration of mechanical ventilation from 124 hours to 68 hours (p=0.001).

The numerous non-randomized controlled clinical trials of weaning [25–33] are generally consistent with the results of the RCTs, demonstrating statistically significant reductions or trends toward reductions in the duration of mechanical ventilation and ICU length of stay. Mortality and reintubation rates do not appear to differ between experimental and control groups. Protocol-based weans are associated with other favorable outcomes such as fewer arterial blood gases and significant cost savings.

Personnel expenses are thought to account for more than 50% of the cost of mechanical ventilation [34], and some investigators have advocated the use of a weaning team [35]. In our study, the total cost of ICU care throughout the study period for the control group was $4,297,024 and for the intervention group was $3,855,001, representing a savings of $442,023. Kollef et al. [22] reported savings of $42,960 in their protocol-directed weaning group. Similarly, Smyrnios et al. [36] reported dramatic savings of $3,440,787 during the course of their recently published prospective, before-and-after intervention trial using their own version of an SBT focused weaning protocol. These savings were the result of only 2 years of protocolized weaning for 518 adult ICU patients. The details of this investigation will be discussed in the protocol section.

What is a 'Spontaneous Breathing Trial' and how is one Performed?

Allowing a patient to breathe spontaneously with minimal or no ventilatory support for a predetermined time during close monitoring is an optimal process to confirm a patient's readiness for extubation. This method of liberation is generally accepted as standard of care for clinicians and researchers alike [2]. We recommend performing a SBT on a daily basis, preferably during the morning hours. Further trials throughout the day may be tolerated, but generally do not reduce ventilator time [19], and always make use of precious ICU resources. The specific definition of an SBT and how to perform one is detailed in Table 5.

Esteban and the Spanish Lung Failure Collaborative Group have defined practical aspects of the SBT. These investigators showed in a RCT of 526 patients that successful extubation was achieved equally effectively with SBTs lasting 30 minutes or 120 minutes [37]. Perren and colleagues [38] recently published a similar RCT involving 98 patients, all of whom were considered ready to wean after 48 hours of mechanical ventilation in 2 medical-surgical adult ICUs. The extubation success rate of a SBT using 7 cmH$_2$O pressure support and lasting only 30 minutes was 93%, with only four (9%) patients requiring reintubation. Comparatively, the success rate of an SBT lasting 2 hours was 88%, with only two (4%) patients requiring re-intubation.

Esteban's group had previously documented that the SBT could be conducted with either a low level of PSV or a T-piece [39]. In our studies, SBTs were performed with either standard T-tube circuits or flow-triggered openings of the demand valve

Table 5. How to conduct a spontaneous breathing trial (SBT)

- A trial of spontaneous breathing for a predetermined amount of time (i.e., 30 to 120 minutes) with ventilator rate set to 0 and pressure support of 0 to 7 (we prefer 0)

- Practical criteria for safety:
  - Absence of agitation (NOT dangerous to self or others)
    Oxygen saturation 88%
  - FiO_2 0.50
  - PEEP 7.5 cmH$_2$O
  - No evidence of active myocardial ischemia
  - No significant use of vasopressors or inotropes (patients may be on dopamine or dobutamine at ≤5 µg/kg/min or norepinephrine ≤2 µg/min, but may not be receiving any vasopressin or milrinone)
  - Patient exhibiting spontaneous inspiratory efforts.
  - No evidence of increased intracranial pressure

Who performs the SBT?

- Registered respiratory therapists and/or registered nurses screen patients for the safety criteria above and initiate or prompt a physician to order an SBT

- Registered respiratory therapists and/or registered nurses initiate the SBT and monitor the patient during the trial, re-initiating mechanical ventilation if criteria for trial termination are met

When is an SBT terminated?

- If the patient successfully tolerates the SBT for 30 minutes to two hours

- When one of the following conditions is met:
  - Any abrupt changes in mental status including but not limited to sustained anxiety, delirium, somnolence, and coma
  - Total RR > 35 or < 8 (5 min at respiratory rate > 35 or <8 may be tolerated).
  - SpO$_2$ < 88% (< 15 min at < 88% may be tolerated).
  - Respiratory distress (two or more of the following):
    - HR > or < 120% of the 0600 rate AND either <60 bpm or >130 bpm.
    - Marked use of accessory muscles.
    - Abdominal paradox.
    - Diaphoresis.
    - Marked subjective dyspnea.

What does it mean if a patient passes an SBT?

- Successful completion of a 2 hour SBT indicates an 85 to 90% chance of successfully staying off the mechanical ventilation for 48 hours [21].

RR = respiratory rate; HR = heart rate; FiO_2 = fraction of inspired oxygen; SpO_2 =oxygen saturation as obtained via a pulse oximeter or an arterial blood gas.

without additional support. Incorporating flow-triggering during the SBT was a convenience that minimized respiratory therapist involvement, and had not been investigated by others. Taken together, these investigations support institutional variations in the specific method of conducting an SBT. In fact, individual physicians may wish to tailor the technique and duration of SBTs for individual patients.

Almost 10 years have passed since publication of the first evidence supporting the process of rapidly removing ventilatory support (e.g., SBTs or PSV tapered quickly) as a means of weaning [18–20]. However, in a recent international utilization review of the actual weaning practices of 412 medical and surgical ICUs in 1,638 patients receiving mechanical ventilation, only 20% of patients were weaned using some form of SBT, and in the United States SBTs were incorporated into weaning in less than 10% of all patients studied [40]. Such a disconnect between daily practice and evidence based medicine is a reality that strongly supports the implementation of widespread protocol-guided weaning algorithms.

Which Data Support 'Real-Life' Implementation of Weaning Protocols?

Smyrnios et al. recently published an interesting prospective before-and-after intervention study [36] examining the effects of a hospital-wide weaning protocol. These investigators recorded data on all adult ICU patients who met criteria for DRG 475 "respiratory system diagnosis with mechanical ventilation", and DRG 483 "tracheotomy except for mouth, laryngeal, or pharyngeal disorder" during a baseline, non-intervention year. They subsequently initiated a multifaceted, multidisciplinary weaning management protocol involving physicians, nurses, and registered respiratory therapists, and included a mandatory pulmonary consult if the primary physician felt that weaning was possible for 3 days, and yet unsuccessful. The once-daily SBT was chosen as the weaning mode of choice, using continuous positive airway pressure (CPAP) at 5 cmH_2O during the trial. This protocol was left in place for 2 years, with frequent monitoring for compliance and continuing educational sessions. The mean APACHE II score actually *increased* from the pre-intervention, baseline year as compared to the second year of the trial (p < 0.0005). However, the endpoints were all significantly reduced (all p < 0.0005) in the post intervention protocol group compared to the pre-protocol group and included mean time on the ventilator (17.5 vs 23.9 days), mean hospital length of stay (24.7 vs 37.5 days), mean ICU length of stay (20.3 vs 30.5 days), and percentage of patients requiring tracheotomy (41 vs 61%). A total cost savings of $3,440,787 was estimated, as total cost per case decreased from $92,933 to $63,687 (p < .0005).

Vitacca et al. published data in regard to patients with chronic respiratory failure [41], which was listed in Krieger's 2002 top ten list in mechanical ventilation [3]. Invasively ventilated COPD patients who remained on the ventilator after 15 days were randomized to either daily SBTs or decreasing levels of pressure support. Both methods were equivocal, and yet both were better than a historical control model of "uncontrolled clinical practice". Again, the influence of protocolized weaning was shown to be superior.

Iregui et al. [42] recently studied the efficacy of a weaning protocol powered by a handheld computer program. This investigation was also designed as a before-and-after prospective study with consecutive control and intervention groups, including all patients in a medical ICU who required invasive ventilation in a single, academic institution. The specific registered respiratory therapist-driven protocol for all patients was identical to that used by Kollef et al. during their 1997 study, hence all patients (n = 176 control/176 intervention) should have undergone SBTs in exactly the same manner. However, patients during the intervention period had a significantly greater likelihood of undergoing an SBT when they first met the protocol criteria, presumably because the handheld computer 'reminded' the registered respiratory therapist to move ahead with the SBT. The registered respiratory therapists were more confident and effective in their bedside management of patients, which allowed for better protocol compliance. This automated methodology, reliant on a small, handheld computer, improved weaning efficiency in a safe manner, and resulted in a reduced length of stay in the ICU, and less ventilator associated pneumonia (VAP).

Written from the perspective of a respiratory therapist, Croft recently published a concise review of protocol recommendations [43] and stated that even the best-planned protocols are only as effective as the registered respiratory therapists (or equivalent non-physician health care provider if outside of the United States) implementing them.

Collectively, these data would suggest that it is the protocol approach to weaning (and the culture change which these protocols represent) that produces benefit in the medical ICU population, rather than any specific modality of weaning. Current data do not support a specific protocol, and the selection of an appropriate protocol is best left to multidisciplinary teams at individual institutions. Importantly, each institution must endorse the fiscal commitment and the staffing modifications necessary for developing and implementing a multidisciplinary weaning protocol team of dedicated health care practitioners. For a list of the seven specific AHCPR recommendations regarding the implementation of weaning protocols, see Table 6.

What Advice can Increase the Success of Implementation?

Specific tips for the implementation of weaning protocols and for avoiding barriers to success, derived from the study of over 15,000 patient days and nearly 2 years of implementation, are presented in Table 7 [44]. Importantly, protocols *per se* should not be viewed as rigid rules, but rather as dynamic tools in evolution, which can be improved upon to address local problems and to accommodate new data. It is imperative that protocols be used not to replace clinical judgment, but rather to complement it.

In our experience, both clinically and from a research perspective, there are 2 important tenants regarding implementation of a weaning algorithm: 1) one must work hard at the outset to attain general consensus about the algorithm among the health care professionals (registered respiratory therapists, nurses, and physicians); and 2) the team must grant reasonable autonomy to the registered respiratory therapists and nurses who will be instrumental in moving patients through the protocol.

To implement a novel protocol, whether in an academic or community based institution, we suggest following the pattern of change known as the "breakthrough method". The concept of this approach is simple; you must first set goals, then implement small changes, measure or quantify the outcome of the changes, and subsequently improve upon the original protocol. Essentially, you must 'plan-do-

Table 6. Seven AHCPR recommendations regarding weaning protocols

1. Non-physician health care professionals should be included in the development and utilization of respiratory care protocols (not confined to liberation from mechanical ventilation).
2. ICU clinicians should utilize protocols for liberating patients from mechanical ventilation in order to safely reduce the duration of mechanical ventilation.
3. At least once daily spontaneous breathing trials should be used to identify patients who are ready for liberation from the ventilator.
4. When patients fail a trial of spontaneous breathing, the following assessments and interventions should be made, based on varying levels of evidence:
   - That all remediable factors be addressed to enhance the prospects of successful liberation from mechanical ventilation (e.g., electrolyte derangements, bronchospasm, malnutrition, patient positioning, excess secretions, etc.).
   - That the patient be placed in an upright position on a comfortable, safe, and well-monitored mode of mechanical vcentilation (such as pressure support ventilation).
   - That a spontaneous breathing test (SBT) be performed at least once daily. Few data support multiple manipulations of ventilator settings each day in an effort to wean or 'train' the patient. For clinicians who prefer step-wise reductions in mechanical ventilation, both multiple daily SBTs and weaning pressure support ventilation appear superior to intermittent mandatory ventilation.
   - In the face of repeated failures at daily trials of spontaneous breathing, clinicians should consider longer-term options, including both tracheotomy and a long-term acute-care or step-down ventilator facility.
5. When patients have passed a spontaneous breathing trial, clinicians should seriously consider prompt extubation.
6. Consideration should be made of protocols that include daily cessation and targeted sedation goals to reduce the duration of mechanical ventilation and ICU stay.
7. Consideration should be made of the following strategies for weaning protocols: development using an evidence-based approach by a multidisciplinary team, and implementation using effective behavior changing strategies such as interactive education, opinion leaders, reminders, audit and feedback.

study-act', as described in detail recently by Brattebo et al. [45]. The initial version of a protocol will have some flaws that mostly relate to the uniqueness of an individual institution. These initial obstacles should not be regarded as failures of the methodology, but rather as opportunities for improvement.

Protocolized care has been advocated in many facets of medicine, but relinquishing control of the patient's management often creates resentment and frustration on the part of physicians. Negative reactions to protocols may be reasonable under some circumstances, since protocols have the potential to do harm. Important considerations that may facilitate behavioral changes include interactive education, timely and specific feedback, participation by physicians in the effort to change, administrative interventions, and even financial incentives [46. Effective implementation also requires adequate staffing. If staffing is reduced below certain thresholds, clinical outcomes may be jeopardized [47, 48]. In the specific context of liberation from mechanical ventilation, reductions in nurse to patient ratios have been associated with prolonged duration of mechanical ventilation [49].

Table 7. How to maximize the likelihood of success in achieving both a change of behavior and long-term protocol implementation[*]

---

1. Identify the patient-care issue as a high priority item (e.g., ventilator weaning and timely extubation)

2. Obtain base-line data (e.g., lengths of stay and complication rates)

3. Base the program on medical evidence, but also reviews of other programs and attain local expert opinion

4. Acknowledge the need for a 'change in culture' on the part of *both* physicians and non-physician healthcare professionals

5. Work hard to attain 'buy-in' and participation of key opinion leaders/physicians

6. Establish a team including the hospital administration, respiratory care practitioners, nurses/nurse practitioners, potentially ethicists, and physicians

7. As a team, establish goals and set objective definitions of success and failure.

8. Structure a graded, staged implementation process which provides all of the following:
   - Education
   - Timely feedback
   - Compliance monitoring (particularly important and yet most often overlooked)
   - Tracking of appropriate outcomes (including cost) via daily data collection
   - Avoid complicated plans aimed at perfection; rather remain practical and useful
   - Consider the entire process to be dynamic not fixed; incorporate innovative changes over time to respond to lessons learned

9. Avoid changing personnel too often

10. Avoid overly rigid interpretation of the 'rules' of the protocol

11. Do not remove clinical judgment on part of any team members

12. Acknowledge the need for and plan to have periodic refresher implementation processes to avoid the otherwise inevitable 'regression to baseline'.

---

[*] These specific tips for the implementation of weaning protocols and for avoiding common barriers to success were derived from the study of over 15,000 patient days and nearly 2 years of implementation [45].

It is clear that guidelines, statements, and protocols have increasingly been considered as part of the standard of care, both by physicians and courts alike. Accordingly, there are some legal implications of clinical practice guidelines, which were recently addressed by Damen et al. [50] with regard to European court standards. The authors are clear that physician autonomy should remain the gold standard for care, and court decisions must be based upon sound clinical judgment. In other words, strict compliance to a protocol does not exclude liability, precisely because protocols and guidelines are designed for a population, rather than an individual patient.

Is there a Relationship Between Weaning Success and Sedation Practices?

Clinical practice guidelines with regard to standardizing sedation protocols within the ICU have recently been published as a collaborative effort among the American College of Critical Care Medicine, the Society of Critical Care Medicine (SCCM), the American Society of Health-System Pharmacists, and the ACCP [51]. Only two of the current 28 recommendations are supported by grade-A evidence. One of the grade-A suggestions reads as follows: "The titration of the sedative dose to a defined endpoint is recommended with systematic tapering of the dose or daily interruption with re-titration to minimize prolonged sedative effects."

Specific support for this statement can be found in the landmark article published by Kress et al. [52]. This study of 150 mechanically ventilated patients implemented a protocol in which the treatment group had sedatives discontinued daily, while the control group's sedation was titrated according to the attending physician's preferences. In the treatment group the duration of mechanical ventilation was reduced by 2 days (p=0.004) and the ICU length of stay was reduced by 3.5 days (p=0.02). Overall complications and length of hospital stay were similar in both groups, and the approach to daily cessation of sedatives appeared safe in this medical ICU population. Kollef et al. [53] showed that delivery of sedation via intermittent bolus was associated with shorter duration of mechanical ventilation than delivery via continuous infusion.

Randolph et al. recently published a RCT comparing a weaning protocol to 'standard care' in 182 critically ill children [54]. The study was stopped early due to an apparent lack of difference between the two groups. After data analysis, however, it was shown that increased sedative use during the first 24 hours of weaning was an important predictor of weaning duration [55]. Whether a sedation protocol could better influence the outcomes of critically ill children in terms of weaning is not known.

The goals of sedation for mechanically ventilated patients usually include the following: 1) alleviation of agitation to a safe, tolerable level of movement by the patient and 2) alleviation of distress (pain, anxiety, dyspnea, and delirium). The pharmacoeconomic impact of clinical practice guidelines for analgesia, sedation, and neuromuscular blockade appear favorable [56]. Following the above-mentioned study by Kollef et al. [53], the same group completed a RCT that incorporated a nursing-implemented protocol to manage the delivery of sedation. They showed a reduction in the duration of mechanical ventilation by 2 days (p=0.008), length of stay in the ICU by 2 days (p<0.0001), and a significantly lower tracheostomy rate among the treatment group (6 vs 13%, p=0.04) [57]. Importantly, the authors report an estimated savings of $349,920 for the 162 patients in the intervention group. Together with the study by Kress et al. [52], these data support that shorter durations of mechanical ventilation and reductions in complication rates can be accomplished by reducing the use of sedative drips and by stopping sedation entirely on a regularly scheduled basis.

Considering the important role that sedatives and analgesics play in causing at least temporary cognitive impairment, we would like to focus the reader's attention on an emerging body of literature that suggests that delirium (or acute brain dysfunction) is independently associated with adverse outcomes in mechanically ventilated patients. Delirium in the ICU, which is a measure of the 'content' of consciousness rather than simply the patient's level of arousal in the ICU, was associated with higher mortality at 6 months and was also found to persist in at least 10% of patients at hospital discharge [58, 59].

We recently undertook a prospective investigation of 275 ventilated patients to determine the relationship between delirium, ventilator free days, and extubation failure [60]. The presence of delirium was identified by the Confusion Assessment Method for the Intensive Care Unit (CAM-ICU) [58, 59], while ventilator-free days were defined as the number of days from initiation of unassisted breathing to day 28 after randomization. After excluding 51 patients who had persistent coma and death in the ICU, the development of at least one episode of delirium (n=183) (median 19 days, interquartile range 5 to 24) during mechanical ventilation was associated with fewer ventilator-free days versus patients without delirium (n=41, 24 days, 21 to 26, p<0.0001). There were trends toward extubation failure among the patients who were delirious within 48 hours following extubation versus those who were not (16 vs 8%, p=0.07).

We have conducted an international survey of 915 ICU health care professionals regarding their opinions about delirum in this setting [61]. The results of this survey suggest that most healthcare professionals consider delirium in the ICU a common and serious problem, most admit it is under-diagnosed, yet few actually monitor adequately for this condition. Data from this survey point to a disconnect between the perceived significance of delirium in the ICU and current practices of monitoring and treatment. However, only through future investigations concerning the prevention of and therapy for delirium will we fully understand the impact of this form of acute brain dysfunction on outcomes of mechanical ventilation.

Conclusion

This chapter has reviewed many of the most important aspects regarding liberating patients from mechanical ventilation, while emphasizing points of uncertainty and those ripe for future research. We have emphasized a simplified approach that focuses on two points: recognizing when patients are able to breath spontaneously, and modifying practice to optimize the use of sedation (e.g., avoiding oversedation). The evidence from multiple randomized trials supports a Grade A, Level I recommendation to implement a standardized/protocolized approach to liberation driven by a team of non-physician health care providers operating in concert with the physician. This protocol should strive to incorporate daily spontaneous breathing trials as the lynchpin of weaning in patients who are clinically improving, rather than placing undue emphasis on specific cut-offs for individual weaning parameters. Each institution must actively adopt an approach that best serves its community. This approach should be evidence-based yet must be adapted so that it will be championed by the local opinion leaders who can continually work to implement, update, and document compliance with *their* protocol.

Perhaps the simplest statement regarding the 'bottom line' on weaning protocols can be stated as previously published in the AHCPR guidelines [2]: "Acknowledging the important nuances in protocols that should be dictated by specific patient populations and institutional preferences, the following two steps in any successful weaning attempt derived from recent RCTs bear repeating: step A should involve minimizing or temporarily discontinuing sedation and analgesia enough to observe patient AWAKENING; and step B should involve an assessment of the patient's ability to spontaneously BREATHE."

References

1. Hess DR (2002) Liberation from mechanical ventilation: Weaning the patient or weaning old-fashioned ideas? Crit Care Med 30:2154–2155
2. MacIntyre NR, Cook DJ, Ely EW, et al (2001) Evidence-based guidelines for weaning and discontinuing ventilatory support a collective task force facilitated by the american college of chest physicians; the american association for respiratory care; and the american college of critical care medicine. Chest 120 (suppl):375S–395S
3. Krieger BP (2002) Top ten list in mechanical ventilation. Chest 122:1797–1800
4. Tobin MJ (2001) Advances in mechanical ventilation. N Engl J Med 344:1986–1996
5. Esteban A, Alia I, Ibanez J, Benito S, Tobin MJ (1994) The Spanish Lung Failure Collaborative Group, Modes of mechanical ventilation and weaning. Chest 106:1188–1193
6. Esteban A, Anzueto A, Frutos F, et al (2002) Characteristics and outcomes in adult patients receiving mechanical ventilation a 28-day international study. JAMA 287:345–355
7. Stroetz RW, Hubmayr RD (1995) Tidal volume maintenance during weaning with pressure support. Am J Respir Crit Care Med 152:1034–1040
8. Listello D, Sessler C (1994) Unplanned extubation: clinical predictors for reintubation. Chest 105:1496–1503
9. Tindol GA, Jr., DiBenedetto RJ, Kosciuk L (1994) Unplanned extubations. Chest 105:1804–1807
10. Boulain T, and the Association des Reanimateurs du Centre-Ouest (1998) Unplanned extubations in the adult intensive care unit: a prospective multicenter study. Am J Respir Crit Care Med 157:1131–1137
11. Betbese AJ, Perez M, Rialp G, et al (1998) A prospective study of unplanned endotracheal extubation in intensive care unit patients. Crit Care Med 26:1180–1186
12. Khamiees M, Raju P, Amoateng-Adjepong Y, Manthous CA (2001) Predictors of extubation outcome in patients who have successfully completed a spontaneous breathing trial. Chest 120:1262–1270
13. Ely EW, Bennett PA, Bowton DL, et al (1999) Large scale implementation of a respiratory therapist-driven protocol for ventilator weaning. Am J Respir Crit Care Med 159:439–446
14. Laghi F, Cattapan SE, Jubran A, et al (2003) Is weaning failure caused by low-frequency fatigue of the diaphragm? Am J Respir Crit Care Med 167:120–127
15. Yang KL, Tobin MJ (1991) A prospective study of indexes predicting the outcome of trials of weaning from mechanical ventilation. N Engl J Med 324:1445–1450
16. Hoo GW, Park L (2002) Variations in the measurement of weaning parameters: a survey of respiratory therapists. Chest 121:1947–1955
17. Sahn SA, Lakshminarayan S (1973) Bedside criteria for discontinuation of mechanical ventilation. Chest 63:1002–1005
18. Brochard L, Rauss A, Benito S, et al (1994) Comparison of three methods of gradual withdrawal from ventilatory support during weaning from mechanical ventilation. Am J Respir Crit Care Med 150:896–903
19. Esteban A, Frutos F, Tobin MJ, et al (1995) A comparison of four methods of weaning patients from mechanical ventilation. N Engl J Med 332:345–350

20. Ely EW, Baker AM, Dunagan DP, et al (1996) Effect on the duration of mechanical ventilation of identifying patients capable of breathing spontaneously. N Engl J Med 335:1864–1869

21. Wood KE, Flaten AL, Reedy JS, Coursin DB (1999) Use of a daily screen and weaning protocol for mechanically ventilated patients in a multidisciplinary tertiary critical care unit. Crit Care Med 27:A94–A94

22. Kollef MH, Shapiro SD, Silver P, et al (1997) A randomized, controlled trial of protocol-directed versus physician-directed weaning from Mechanical Ventilation. Crit Care Med 25:567–574

23. Strickland JH Jr, Hasson JH (1993) A computer-controlled ventilator weaning system: a clinical trial. Chest 103:1220–1226

24. Marelich GP, Murin S, Battistella F, et al (2000) Protocol weaning of mechanical ventilation in medical and surgical patients by respiratory care practitioners and nurses: Effect on weaning time and incidence of ventilator-associated pneumonia. Chest 118:459–467

25. Foster GH, Conway WA, Pamulkov N, et al (1984) Early extubation after coronary artery bypass: brief report. Crit Care Med 12:994–996

26. Tong DA (1991) Weaning patients from mechanical ventilation. A knowledge-based system approach. Comput Methods Programs Biomed 35:267–278

27. Rotello LC, Warren J, Jastremski MS, et al (1992) A nurse-directed protocol using pulse oximetry to wean mechanically ventilated patients from toxic oxygen concentrations. Chest 102:1833–1835

28. Wood G, MacLeod B, Moffatt S (1995) Weaning from mechanical ventilation: physician-directed vs a respiratory-therapist-directed protocol. Respir Care 40:219–224

29. Saura P, Blanch L, Mestre J, et al (1996) Clinical consequences of the implementation of a weaning protocol. Intensive Care Med 22:1052–1056

30. Djunaedi H, Cardinal P, Greffe-Laliberte G, et al (1987) Does a ventilatory management protocol improve the care of ventilated patients? Respir Care 42:604–610

31. Burn SM, Marshall M, Burns JE, et al (1998) Design, testing, and results of an outcomes-managed approach to patients requiring prolonged mechanical ventilation. Am J Crit Care 7:45–57

32. Horst HM, Mouro D, Hall-Jenssens RA, et al (1998) Decrease in ventilation time with a standardized weaning process. Arch Surg 133:483–488

33. Kollef MH, Horst HM, Prang L, et al (1998) Reducing the duration of mechanical ventilation: three examples of change in the intensive care unit. New Horiz 6:52–60

34. Cohen IL, Booth FV (1994) Cost containment and mechanical ventilation in the United States. New Horiz 2:283–290

35. Cohen IL (1994) Weaning from mechanical ventilation —the team approach and beyond. Intensive Care Med 20:317–318

36. Smyrnios NA, Connolly A, Wilson MM, et al (2002) Effects of a multifaceted, multidisciplinary, hospital-wide quality improvement program on weaning from mechanical ventilation. Crit Care Med 30:1224–1230

37. Esteban A, Alia I, Tobin M, et al (1999) Effect of spontaneous breathing trial duration on outcome of attempts to discontinue mechanical ventilation. Am J Respir Crit Care Med 159:512–518

38. Perrren A, Domenighetti G, Mauri S, Genini F, Vizzardi N (2002) Protocol-driven weaning from mechanical ventilation: clinical outcome in patients randomized for a 30-min or 120-min trial with pressure support ventilation. Intensive Care Med 28:1058–1063

39. Esteban A, Alia I, Gordo F, et al (1997) The Spanish Lung Failure Collaborative Group. Extubation outcome after spontaneous breathing trials with T-tube or pressure support ventilation. Am J Respir Crit Care Med 156:459–465

40. Esteban A, Anzueto A, Alia I, et al (2000) How is mechanical ventilation employed in the intensive care unit. Am J Respir Crit Care Med 161:1450–1458

41. Vitacca M, Vianello A, Colombo D, et al (2001) Comparison of two methods for weaning patients with chronic obstructive pulmonary disease requiring mechanical ventilation for more than 15 days. Am J Respir Crit Care Med 164:225–230

42. Iregui M, Ward S, Clinikscale D, Clayton D, Kollef MH (2002) Use of a handheld computer by respiratory care practitioners to improve the efficiency of weaning patients from mechanical ventilation. Crit Care Med 30:2038–2043

43. Croft B (2002) Ventilator weaning protocols. Journal for Respiratory Care Practitioners. Aug/Sept, pp:26–30

44. Ely EW (2000) The utility of weaning protocols to expedite liberation from mechanical ventilation. Respir Care Clin N Am 6:303–319

45. Brattebo G, Hofoss D, Flaatten H, Muri AK, Gjerde S, Plsek P (2002) Effect of a scoring system and protocol for sedation on duration of patient's need for ventilator support in a surgical intensive care unit. Br Med J 324:1386–1389

46. Main DS, Cohen SJ, DiClemente CC (1995) Measuring physician readiness to change cancer screening: preliminary results. Am J Prev Med 11:54–58

47. Fridkin SK, Pear SM, Williamson TH, et al (1996) The role of understaffing in central venous catheter-associated bloodstream infections. Infect Control Hosp Epidemiol 17:150–158

48. Archibald LK, Manning ML, Bell LM, et al (1997) Patient density, nurse-to-patient ratio and nosocomial infection risk in a pediatric cardiac intensive care unit. Pediatr Infect Dis 16:1045–1048

49. Thorens JB, Kaelin RM, Jolliet P, et al (1995) Influence of the quality of nursing on the duration of weaning from mechanical ventilation in patients with chronic obstructive pulmonary disease. Crit Care Med 23:1807–1815

50. Damen J, van Diejen D, Bakker J, van Zanten ARH (2003) Legal implications of clinical practice guidelines. Intensive Care Med 29:3–7

51. Jacobi J, Fraser GL, Coursin DB, et al (2002) Clinical practice guidelines for the susstained use of sedatives and analgesics in the critically ill adult. Crit Care Med 30:119–140

52. Kress JP, Pohlman AS, O'Connor MF, Hall JB (2000) Daily interruption of sedative infusions in critically ill patients undergoing mechanical ventilation. N Engl J Med 342:1471–1477

53. Kollef MH, Levy NT, Ahrens TS, Schaiff R, Prentice D, Sherman G (1998) The use of continuous iv sedation is associated with prolongation of mechanical ventilation. Chest 114:541–548

54. Randolph AG, Wypij D, Venkataraman ST, et al (2002) Effect of mechanical ventilator weaning protocols on respiratory outcomes in infants and children a randomized controlled trial. JAMA 288:2561–2568

55. O'meade MO, Ely EW (2002) Protocols to improve the care of critically ill pediatric and adult patients. JAMA 288:2601–2603

56. Mascia MF, Koch M, Medicis JJ (2000) Pharmacoeconomic impact of rational use guidelines on the provision of analgesia, sedation, and neuromuscular blockade in critical care. Crit Care Med 28:2300–2306

57. Brook AD, Ahrens TS, Schaiff R, et al (1999) Effect of a nursing-implemented sedation protocol on the duration of mechanical ventilation. Crit Care Med 27: 2609–2615

58. Ely EW, Margolin R, Francis J, May L, et al (1999) Delirium in the ICU: measurement and outcomes. Am J Respir Crit Care Med 161:A506 (abst)

59. Ely EW, Inouye SK, Bernard GR, et al (2001) Delirium in mechanically ventilated patients: validity and reliability of the confusion assessment method for the intensive care unit (CAM-ICU). JAMA 286:2703–2710

60. Thomason JWW, Truman B, Ely EW, et al (2003) The impact of delirium in the ICU on outcomes of mechanical ventilation. Am J Respir Crit Care Med 167:A970 (abst)

61. Ely EW, Stephens R, Jackson JC, et al (2003) Current opinions regarding delirium in the ICU: A survey of 915 healthcare professionals. Crit Care Med (in press)

62. Vallverdu I, Calaf N, Subirana M, Net A, Benito S, Mancebo J (1998) Clinical characteristics, respiratory functional parameters, and outcome of a two-hour T-piece trial of patients weaning from mechanical ventilation. Am J Respir Crit Care Med 158:1855–1862

Novel Approaches to Monitoring Mechanical Ventilatory Support

N. MacIntyre

Introduction

Routine monitoring of patients receiving mechanical ventilatory support includes pressure/flow/volume measurements in the ventilator circuitry and arterial blood gas measurements/pulse oximetry [1–3] (Table 1). This monitoring is designed to assure safe ventilator operations, effective gas exchange and help guide clinical decision-making. These common monitoring techniques, however, provide little information about a number of other important physiologic variables. For example, lung stretch is only superficially assessed by measurements of circuit pressure and tidal volume (V_T), lung recruitment is only indirectly assessed by arterial oxygenation, and mechanical loads on patient muscles have no direct monitoring technique. Clinical decisions may thus be made suboptimally.

In recent years, a number of new techniques have become available that may address some of these shortcomings. These innovations are of two types: a) more sophisticated analyses of existing monitored signals; and b) new monitored signals. These are summarized in Table 2. Reviewed in this chapter are tracheal/esophageal pressure monitoring and inert/soluble gas measurements of lung function, two of these innovations with particular clinical potential.

Assessing Mechanics with Tracheal and Esophageal Pressure Measurements

Rationale

The respiratory system receiving positive pressure mechanical ventilation (PPV) can be represented as having two resistive elements (Ret: endotracheal tube resistance and Raw: patient airway resistance) in series with two compliance elements (Cl: lung compliance and Ccw: chest wall compliance). These four mechanical elements are sometimes combined into two: total resistance (Rtot = Ret + Raw) and respiratory system compliance (Crs = 1/(1/Cl + 1/Ccw)) [4, 5].

During gas flow (V'), Ret produces a pressure gradient between pressure in the ventilator circuit at the airway opening (Paw) and pressure in the trachea (Ptr); and Raw produces a pressure gradient between Ptr and alveolar pressure (Palv) (Figure 1). At any lung volume above the resting lung volume (V), Cl produces a pressure

Table 1. AARC Consensus Group recommendations on monitoring and alarm systems for mechanical ventilators. From [3] with permission

Variable	Principal Ventilator Application		
	Critical Care	Transport	Home Care
Pressure			
P_{PEAK}	Essential	Essential	Essential
P_{MEAN}	Essential	Optional	Optional
P_{PLAT}	Essential	Optional	Optional[3]
Instrinsic PEEP (auto-PEEP)	Essential	Optional	Optional
Volume[5]			
V_T expired machine	Essential	Recommended	Optional
$\dot{V}_E$ machine	Essential	Optional	Optional
V_T expired spontaneous	Essential	Recommended	Optional
$\dot{V}_E$ spontaneous	Essential	Optional	Optional
V_T inspired spontaneous	Recommended	Optional	Optional
Timing			
Flow mechanical	Recommended	Optional	Optional
Flow spontaneous	Optional	Optional	Optional
I:E ratio	Essential	Recommended	Optional
Rate mechanical	Essential	Recommended	Optional
Rate spontaneous	Essential	Recommended	Optional
Gas Concentration			
F_{DO2}[4]	Essential	Optional[3]	Optional[3]
Lung mechanics			
Effective compliance	Optional	Optional	Optional
Inspiratory airways resistance	Optional	Optional	Optional
Expiratory airways resistance	Optional	Optional	Optional
Maximal inspiratory pressure	Optional	Optional	Optional
Circuit characteristics			
Tubing compliance	Recommended	Optional	Optional

[1] Essential, considered necessary for safe and effective operation in most patients in the specified in the specified setting; recommended, considered necessary for optimal management of virtually all patients in the specified; optional, considered possibly useful in limited but not necessary for most patients inthe specified setting.

[2] Monitors need not be integral part of ventilator.

[3] Essential if feature is used on a specific patient.

[4] F_{DO2}, Oxygen concentration delivered by device; FiO_2 when patient demand (inspiratory flowrate) is met.

[5] I:E, inspiratory:expiratory time; PEEP, positive end-expiratory pressure; V_E, minute volume; V_T tidal volume.

Table 2. Newer approaches to monitoring mechanically ventilated patients

More sophisticated analyses of existing signals:

Pressure/flow/ volume signals in the airway to assess spontaneous
  ventilatory patterns to various stimuli (e.g., CO_2, loads)

Circuit occlusion pressure at 100 msec (P0.1) to assess ventilatory drive
  and muscle strength

Continuous assessment of arterial blood gases

New signals

Exhaled O_2 and CO_2 to assess metabolic activity

Tracheal and esophageal pressure monitoring to assess mechanics, interactions

Chest impedance bands for lung volumes

Indicator dilution methods to assess lung water

Exhaled soluble gas behavior to assess relationship of alveolar volume to blood flow

Exhaled nitric oxide to assess inflammatory processes

EMGs to assess neuromuscular component of ventilation

Transcutaneous, gastric pH, near infra-red spectroscopy and other approaches to assess
  tissue oxygenation

gradient between Palv and pleural pressure (estimated by esophageal pressure: Pes); and Ccw produces a pressure gradient between Pes and atmospheric pressure. The relationships among these various pressure measurements and mechanical properties can be represented by the equation of motion:

Total pressure across respiratory system = (Ret x V') + (Raw x V') + (Cl/V) + (Ccw/V).

From this relationship and consideration of Figure 1, the factors impacting the various pressures can be determined and are summarized in Table 3. Note that in Table 3, all pressures except Palv can be measured directly from appropriate pressure sensing sites. Palv, however, can be approximated by either Paw or Ptr under no-flow conditions (so called plateau pressures or Pplat).

The various respiratory system mechanical properties can be calculated for a given flow (V'), volume delivery (V) and driving pressure (Paw) using the equations in Table 4. Although many of these require only circuit pressure measurements, important parameters specific to lung mechanics also require Ptr and Pes. Specific clinical scenarios are described below to illustrate this point.

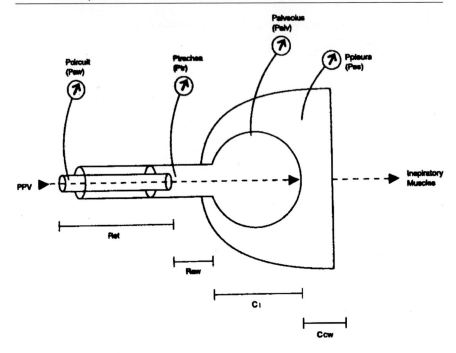

Fig. 1. A schematic illustrating that the respiratory system behaves as four mechanical elements in series: Endotracheal tube resistance (Ret), airway resistance (Raw), lung compliance (Cl), and chest wall compliance (Ccw). Pressure monitoring at various sites depends upon these various elements as they interact with delivered flow/volume and the source of the driving pressure.

Table 3. Pressure determinants

	Pressure Measurement	Mechanical Determinants
Paw	- during flow - with volume, no flow	- Ret, Raw, Cl, Ccw - Cl, Ccw
Ptr	- during flow - with volume, no flow	- Raw, Cl, Ccw - Cl, Ccw
Palv	- during flow - with volume, no flow	- Cl, Ccw - Cl, Ccw
Pes	- during flow - with volume, no flow - during spontaneous effort with flow - during spontaneous effort, no flow	- Ccw - Ccw - Ret, Raw, Cl - Cl

Paw: airway opening pressure; Ptr: tracheal pressure; Palv: alveolar pressure; Pes: esophageal pressure; Ret: endotracheal tube resistance; Raw: patient airway resistance; Cl: lung compliance; Ccw: chest wall compliance

Table 4. Mechanics calculations

During positive pressure venatilation, Paw is the driving pressure such that:
$$Ret = (Paw \ Ptr)/V'$$
$$Raw = (Ptr \ Palv)/V'$$
$$Crs = V/Palv$$
$$Ccw = V/Pes$$
$$Cl = V/(Palv\text{-}Pes) = 1(1/Crs \ 1/Ccw)$$

During spontaneous breaths, Pes is the driving pressure such that:
$$Cl = V/Pes \text{ (no flow conditions)}$$

Paw: airway opening pressure; Ptr: tracheal pressure; Palv: alveolar pressure; Pes: esophageal pressure; Ret: endotracheal tube resistance; Raw: patient airway resistance; Cl: lung compliance; Ccw: chest wall compliance; Crs: respiratory system compliance; V: lung volume; V': gas flow

Using Pes to Separate Lung and Chest Wall Mechanical Properties

The 'stretch' across the lung at end inspiration is commonly assessed by the measurement of Palv as reflected in the airway opening Pplat [4, 5]. An important assumption made during this standard approach is that this Palv is primarily determined by alveolar distension. Recall, however, that chest wall compliance can also affect Paw and Palv. In many patients, Ccw is usually several times greater than Cl such that it has little impact on airway opening Pplat. In patients with abnormal chest wall mechanics (e.g., massive obesity, anasarca, chest wall injury, surgical dressings), however, Ccw can be quite poor and can have profound effects on Palv [6, 7]. Under these conditions, the assumption that Palv represents only lung properties does not hold.

Pes measurements can address this problem [8–13]. During a passive positive pressure inflation, Pes reflects pressure on the `other side' of the alveolus and in front of the chest wall. It thus can be used as a reference value for Palv to give true transalveolar `lung stretching' pressure.

Using Ptr to Estimate a Static Pressure-volume Plot

Static pressure volume (PV) plots are thought to be good representations of Crs and Palv throughout a positive pressure breath [14, 15]. Unfortunately, static PV plots require measurements of airway opening Pplat at multiple different inflation volumes. This is time consuming and often requires patient sedation or paralysis to accomplish. Conceivably, a single breath dynamic PV plot could be utilized to approximate the static PV plot if the effects of Ret and Raw could be eliminated. One approach to this is the 'slow flow' single inflation (i.e., inspiratory flow of 10 l/min) which requires minimal flow related inflation pressure [16]. This approach can be further enhanced if the effect of Ret is completely eliminated by using a direct measurement of Ptr (Fig. 2).

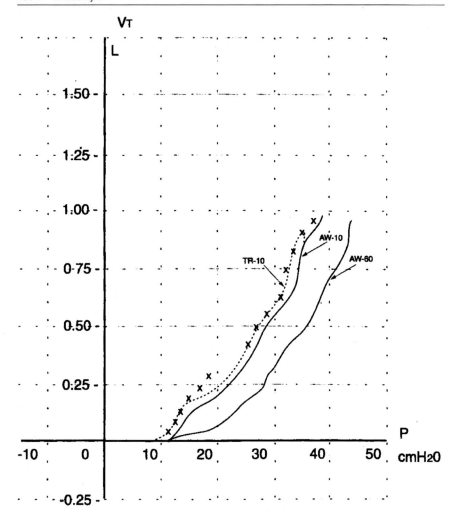

Fig. 2. Pressure volume (PV) curves plotted by different techniques. The 'X' points indicate a static PV plot. The AW-60 curve is a PV curve using airway pressure determinations done during a single constant flow breath delivered at 60 l/min. Note the substantial displacement of this curve to the right reflecting the pressure required for flow through the endotracheal tube and airway resistances during the inspiration. The AW-10 curve is a PV curve using airway pressure determinations during a single constant flow breath delivered at 10 l/min. This curve is now closer to the static curve because the slower flow delivery requires less pressure. The TR-10 curve is a PV curve using tracheal pressure determinations during a single constant flow breath at 10 l/min. This curve is the closest approximation to the static curve since endotracheal tube resistance has been eliminated from the pressure measurement.

Paw, Ptr, and Pes to Calculate Mechanical Loads

Energy demands for ventilation that are borne by either the patient or the ventilator can be expressed as a mechanical load [4, 5, 17–19]. Load is determined by the actual amount of ventilation and by the various resistance and compliance elements of the respiratory system. Mechanical load can be expressed as a pressure time product (PTP) or work (W) value. The pressure time product is the integral of pressure change over (PTP = PdT); the work is calculated as the integral of pressure change over (W = PdV).

In Figure 3, pressure is plotted over time for three breaths (spontaneous, controlled and interactive). In breath A, the integral of Pes over time (the two hatched areas) reflects the PTP borne by the ventilatory muscles to overcome Cl, Raw and Ret in delivering the tidal volume. In breath B, the integral of Paw over time (the 3 shaded areas) reflects the PTP borne by the ventilator to overcome Cl, Ccw, Raw and Ret in delivering the V_T. Note that in breath B, the integral of Pes over time (dotted area) reflects only the load imposed by Ccw on the ventilator and this can be used to separate Ccw from other components of load. In breath C the PTP components borne by the patient and the ventilator during an interactive breath can be displayed by superimposing a ventilator controlled breath of the same volume and flow and subtracting the patient component. These same mechanical properties can be depicted by integrating pressure over volume as work (W). Note also that the use of Ptr eliminates the load imposed by Ret in all of the calculations.

Using Ptr and Pes as a Target for Interactive Pressure Targeted Breaths

Pressure targeted breaths deliver gas flow in accordance to a set inspiratory pressure. The measured pressure that serves as the target for the ventilator's flow delivery is usually from the proximal airway or ventilator circuitry. Because of the high flow resistance imposed by the endotracheal tube, a targeted square wave of pressure in the proximal airway/ventilator circuitry is deformed into a slow rising pressure waveform in the patient's tracheobronchial system (Fig. 4 left panel). This slow rise in pressurization may impose discomfort on the part of a patient who has a very active respiratory drive. A solution to this is to use the pressure actually in the trachea (Ptr) as a target for the ventilator [20, 21]. Pressure targeted breaths using Ptr create a more square wave of pressure in the airway which conceivably would keep up with an active patient flow demand more readily. The simultaneous Paw tracing under these conditions becomes more of a peak and decelerating pattern (Figure 4 right panel).

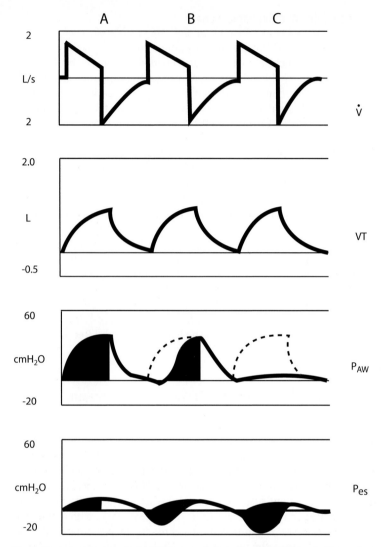

Fig. 3. Pressure time products (PTP) as an index of mechanical load. Pictured are three breaths of similar flow/volume with both airway and pleural (esophageal) pressure plotted over time. The integral of pressure over time is the PTP (shaded area). During a controlled breath (no patient activity - left panel A), all of the load is borne by the ventilator. The PTP from the airway reflects the load imposed by the total respiratory system and the PTP from the esophagus reflects that portion of the respiratory system load imposed by the chest wall. During a spontaneous breath (unassisted patient activity - right panel C), all of the load is borne by the patient. The pressure from the esophagus under these conditions can either be referenced to atmospheric pressure (the end expiratory value) or to a passive esophageal pressure tracing from a controlled breath of similar flow/volume (dotted line). The PTP from the former approach reflects only the load imposed by the lungs; the PTP from the latter approach reflects the loads from the total respiratory system. Note that given the same compliances, resistances and breath flow/volume, the respiratory system PTP from the control breath A is equal to the respiratory system PTP from the

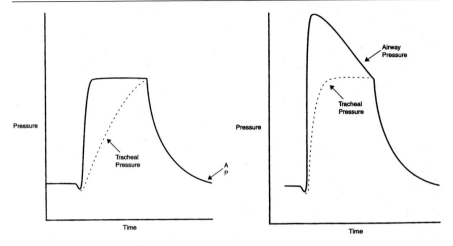

Fig. 4. *Left:* A typical pressure supported breath with airway pressure targeting is depicted. Note that tracheal pressure beyond the endotracheal tube lags behind the airway pressure tracing because of the resistance of the endotracheal tube. The 'square wave' pressure target in the airway is thus distorted to a rising 'triangular wave' in the trachea. *Right:* A pressure supported breath with tracheal pressure targeting creates a 'square wave' in the trachea. The simultaneous airway pressure must of necessity be higher at the beginning of inspiration and then taper to the pressure target.

Using Pes to Assess and Manage Triggering Loads Imposed by Intrinsic PEEP

In a patient with severe obstructive lung disease, flow limited segments can produce significant intrinsic positive end-expiratory pressure (PEEPi) [22, 23]. This high end expiratory alveolar pressure can then serve as an inspiratory threshold load for triggering the next breath [22–25]. The amount of the PEEPi triggering load can be readily estimated from esophageal pressure tracing. In a patient with no PEEPi, the initiation of effort (i.e., the drop in the esophageal pressure) is accompanied by a simultaneous drop in airway pressure and increase in flow from the circuitry. In contrast, in a patient with PEEPi (Fig. 5 left panel), a similar effort reflected by a drop in the esophageal pressure tracing is not accompanied by a simultaneous drop in airway pressure or increase in flow until the PEEPi level (in this case 20 cmH2O) has been exceeded by the effort. Note that under these circumstances, additional PEEP (Fig. 5 right panel), by balancing the PEEPi, reduces the inspiratory threshold load.

---

spontaneous breath C. During interactive breaths (patients and ventilator both active - middle panel B), load is shared by the patient and the ventilator. The proportion of load borne by the patient and by the ventilator can be determined by superimposing a controlled breath (dotted lines) of similar flow/volume on the interactive breath (solid lines). From [2] with permission

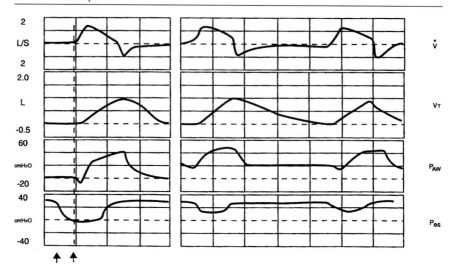

Fig. 5. Intrinsic PEEP from flow limited airways producing an inspiratory threshold triggering load, In the left panel, a patient effort is reflected by the drop in esophageal pressure (left arrow), Note, however, that no simultaneous drop in circuit pressure or flow occurs until almost 1/2 sec, has passed and the Pes has dropped almost 25 cmH$_2$0 (right arrow). This represents an intrinsic PEEP level of at least 25 cmH$_2$0 that must be overcome by the inspiratory muscles before this patient demand can be sensed in the ventilator circuitry (triggering threshold load). In the right panel, 20 cmH$_2$0 applied PEEP has been given. This level of PEEP does not eliminate the trapped gas in the lung but it does help equilibrate the expiratory pressures throughout the lung and circuitry. Because of this, the patient effort to change circuit pressure/flow to trigger an assisted breath becomes considerably less.

Assessing Lung Recruitment and Distention with Exhaled Soluble Gas Analyses

Rationale

End-expiratory lung volume (EELV) and functional residual capacity (FRC) are conceptually important physiologic parameters to monitor during mechanical ventilation. This may be particularly true when parenchymal lung injury or atelectasis and inflammation creates low EELV with consequent low ventilation perfusion (V/Q) relationships and shunts. These abnormalities in turn compromise oxygen transport across the alveolar capillary interface and may contribute to ventilator-induced injury in units where there is repetitive open and collapsing during positive pressure ventilation [26–28].

Raising the EELV with PEEP (either applied or intrinsic) has long been the major focus of therapy for lung collapse and infiltrates [29]. Conceptually, the end expiratory pressure is applied following a positive pressure breath which has opened the alveolar units. The expiratory pressure thus prevents, in effect, the re-collapse. As a consequence, V/Q relationships are improved and there is less of a shear stress phenomenon in that particular unit. Indeed, it is the V/Q improvement with improvement in PO_2 that often guides expiratory pressure therapy.

This simple gas exchange approach to expiratory pressure setting, however, ignores an important pathophysiologic effect of parenchymal lung injury. Because parenchymal lung injury is often quite heterogeneous, an optimal expiratory pressure setting with appropriate restoration of EELV in one unit may be an excessive expiratory pressure application with over-distension in a healthier regions [30, 31]. Minimizing ventilator-induced lung injury (VILI) and still providing adequate gas exchange may thus involve expiratory pressure settings that are not associated with the best values for PO_2. Supporting this concept is the observation in the NIH ARDS Network trial of positive pressure ventilation management strategies which showed that the small V_T approach, which produced the best mortality outcome, was associated with less recruitment and a lower PAO_2/FiO_2 ratio than the higher V_T approach [32].

Techniques to Assess EELV and Lung Mechanics

Because PO_2 may not be the best way to assess optimal lung recruitment, other approaches would seem desirable. One simple technique is to directly measure EELV with inert gas dilution technology [33]. This, however, only measures a 'global' EELV and tells nothing of regional behavior. Moreover, it is not at all clear what the ideal EELV would be with this approach. Radiologic approaches using computerized tomography offer more appeal as regional recruitment and/or overdistention can be visualized [31, 32]. This type of assessment, however, is complex and expensive and thus does not lend itself as an intensive care unit (ICU) monitoring tool. Another approach might be to measure static PV relationships during a positive pressure breath as described above. Conceptually, the ideal ventilator settings should place the lung on the steepest part of the PV curve [34]. As noted above, however, the static PV curve is technically difficult to do properly and again it is an assessment of 'global' rather than regional behavior.

Soluble Gas Behavior

The behavior of various test gases delivered to the lungs has been used for decades to better understand lung function. The underlying concept is that analysis of the uptake/exhalation of gases with different blood solubilities and/or hemoglobin binding can be used to define the relationships between EELV, ventilation, and perfusion. Conceivably these techniques might be used to better provide positive pressure ventilation and PEEP.

A very sophisticated way of assessing ventilation perfusion relationships is the multiple inert gas elimination technique (MIGET) [35]. This involves the administration of six inert gases of different solubilities and analyzing gas and blood samples over a period of time. The retention and excretion of these gases can then be used to construct a 50-unit lung model having ventilation perfusion relationships ranging from 0 (shunt) to infinity (dead space). This technique has been used in a number of physiologic experiments both in animals and humans to quantify V/Q distribution changes as a function of various interventions. For example, the MIGET technique has been used in models of respiratory failure to demonstrate how V/Q distributions will change with different positive pressure ventilatory patterns [36–39], different PEEP settings [40], application of perflubron [41], and other techniques.

In concept, this technique might be used to help assess the optimal EELV. The goal would be to apply expiratory pressure and increase lung volume as long as V/Q relationships were being made better. When regions of over-distension were beginning to occur, high V/Q units would start to appear.

Although physiologically fascinating and conceptually attractive, this technique is very cumbersome to use, requires expensive equipment and is not, therefore, suitable for true monitoring. Moreover, the ventilator settings established with this technique have not been studied in any meaningful outcome way.

A simpler approach might be to use a three-gas system to simultaneously measure lung volume, pulmonary capillary blood flow, and pulmonary diffusing capacity [42]. This technique uses methane (CH_4) as the inert insoluble gas for determining lung volume, acetylene (C_2H_2), a very soluble gas whose uptake is determined primarily by pulmonary capillary blood flow through ventilated regions, and carbon monoxide, a gas avidly bound to hemoglobin and whose uptake is primarily determined by the pulmonary capillary blood volume in proximity to ventilated regions.

The behavior of these gases during a single inspiration and expiration can be assessed with a readily available infrared analyzer (Fig. 6). The simple dilution of CH_4 allows for the calculation of the absolute lung volume at end inspiration and the slope of the C_2H_2 and the carbon monoxide disappearance curve allows for the calculation of pulmonary capillary blood flow and diffusing capacity respectively (Table 5) [42].

This technique has been used in pulmonary function labs for a number of years to measure FRC and carbon monoxide diffusing capacity [42, 43]. The acetylene channel is easily added with appropriate filtering systems and has been used at rest and during exercise in both healthy and diseased populations [44]. Although no current interface exists with mechanical ventilators, this should not be difficult to make.

In the mechanically ventilated patient, one can conceive of using these measurements in the following way. As PEEP is increased, EELV will increase accordingly. If recruitment is taking place, there should be increased exposure of pulmonary capillary blood thereby increasing pulmonary capillary blood flow and pulmonary

Table 5. Equations for calculating diffusing capacity and pulmonary capillary blood flow and diffusing capacity during a single inspiration:expiration of carbon monoxide (CO) and acetylene (C_2H_2) (DLexh and Qcexh respectively).

$$DLexh = Vex\{\ln(CO_1/CO_0)/\ln(VA_1/VA_0)\} \times \{60 \times 1000/(PB-47)\}$$

$$Qcexh = (Vex/_{blood}) \times \{\ln(C2H2_1/C2H2_2)/\ln\{(VA_1+_{tissue}Vt)/(VA_0+_{tissue}Vt)\} \times \{60 \times 1000/(PB-47)\}$$

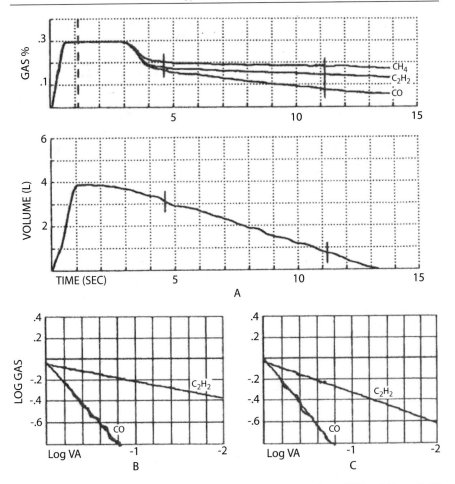

Fig. 6. The single exhalation technique. A. A representative tracing of CH_4, C_2H_2, and CO concentrations (upper panel) and lung volume (middle panel) during a single inhalation and exhalation. The expiratory flow is kept relatively constant. The regression method is applied to C_2H_2 and CO at rest (B) and during exercise (C). Note that the slopes of the regression lines for both C_2H_2 and CO during exercise are steeper than those at rest. DLexh and Qcexh are 23.5 ml/min/mm Hg and 3.73 l/min, respectively, at rest. During exercise, DLexh and Qcexh increase to 29.6 ml/min/mm Hg and 7.86 l/min, respectively. From [44] with permission

diffusing capacity to ventilated regions accordingly. Conversely, if the increase in EELV is serving primarily to over-distend already recruited lung units, it will not be accompanied by additional increases in either pulmonary capillary blood flow or diffusing capacity. It must be emphasized that these ideas are only speculative at the present time as this technique has not been tried in mechanically ventilated patients. How it might compare with other techniques or whether it will impact outcome remains to be answered.

Conclusion

Manipulations of EELV can be critically important to mechanically ventilated patients. If these manipulations facilitate lung recruitment, then improved gas exchange and perhaps less VILI should occur. Because of the heterogeneity of lung disease, however, optimal changes in EELV in one lung unit may be suboptimal in others. Since ventilator manipulations apply to the lung as a whole (i.e.; they are not regionalized) ventilator settings must strike a balance between beneficial effects and detrimental effects. To optimize this, clinicians need to assess both the beneficial effects of their manipulation as well as the detrimental. To this end, simple measurements of gas exchange or simple global measurements of lung volume are not sufficient. Instead, techniques to assess physiologic parameters that reflect both recruitment and over-distension would seem to be important.

References

1. Tobin MJ (2000) Principles and Practice of Intensive Care Monitoring. McGraw Hill, New York
2. MacIntyre NR (2000) Ventilator monitors, displays and alarms. In: MacIntyre NR, Branson RD (eds) Mechanical Ventilation. WB Saunders, Philadelphia, pp 131–145
3. American Association for Respiratory Care Consensus Group (1992) Essentials of mechanical ventilation. Respir Care 37:1001–1009
4. Truwit JD, Marini JJ (1988) Evaluation of thoracic mechanics in the ventilated patient: part I, primary measurements. J Crit Care 3:133–150
5. Truwit JD, Marini JJ (1988) Evaluation of thoracic mechanics in the ventilated patient: part II, applied mechanics. J Crit Care 3:192–213
6. D'Angelo E, Robatto FM, Calderini E, et al (1991) Pulmonary and chest wall mechanics in anesthetized paralyzed humans. J Appl Physiol 70:2602–2610
7. LeSouëf PN, Lopes JM, England SJ, et al (1983) Influence of chest wall distortion on esophageal pressure. J Appl Physiol 55:353–358
8. Mead J, Mellroy MB, Selverstone NJ, Kriete BC (1955) Measurement of intraesophageal pressure. J Appl Physiol 7:491–495
9. Schilder DP, Hyatt RE, Fry DL (1959) An improved balloon system for measuring intraesophageal pressure. J Appl Physiol 14:1057–1058
10. Knowles JH, Hong SK, Rahn H (1959) Possible errors using esophageal balloon in determination of pressure-volume characteristics of the lung and thoracic cage. J Appl Physiol 14:525–530
11. Hurewitz AN, Sidhu U, Bergofsky EH, Chanana AD (1984) How alterations in pleural pressure influence esophageal pressure. J Appl Physiol 56:1162–1169
12. Cherniack RM, Fahri LF, Armstrong RW, Proctor DF (1955) A comparison of esophageal and intrapleural pressures in man. J Appl Physiol 8:203–211
13. Milic-Emili J, Mead J, Turner JM, Glauser EM (1964) Improved technique for estimating pleural pressure from esophageal balloons. J Appl Physiol 19:207–211
14. Metamis D, LeMaire F, Harf A, et al (1984) Total respiratory pressure-volume curves in the adult respiratory distress syndrome. Chest 86:58–66
15. Field S, Sanci S, Grassino A (1984) Respiratory muscle oxygen consumption estimated by the diaphragm pressure-time index. J Appl Physiol 57:44–51
16. Servillo G. Svantesson C Beydon, et al (1997) Pressure-volume curves in acute respiratory failure: automated low flow inflation versus occlusion. Am J Respir Crit Care Med 155:1629–1636

17. Fleury B, Murciano D, Talamo C, et al (1985) Work of breathing in patients with chronic obstructive pulmonary disease in acute respiratory failure. Am Rev Respir Dis 131:822–827
18. Marini JJ, Rodriguez M, Lamb V (1986) Bedside estimation of the inspiratory work of breathing during mechanical ventilation. Chest 89:56–63
19. Banner MJ, Kirby RR, MacIntyre NR (1991) Patient and ventilator work of breathing and ventilatory muscle loads at different levels of pressure support ventilation. Chest 100:531–533
20. Guttmann J, Haberthur C, Mols G (2001) Automatic tube compensation. Respir Care Clin N Am 7:475–501
21. Cohen JD, Shapiro M, Grozovski E, Singer P (2002) Automatic tube compensation-assisted respiratory rate to tidal volume ratio improves the prediction of weaning outcome. Chest 122:980–984
22. Pepe PE, Marini JJ (1982) Occult positive end-expiratory pressure in mechanically ventilated patients with airflow obstruction: the auto-PEEP effect. Am Rev Respir Dis 126:166–170
23. Romand JA, Suter PM (1994) Dynamic hyperinflation and intrinsic PEEP during mechanical ventilation. Eur J Anaesthesiol 11:25–28
24. Petrof BJ, Legaré M, Goldberg P, et al (1990) Continuous positive airway pressure reduces the work of breathing and dyspnea during weaning from mechanical ventilation in severe chronic obstructive pulmonary disease. Am Rev Respir Dis 141:281–289
25. MacIntyre NR, Cheng KC, McConnell R (1997) Applied PEEP during pressure support reduces the inspiratory threshold load of intrinsic PEEP. Chest 111:188–193
26. Webb HH, Tierney DF (1974) Experimental pulmonary edema due to intermittent positive pressure ventilation with high inflation pressures. Protection by positive end-expiratory pressure. Am Rev Respir Dis 110:556–565
27. Dreyfuss D. Saumon G (1998) Ventilator-induced lung injury: lessons from experimental studies. Am J Respir Crit Care Med 157:294–323
28. Dos Santos CC, Slutsky AS (2000) Invited review: mechanisms of ventilator-induced lung injury: a perspective. J Appl Physiol 89:1645–1655
29. American Association of Respiratory Care State of the Art Panel (1988) Positive end expiratory pressure. Respir Care 33:487–492
30. Gattinoni L, Caironi P, Pelosi P, Goodman LR (2001) What has computed tomography taught us about the acute respiratory distress syndrome? Am J Respir Crit Care Med 164:1701–1711
31. Macklen PT (1973) Relationship between lung mechanics and ventilation distribution. Physiology 16:580–588
32. NIH ARDS Network (2000) Ventilation with lower tidal volumes as compared to traditional tidal volumes in acute lung injury and acute respiratory distress syndrome. N Engl J Med 342:1301–1308
33. Dahlqvist M, Hedenstierna G (1985) Lung volumes measured by He dilution and by body-plethysmograph with mouth and esophageal pressures. Clin Physiol (Oxford) 5:179–187
34. Suter PM, Fairley B, Isenberg MD (1975) Optimum end-expiratory airway pressure in patients with acute pulmonary failure. N Engl J Med 292:284–289
35. Ferrer M, Zavala E, Diaz O, et al (1998) Assessment of ventilation-perfusion mismatching in mechanically ventilated patients. Eur Respir J 12:1172–1176
36. Neumann P, Berglund JE, Andersson LG, et al (2000) Effects of inverse ratio ventilation and positive end-expiratory pressure in oleic acid-induced lung injury. Am J Respir Crit Care Med 161:1537–1545
37. Dembinski R, Max M, Bensberg R, et al (2002) High-frequency oscillatory ventilation in experimental lung injury: effects on gas exchange. Intensive Care Med 28:768–774
38. Santak B, Radermacher P, Sandmann W, Falke KJ (1991) Influence of SIMV plus inspiratory pressure support on VA/Q distributions during postoperative weaning. Intensive Care Med 17:136–40
39. Valentine DD, Hammond MD, Downs JB, et al (1991) Distribution of ventilation and perfusion with different modes of mechanical ventilation. Am Rev Respir Dis 143:1262–1266

40. Matamis D, Lemaire F, Harf A, et al (1984) Redistribution of pulmonary blood flow induced by positive end-expiratory pressure and dopamine infusion in acute respiratory failure. Am Rev Respir Dis 129:39–44
41. Lim CM, Domino KB, Glenny RW, Hlastala MP (2001) Effect of increasing perfluorocarbon dose on VA/Q distribution during partial liquid ventilation in acute lung injury. Anesthesiology 94:637–642
42. Graham BL. Dosman JA. Cotton DJ (1980) A theoretical analysis of the single breath diffusing capacity for carbon monoxide. IEEE Trans Biomed Eng 27:221–227
43. Huang YC, O'Brien SR, MacIntyre NR (2002) Intrabreath diffusing capacity of the lung in healthy individuals at rest and during exercise. Chest 122:177–185
44. Huang YC, Helms MJ, MacIntyre NR (1994) Normal values for single exhalation diffusing capacity and pulmonary capillary blood flow in sitting, supine positions, and during mild exercise. Chest 105:501–508

Non-invasive Ventilation

Indications for Non-invasive Ventilation

N. S. Hill, T. Liesching, and H. Kwok

Introduction

Non-invasive ventilation (NIV), the provision of ventilatory assistance without the need for airway invasion, has seen increasing use in critical care units to avoid endotracheal intubation and its attendant complications [1-3]. Evidence has been rapidly accumulating to support many applications of NIV in the acute setting. NIV is also widely applied in the long-term setting, but a discussion of these applications is beyond the scope of this chapter. The following will make recommendations on current indications of NIV in the acute setting, based on the supporting evidence (Table 1).

Table 1. Evidence to support use of non-invasive positive pressure ventilation (NPPV) for different types of acute respiratory failure

Strong Evidence (multiple controlled trials) (Level 'A')
    COPD Exacerbations
    Acute cardiogenic pulmonary edema[*]
    Immunocompromised Patients

Less Strong Evidence (single controlled trial or multiple case series) (Level 'B')
    Asthma
    Community-acquired pneumonia (COPD patients)
    Post-operative respiratory failure
    Facilitation of weaning in COPD patients
    Avoidance of extubation failure
    Do-not-intubate patients

Weak Evidence (few case series, case reports, or failure to demonstrate benefit in controlled trials) (Level 'C')
    Cystic fibrosis
    Community-acquired pneumonia in non-COPD patients
    Upper airway obstruction
    Obstructive sleep apnea, obesity hypoventilation
    Acute respiratory distress syndrome (ARDS)
    Trauma

* Evidence strongest for CPAP

Strong Recommendation

Chronic Obstructive Pulmonary Disease (COPD)

The best established application of NIV is to treat acute exacerbations of COPD. A dozen years ago, Brochard et al. [4] showed that pressure support ventilation (PSV), administered via a face mask, significantly reduced the need for intubation, duration of mechanical ventilation and ICU length of stay compared to historically-matched controls. Subsequently, six randomized controlled trials have confirmed these findings [5-11]. Bott et al. [5] observed significantly greater improvements in $PaCO_2$ as well as dyspnea scores within the first hour in a group of NIV-treated patients compared to controls. Also, there was a 10% mortality rate in the NIV group compared to 30% in controls, but this was not statistically significant unless four patients who were randomized to NIV, but did not actually receive it, were excluded from the analysis. Kramer et al. [6] subsequently found that NIV reduced the rate of endotracheal intubation to 9% from 67% in controls in a subgroup of COPD patients. This study also showed more rapid improvements in respiratory rates and blood gases in the NIV group but no significant differences in hospital lengths of stay or mortality rates, perhaps because of the small sample size. In their multicenter randomized trial, Brochard et al. [7] found not only that vital signs, blood gas values, and encephalopathy scores improved more rapidly in the NIV-treated group than in controls, but also that intubation rates (from 74-26%), complication rates (notably pneumonia and other complications from endotracheal intubation), hospital lengths of stay (from 35 to 17 days) and mortality rates (from 31 to 9%) fell significantly. A subsequent smaller trial by Celikel et al. [9] also found that NIV significantly reduced intubation rates and hospital lengths of stay (from 14.6 to 11.7 days, p<0.05) compared to controls. Plant et al. [10] randomized 236 patients with acute exacerbations of COPD to receive NIV or standard therapy administered by nurses in general medical respiratory wards. The intubation and mortality rates were significantly lower in the NIV group compared to controls (15 vs. 27%, p=0.02 and 10 vs. 20%, p=0.05, respectively). The authors confirmed earlier findings of more rapid improvements in arterial pH, respiratory rate and breathlessness in the NIV compared to the control group. Of note, the mortality benefit was not apparent in patients with pH < 7.30, and the authors surmised that this more severely ill subgroup would have fared better in a more closely monitored setting such as an ICU.

The only negative study [12] found that NIV failed to lower intubation or mortality rates or hospital lengths of stay, but it is notable that no intubations or mortalities occurred in the control group. Furthermore, the hospital length of stay was only one third that of the control group in the Brochard study [7]. Thus, the enrolled patients were less severely ill than those included in other randomized trials and were less likely to benefit from NIV. The most important finding of this study is that patients with relatively mild COPD exacerbations are not likely to benefit from NIV.

Taken together, the above studies demonstrate that NIV is effective in acute COPD exacerbations, not only bringing about rapid symptomatic and physiologic improvements, but also significantly reducing the need for intubation, complication and mortality rates, and, in some studies, hospital lengths of stay. A meta-analysis [13] combining the results of some of these studies came to a similar conclusion about the need for intubation and mortality rate. Based on this evidence, consensus groups have opined that NIV is indicated as the ventilator mode of first choice in selected patients with COPD exacerbations [14].

Cardiogenic Pulmonary Edema

Along with COPD exacerbation, cardiogenic pulmonary edema is one of the two most common indications for non-invasive positive pressure techniques in the acute setting [15]. The evidence supporting the use of positive pressure in pulmonary edema, however, is stronger for the use of continuous positive airway pressure (CPAP) than for NIV (in which air pressure is increased during inspiration). CPAP has been used for many decades to treat cardiogenic pulmonary edema and the rationale for its application is quite strong. CPAP rapidly improves oxygenation by re-expanding flooded alveoli. It also increases functional residual capacity (FRC), thus more favorably positioning the lung on its compliance curve [16], reducing the work of breathing. Further, it can improve cardiac performance by raising pericardial pressure [16-18], lowering transmural pressure and thereby decreasing afterload [19, 20]. This favorable hemodynamic effect is most likely to occur when filling pressures are high and ventricular performance is poor. However, in patients with relatively low filling pressures and good ventricular performance, the hemodynamic effects of CPAP can be adverse, by diminishing venous return [17].

Several randomized studies have demonstrated that CPAP is effective in treating acute pulmonary edema [21-25]. Rasanen et al. [21] randomized 40 patients with cardiogenic pulmonary edema to either face mask CPAP (10 cmH2O) or standard medical therapy and demonstrated a rapid improvement in oxygenation and respiratory rate. Lin and Chiang [23] randomized 55 patients to face mask CPAP adjusted along with the inspired oxygen fraction (FiO2) to maintain PaO2 = 80 mmHg. CPAP significantly lowered the rate of intubation (17.5 vs. 42.5%, p<0.05), but no significant difference in mortality rate was observed. Bersten et al. [24] and Lin et al. [25] subsequently performed similar randomized studies on 39 and 100 patients, respectively, demonstrating the same favorable effects on oxygenation, respiratory rates and the need for intubation. The Bersten et al. study [24] also showed a significant reduction in ICU stay among CPAP-treated patients and the Lin et al. study [25] showed trends for improved hospital mortality rates.

Fewer controlled trials have been performed to determine whether NIV (usually pressure support plus positive end-expiratory pressure [PEEP]) is effective for acute pulmonary edema. Hypothetically, this approach might be more effective than CPAP alone, because a greater reduction in the work of breathing and more rapid alleviation of hypercapnia and dyspnea might be superimposed on the benefits achieved with CPAP.

Several uncontrolled trials have demonstrated low intubation and complication rates [26-30], supporting the contention that NIV is an effective therapy for acute pulmonary edema. However, one of these studies noted a high mortality rate in patients with acute myocardial infarction and cautioned about the use of NIV in such patients [30, 31]. In a randomized, prospective trial of 40 patients treated with mean inspiratory and expiratory pressures of 15 and 5 cmH2O, respectively, Masip et al. [32] found a significantly lower rate of intubation in NIV-treated patients (5%) compared to oxygen-treated controls (33%) (p=0.037). While oxygenation improved more rapidly in the NIV treated group compared to control, hospital lengths of stay and mortality rates were similar in the two groups. Sharon and colleagues [33] also performed a randomized trial that compared NIV plus low dose nitroglycerin versus high dose nitroglycerin in 40 patient with acute pulmonary edema. Patients treated with NIV had higher intubation (80 vs. 20%), myocardial infarction (55 vs. 10%) and death (10% vs. none) rates compared to controls (all p<0.05), leading the authors to conclude that NIV was less effective and potentially harmful compared to high dose nitroglycerin. However, this inference is unjustified because the groups were not comparable and the inordinately high intubation rate in the NIV group (80%) is difficult to explain.

Superiority of NIV over standard therapy for acute pulmonary edema is not surprising, but the question of most interest is whether NIV is superior to CPAP alone. If not, then the simpler and less expensive CPAP devices could be used to treat acute pulmonary edema. Only one randomized trial has thus far compared CPAP to NIV to treat acute pulmonary edema [34]. Although this trial showed significantly more rapid reductions in respiratory rate, dyspnea scores and hypercapnia in the NIV compared to the CPAP-treated group, the study was stopped prematurely after enrollment of 27 patients because of a greater myocardial infarction rate in the NIV group. This difference may have been attributable to unequal randomization because more patients in the NIV group presented with chest pain, but the results nonetheless raise concerns about the safety of ventilatory techniques used to treat acute pulmonary edema complicated by cardiac ischemia or infarction.

A more recent randomized controlled trial compared NIV to high flow oxygen by mask and demonstrated no statistically significant difference in the myocardial infarction rate between the two groups [35]. However, this study had limitations including a small number of patients and possibly inadequate pressures, considering that respiratory rate was not lowered more significantly by NIV. Presently, evidence on whether NIV is superior to CPAP is inconclusive; NIV lowers PaCO2 and dyspnea scores more rapidly, but it is unclear whether outcomes like intubation or mortality rate, or hospital length of stay differ between the modalities. Pending further studies, the most sensible current recommendation is to use CPAP (10 cmH2O) initially and consider switching to NIV if the patient is found to have substantial hypercapnia or unrelenting dyspnea. This is in line with the conclusion of a meta-analysis that found insufficient evidence to support the use of NIV in preference to CPAP to treat acute pulmonary edema [36].

Immunocompromised Patients

Evidence is accumulating to support the use of NIV in immunocompromised patients with acute respiratory failure. Antonelli et al. randomized 40 patients who developed acute respiratory failure following solid organ transplant to NIV vs.

conventional therapy. Patients treated with non-invasive positive pressure ventilation more often had increases in PaO_2/FiO_2 ratios (60 vs. 25%, p=0.03) and lower intubation (20 vs. 70%, p=0.05) and mortality rates (20 vs. 50%, p=0.05) [37]. In addition, the incidence of severe sepsis and shock was significantly reduced in the NIV group. More recently, another randomized trial of 52 patients with various immunocompromised states, mainly related to hematological malignancy, demonstrated reductions in the need for intubation (46 vs. 76%, p=0.03) and serious complication and mortality rates (both 50 vs. 80%, p=0.02) in NIV-treated patients compared with conventionally-treated controls [38]. The mortality of patients with hematological malignancies requiring intubation has been reported to exceed 80% in some series [39-45], largely because of septic and hemorrhagic complications. Thus, the avoidance of intubation in this patient population is a desirable outcome and the use of NIV is, therefore, justifiable in selected patients with immunocompromised states. It is important to note, however, that the authors of these studies stress the importance of early initiation, before progression to severe compromise [38].

Recommended with Reservations

Asthma

The success of NIV in treating COPD raises the possibility that it would also be beneficial in acute asthma. However, the lack of randomized controlled trials to confirm this hypothesis weakens the indication. Furthermore, the pathophysiologies and natural histories of COPD and asthma differ markedly and, thus, it is not fair to assume that one would respond to NIV in the same way as the other. However, cohort studies have reported successful outcomes with NIV in severe status asthmaticus complicated by CO_2 retention [27, 46]. In one study, only two of 17 asthmatics required intubation after starting NIV, with $PaCO_2$ falling from an average of 65 to 52 mmHg and respiratory rate from 29 to 20/min (p=0.002 and 0.0001, respectively), after 2 hours of therapy [46]. In a retrospective analysis of 33 asthmatic patients who were deemed to be candidates for NIV, the outcomes of 11 patients managed with invasive mechanical ventilation were compared with 22 managed non-invasively [47]. Gas exchange and vital signs improved rapidly in the NIV group and only 3 patients eventually required endotracheal intubation. A recent randomized, controlled trial on the use of NIV in acute asthma found no significant advantages attributable to the use of NIV [48]. However, the study was severely under-powered and the authors reported that bias on the part of emergency room physicians favoring NIV interfered with enrollment because of the concern that enrolled patients might become controls and not receive NIV therapy [48].

Despite the lack of convincing evidence to support the use of NIV in acute severe asthma, a trial of NIV in carefully selected and monitored patients is justifiable based on the anecdotal evidence. While no selection guidelines have been established, a reasonable approach would be to use NIV in patients who fail to respond promptly to standard initial medical therapy (i.e., within the first hour), but who have not developed contraindications to NIV (see patient selection section). Caution is advised because asthmatics may deteriorate abruptly and delay of needed intubation is a risk. Some studies indicate that aerosolized medication may be more effectively delivered via the NIV circuit compared to a standard nebulizer [49] and, anecdotally, NIV has been combined with heliox to treat status asthmaticus (personal observation), although no data are available to support this practice.

Cystic Fibrosis

Like asthmatics, patients with cystic fibrosis have airway obstruction and might be expected to respond to NIV like COPD patients. However, only a few anecdotal reports support the use of NIV in acute exacerbations of cystic fibrosis [50, 51]. Hodson et al. [50] used NIV to treat six cystic fibrosis patients with baseline forced expiratory volume in one second (FEV_1) ranging from 350 to 800 ml who developed acute superimposed on chronic CO_2 retention. These patients, with initial $PaCO_2$ ranging from 63 to 112 mm Hg, were supported for periods ranging from 3 to 36 days. Four patients survived until heart-lung transplantation could be performed. These same investigators recently reported their experience using NIV in 113 cystic fibrosis patients suffering acute deteriorations [51]. Of the 90 patients (median FEV_1/FVC ratio 0.51) who were either on, or being evaluated for, the lung transplant waiting list, 28 patients had successfully received lung transplantation and 10 others were still on the list. The authors noted that NIV improved hypoxia but not hypercapnia. These case series suggest that NIV is helpful as a rescue therapy in supporting acutely deteriorating cystic fibrosis patients providing a 'bridge to transplantation'. Despite the lack of evidence from randomized, controlled trials, using NIV to avoid intubation in appropriately selected patients with acute exacerbations or with deteriorating disease who have increasing CO_2 retention is sensible, particularly in view of the practice at some lung transplantation centers to remove intubated patients from the transplant list.

Pneumonia

The application of NIV to treat acute pneumonia has generated conflicting reports. Early on, pneumonia was associated with a poor outcome in patients treated with NIV [52]. A more recent study demonstrated that outcomes are significantly worse for patients with acute pneumonia compared to those with acute pulmonary edema who have a similar degree of hypoxemia (intubation rate 38 vs. 6.6%, p<0.05). In some of the early studies, part of the difficulty in assessing the efficacy of NIV in patients with 'pneumonia' was a failure to offer clear diagnostic criteria.

One randomized trial has been performed on patients with 'severe community-acquired pneumonia', defined as patients with severe hypoxemia (PaO_2/FiO_2 < 200 mmHg) and respiratory distress (respiratory rate > 35/min). In this study, NIV reduced the need for intubation (21 vs. 50%, p=0.03), shortened ICU length of stay (1.8 vs. 6 days, p=0.04), and reduced mortality rate among the COPD subgroup of patients two months after hospital discharge [53]. However, further analysis showed that the COPD subgroup was the only one to benefit from NIV. More recently, a prospective trial focusing on NIV use in non-COPD patients with severe community-acquired pneumonia observed that 22 of 24 patients had initial improvements in oxygenation and respiratory rates after starting NIV, but 66% eventually required intubation [54].

Although the authors of these trials concluded that NIV should be used routinely in patients with community-acquired pneumonia, the lack of controls in the latter study, and the failure to demonstrate benefit in the non-COPD subgroup in the controlled trial, undermine this recommendation. Presently, NIV is indicated in appropriate COPD patients with community-acquired pneumonia, but the benefit of NIV in pneumonia patients without COPD has not been established and, as such, NIV should be used with caution in such patients.

Facilitation of Extubation and Weaning

NIV has been used to facilitate early extubation after bouts of acute respiratory failure and to avoid extubation failure when patients deteriorate following extubation. In the first instance, NIV is used as a 'crutch' to permit early extubation in patients who fail to meet standard extubation criteria. The rationale is that outcomes can be improved by avoiding the complications of prolonged intubation such as nosocomial infection and upper airway trauma. The first controlled trial to test this idea enrolled 50 COPD patients who had been intubated for 48 hours and failed a T-piece trial [55]. They were randomized to prompt extubation and NIV or continued intubation with standard weaning. The NIV group had higher overall weaning rates after 60 days (88 vs. 68%), shorter durations of mechanical ventilation (10.2 vs. 16.6 days), briefer stays in the ICU (15.1 vs. 24 days) and improved 60 day survival rates (92 vs. 72%) compared to controls, respectively (all $p<0.05$). In addition, NIV-treated patients had no nosocomial pneumonias compared to seven in the control group.

A second trial of 33 patients randomized to early extubation and NIV or conventional intubation with standard weaning addressed the question of whether NIV should be used as a 'systematic' extubation technique [56]. NIV-treated patients had shorter durations of invasive mechanical ventilation than the control group (4.56 vs. 7.69 days, $p<0.05$), but the total duration of mechanical ventilation (including NIV) was actually greater in the NIV group (16.1 vs. 7.69 days, p= 0.0001). Furthermore, patients in the NIV group had similar eventual weaning and mortality rates, and although they had a tendency toward fewer complications (9 vs. 16%), the difference was not statistically significant. The authors concluded that NIV shortens the duration of invasive mechanical ventilation, but they were unable to demonstrate significant improvements in other outcomes. A third controlled, preliminary trial of 25 patients with various etiologies for their acute respiratory failure also found a significantly shorter duration of invasive mechanical ventilation, but extubation failure rate was higher (41% vs. none in controls, $p<0.05$) among patients extubated early to NIV [57].

Although the randomized controlled trials support the idea that early extubation to NIV can improve some outcomes of some mechanically ventilated patients, the results are mixed, raising questions about whether NIV should be used routinely to shorten the duration of invasive mechanical ventilation. Clinicians are advised to exert caution when selecting patients for early extubation, reserving the technique mainly for patients with acute on chronic respiratory failure (i.e., COPD patients) who are unable to meet standard extubation criteria but are otherwise good candidates for NIV. Those with prior difficult intubations, multiple co-morbidities, copious secretions, weakened cough, or the need for high levels of pressure support (>20 cmH2O) should not be considered for early extubation.

NIV can also potentially be used to avoid re-intubation in patients who fail extubation. Extubation failure occurs after 5-20% of planned [58] and 40-50% of unplanned extubations [59] and has been associated with a mortality of 43% compared to only 12% in those who succeed after extubation [58]. Several non-randomized studies support the idea that NIV can be used to avert the need for re-intubation in patients with extubation failure, thereby avoiding the complications and mortality of prolonged intubation [27, 60-62]. One of these studies found that 30 COPD patients with post-extubation hypercapnic respiratory insufficiency treated with NIV required re-intubation less often (20 vs. 67%, p<0.05) and had shorter ICU lengths of stay than 30 historically matched controls [62]. In a subsequent randomized trial of patients at high risk for extubation failure and who developed respiratory distress within 48 hours of extubation, however, NIV did not reduce the need for intubation, duration of mechanical ventilation, length of hospital stay or mortality [63].

To date, only one randomized trial has examined NIV as a 'prophylactic' technique; i.e., using it in all extubated patients to see if it lowers the extubation failure rate [64]. Ninety-three consecutive patients were enrolled, 56 after planned and 37 after unplanned extubations. Thirteen (28%) of the 47 patients randomized to NIV required re-intubation compared to only 7 (15%) of the 46 controls who received oxygen supplementation alone (p > 0.05). Although there was a problem with randomization in that more patients with unplanned extubations were assigned to the NIV group and these constituted most of the failures, the authors concluded that their results did not support the "indiscriminate" use of NIV to avoid post-extubation failure. Although NIV should certainly not be used routinely in post-extubation patients, just which patients with extubation failure should receive NIV to avoid re-intubation is unclear, considering the conflicting trial results. The most reasonable approach currently is to evaluate each patent individually, applying the selection criteria discussed below. The criteria are applicable to those patients who have underlying pulmonary edema or COPD as the cause of their respiratory distress, and should be applied with caution in other patients. Further studies must be done to determine which subcategories of patients might respond favorably to NIV.

Postoperative Patients

Some early case series reported the use of NIV to treat respiratory insufficiency after surgery in patients with $PaCO_2 > 50$ mmHg, $PaO_2 < 60$ mmHg, or evidence of respiratory muscle fatigue [65-68]. Using nasal bilevel positive airway pressure

(BiPAP®), these studies reported prompt reductions in respiratory rate and dyspnea scores, improvements in gas exchange, and high success rates in avoiding the need for reintubation. Subsequently, prophylactic postoperative use of NPPV in lung resection [69] and post-gastroplasty patients [70] has been shown to improve gas exchange and pulmonary function, respectively, compared to controls treated with oxygen alone. More recently, a randomized trial of NIV in post lung resection patients with acute respiratory insufficiency showed significant reductions in the need for intubation, ICU length of stay and mortality rate compared to conventionally-treated controls [71]. Thus, accumulating evidence now supports the use of NIV in selected postoperative patients to maintain improved gas exchange and avoid re-intubation and its attendant complications. NIV should not be used in patients with recent neck, upper airway or esophageal surgery, and caution should be exercised after recent upper gastrointestinal surgery that penetrates the mucosal barrier.

Do-Not-Intubate (DNI) Patients

The use of NIV to treat respiratory failure in patients who have declined intubation is common in some centers, accounting for some 10% of acute applications in a recent survey [72]. Some have argued that there is little to lose with this approach, as it may reverse the acute deterioration or, at least, provide relief of dyspnea and a few extra hours to finalize affairs [73]. However, others have argued that this merely prolongs the dying process, consumes resources inappropriately, and may add to discomfort or counter patients' wishes about avoidance of life-prolonging measures [74]. In one study of 30 patients, mostly with COPD, in whom endotracheal intubation was "contraindicated or postponed," eighteen (60%) patients were successfully supported with NIV and weaned [75]. Another uncontrolled series [76] observed a similar response to NIV among 26 patients with acute hypercapnic and hypoxemic respiratory failure who refused intubation. In a more recent prospective survey of 113 DNI patients treated with NIV, survival to hospital discharge was 72% and 52% for acute pulmonary edema and COPD patients, respectively, whereas it was less than 25% for those with diagnoses of pneumonia or cancer [72]. Thus, NIV is indicated in DNI patients with acutely reversible processes that are known to respond well, such as acute pulmonary edema or COPD exacerbation. However, if NIV is to be used for DNI patients, patients and/or their families should be informed that NIV is being used as a form of life support that may be uncomfortable and can be removed at any time.

Recommended with Caution

Upper Airway Obstruction

NIV can be used to treat patients with upper airway obstruction such as that caused by glottic edema following extubation. In this situation, NIV can be combined with aerosolized medication and/or heliox, but to date no controlled trials have confirmed the efficacy of this approach. If NIV is considered, patients should be selected with great caution and monitored closely because upper airway obstruction can lead to precipitous deteriorations. The inappropriate use of NIV in patients with tight, fixed upper airway obstruction should be avoided so as not to delay the institution of definitive therapy.

Decompensated Obstructive Sleep Apnea or Obesity-Hypoventilation Syndrome

Patients with acute on chronic respiratory failure caused by sleep apnea syndrome have been treated with NIV and transitioned to CPAP once stabilized [77], but no controlled trials have evaluated this application. NIV is indicated for such patients if they have acute worsening of CO_2 retention and are otherwise good candidates for NIV.

Hypoxemic Respiratory Failure

Hypoxemic respiratory failure refers to a broad subgroup of patients whose acute respiratory failure is characterized by severe hypoxemia (PaO_2/FiO_2 200), severe respiratory distress (respiratory rate > 35) and a non-COPD diagnosis including pneumonia, acute respiratory distress syndrome (ARDS), trauma or cardiogenic pulmonary edema [27]. Studies on this subgroup of patients have yielded conflicting results. Meduri et al. [26] reported success with NIV in all four patients with hypoxemic respiratory failure in their early trial. Later, however, Wysocki observed no significant benefit attributable to NIV among patients with hypoxemic respiratory failure, unless patients were hypercapnic [78]. In a large, uncontrolled series of 158 patients with various forms of respiratory failure treated with NIV, Meduri et al. [27] identified 41 with hypoxemic respiratory failure, 66% of whom avoided endotracheal intubation. Subsequently, Antonelli et al. [79] randomized 64 patients with hypoxemic respiratory failure to receive NIV or prompt intubation. NIV was as effective as invasive mechanical ventilation in improving oxygenation within the first hour, and only 10 of the 32 NIV patients required intubation. Patients in the NIV group had significantly fewer septic complications and strong trends toward shorter stays in the ICU and lower mortality rates. In another randomized trial of patients with various forms of respiratory failure [80], NIV lowered intubation and mortality rates in the subgroup with hypoxemic respiratory failure.

Thus, NIV can improve gas exchange, lower the need for intubation, and reduce mortality rates in patients with hypoxemic respiratory failure [79, 80]. However, results have been inconsistent between studies and the wide variety of patients that fall into this very broad diagnostic category makes it difficult to apply results to individual patients. For this reason, clinicians are discouraged from using this diagnostic grouping when applying NIV to individual patients, but rather to select patients based on more specific diagnoses. For example, two diagnostic categories that fall into the hypoxemic respiratory failure grouping are acute pulmonary edema, for which positive pressure techniques are strongly recommended, and ARDS, for which NIV should not be used routinely.

NIV has been reported to maintain adequate oxygenation and avert intubation in 6 of 12 episodes of ARDS in 10 patients [81]. However, no controlled trials have been performed to assess the effect of NIV on morbidity or mortality rates in ARDS. Thus, although NIV can be tried in patients with early, uncomplicated ARDS in an attempt to avoid intubation, routine use is not advised, particularly in patients with multiorgan system failure who are likely to require prolonged ventilatory support using sophisticated ventilator modes. If a trial of NIV is initiated, patients should be closely monitored and promptly intubated if they deteriorate, so that inordinate delays in needed interventions are avoided.

Trauma

Trauma patients develop respiratory failure for a multitude of reasons, but some have chest wall injuries such as flail chest or mild acute lung injury (ALI) that might respond favorably to NIV. In a retrospective survey on 46 trauma patients with respiratory insufficiency treated with NIV, Beltrame et al. [82] found rapid improvements in gas exchange and a 72% success rate; however, those patients with burns responded poorly. Despite these promising results, the uncontrolled design of the study limits the ability to draw conclusions or make recommendations on the use of NIV in trauma patients.

Restrictive Diseases

NIV is considered the ventilatory mode of first choice to treat chronic respiratory failure in patients with thoracic restriction caused by neuromuscular disease or chest wall deformity [83]. However, few studies have examined the role of NIV when these patients become acutely ill, partly because they constitute a very small portion of patients with respiratory failure entering acute care hospitals [27]. Some retrospective series suggest that NIV alleviates gas exchange abnormalities and avoids intubation in neuromuscular disease [84] and kyphoscoliotic [85] patients with acute respiratory failure. For managing acute deteriorations in patients already using NIV at home for chronic respiratory failure due to neuromuscular disease, Bach et al. [86] recommend increasing the duration of use to 24h/day while continuously monitoring pulse oximetry. If oxygen saturation falls below 90%, aggressive removal of secretions is undertaken using manually assisted coughing and mechanical aids such as the cough insufflator-exsufflator [86] until oxygen saturation returns to above 90%. No controlled studies have established the efficacy of this approach, but Bach's data [86] suggest that its use during acute exacerbations dramatically reduces the need for hospitalization. When such patients are hospitalized, clearance of retained secretions poses a major challenge; they should be placed in a closely monitored setting where aggressive techniques can be applied to assist with mobilization of secretions and intubation can be promptly performed if indicated.

Patient Selection

Selection of appropriate patients is an important part of the success of NIV. The selection process takes into consideration a number of factors including the patient's diagnosis, clinical characteristics, risk of failure and ultimately becomes a clinical judgment depending largely on physician experience. The etiology and reversibility of the respiratory failure are key, and clinicians should consider the evidence supporting the use of NIV for a particular diagnosis, as discussed above.

Predictors of success of NIV have been identified by some studies [52, 60, 87, 88] and are outlined in Table 2. As might be anticipated, these studies show that patients with a better neurologic status (and hence more cooperative) who are able to adequately protect their airway and who have not developed severe acid-base or gas exchange derangements are more likely to succeed. Several studies have also found that a patient's initial response to NIV after one hour of treatment (demonstrated by improvements in pH, $PaCO_2$ and level of consciousness) are associated with success [87–89]. These studies [52, 60, 87, 89] also indicate that there is a 'window of opportunity' when initiating NIV. The window opens when patients become distressed enough to warrant ventilatory assistance but closes if they progress too far and become severely acidemic. Thus, early initiation of NIV is recommended so that patients have time to adapt and respiratory crises can be averted. Contrariwise, NIV begun too early might be unhelpful and wasteful of resources because many treated patients might do well without any ventilatory assistance. For this reason, selection guidelines recommend first establishing the need for ventilatory assistance according to clinical and blood gas criteria and exclusion of patients in whom NIV is contraindicated or likely to fail (Table 3).

Summary and Conclusions

Indications for NIV in the acute setting have been broadening over the past decade, based on accumulating evidence and experience. The best-established indications remain acute exacerbations of COPD and acute pulmonary edema, with non-invasive CPAP being the positive pressure mode supported by the strongest evidence for the latter diagnosis. However, NIV can be used for numerous other diagnoses, as long as selection guidelines are observed. Strong evidence supports the use of NIV for immunocompromised patients with acute respiratory failure, largely because of the risk of invasive ventilation in these patients. NIV can also be used to facilitate extubation with the aim of reducing the complications of prolonged intubation, and to avoid re-intubation in patients with post-extubation failure. Weaker evidence supports use in selected patients with acute exacerbations of asthma, cystic fibrosis, and deteriorating obstructive sleep apnea and obesity hypoventilation syndrome. Recent evidence supports use in selected patients with post-operative respiratory failure and in patients who have decided to forego intubation, as long as they or their proxies are informed and given the option to decline all potentially life-prolonging therapies. NIV should be used only with caution and very selectively in patients with ARDS, trauma or upper airway

Table 2. Determinants of success for non-invasive positive pressure ventilation (NPPV) in the acute setting. Modified from [90]

Synchronous breathing [87]	No pneumonia [52, 87]
Dentition [87]	pH > 7.10 [52]
Lower APACHE score [52, 87]	$PaCO_2 < 92$ [52]
Less air leaking [87]	Better neurologic score [52, 89]
Less secretions [87]	Better 'compliance'*[52]

Good initial response to NPPV: [52, 87, 89]
    Correction of pH [89]
    Reduction in respiratory rate
    Reduction in $PaCO_2$ [89]	

* 'Compliance' refers to the clinician's assessment of the patient's acceptance of the technique.

Table 3. Selection criteria for non-invasive positive pressure ventilation (NPPV) in the acute setting. Modified from [90]

1. Appropriate diagnosis with potential reversibility

2. Establish need for ventilatory assistance
   a. Moderate to severe respiratory distress
   b. Tachypnea
   c. Accessory muscle use or abdominal paradox
   d. Blood gas derangement
      1. pH < 7.35, $PaCO_2 > 45$, or
      2. $PaO_2/FiO_2 < 200$

3. Exclude patients with contraindications to NPPV
   a. Respiratory arrest
   b. Medically unstable
   c. Unable to protect airway
   d. Excessive secretions
   e. Uncooperative or agitated
   f. Unable to fit mask
   g. Recent upper airway or gastrointestinal surgey

obstruction. The modality has assumed an important role in the ventilatory management of patients in critical care units and if applied optimally, should improve patient outcomes as well as efficiency of care.

References

1. Pingleton SK (1988) Complications of acute respiratory failure. Am Rev Respir Dis 137:1463–1493
2. Stauffer JL, Olson DE, Petty TL (1981) Complications and consequences of endotracheal intubation and tracheotomy. A prospective study of 150 critically ill adult patients. Am J Med 70:65–76
3. Fagon JY, Chastre J, Hance AJ, et al (1993) Nosocomial pneumonia in ventilated patients: a cohort study evaluating attributable mortality and hospital stay. Am J Med 94:281–288
4. Brochard L, Isabey D, Piquet J, et al (1990) Reversal of acute exacerbations of chronic obstructive lung disease by inspiratory assistance with a face mask. N Engl J Med 323:1523–1530
5. Bott J, Carroll MP, Conway JH, et al (1993) Randomised controlled trial of nasal ventilation in acute ventilatory failure due to chronic obstructive airways disease. Lancet 341:1555–1557
6. Kramer N, Meyer TJ, Meharg J, et al (1995) Randomized, prospective trial of noninvasive positive pressure ventilation in acute respiratory failure. Am J Respir Crit Care Med 151:1799–1806
7. Brochard L, Mancebo J, Wysocki M, et al (1995) Noninvasive ventilation for acute exacerbations of chronic obstructive pulmonary disease. N Engl J Med 333:817–822
8. Angus RM, Ahmed AA, Fenwick LJ, et al (1996) Comparison of the acute effects on gas exchange of nasal ventilation and doxapram in exacerbations of chronic obstructive pulmonary disease. Thorax 51:1048–1050
9. Celikel T, Sungur M, Ceyhan B, et al (1998) Comparison of noninvasive positive pressure ventilation with standard medical therapy in hypercapnic acute respiratory failure. Chest 114:1636–1642
10. Plant PK, Owen JL, Elliott MW (2000) Early use of non-invasive ventilation for acute exacerbations of chronic obstructive pulmonary disease on general respiratory wards: a multicentre randomised controlled trial. Lancet 355:1931–1935
11. Boyd RL, Fisher MJ, Jaeger MJ (1980) Non-invasive lung function tests in rats with progressive papain-induced emphysema. Respir Physiol 40:181–190
12. Barbe F, Togores B, Rubi M, et al (1996) Noninvasive ventilatory support does not facilitate recovery from acute respiratory failure in chronic obstructive pulmonary disease. Eur Respir J 9:1240–1245
13. Keenan SP, Kernerman PD, Cook DJ, et al (1997) Effect of noninvasive positive pressure ventilation on mortality in patients admitted with acute respiratory failure: a meta-analysis. Crit Care Med 25:1685–1692
14. International Consensus Conferences in Intensive Care Medicine (2001) Noninvasive positive pressure ventilation in acute respiratory failure. Am J Respir Crit Care Med 163:283–291
15. Carlucci A, Richard JC, Wysocki M, et al (2001) Noninvasive versus conventional mechanical ventilation. An epidemiologic survey. Am J Respir Crit Care Med 163:874–880
16. Katz JA, Marks JD (1985) Inspiratory work with and without continuous positive airway pressure in patients with acute respiratory failure. Anesthesiology 63:598–607
17. Bradley TD, Holloway RM, McLaughlin PR, Ross BL, Walters J, Liu PP (1992) Cardiac output response to continuous positive airway pressure in congestive heart failure. Am Rev Respir Dis 145:377–382
18. Baratz DM, Westbrook PR, Shah PK, et al (1992) Effect of nasal continuous positive airway pressure on cardiac output and oxygen delivery in patients with congestive heart failure. Chest 102:1397–1401
19. Fessler HE, Brower RG, Wise RA, Permutt S (1988) Mechanism of reduced LV afterload by systolic and diastolic positive pleural pressure. J Appl Physiol 65:1244–1250
20. Fessler HE, Brower RG, Wise RA, Permutt S (1992) Effects of systolic and diastolic positive pleural pressure pulses with altered cardiac contractility. J Appl Physiol 73:498–505

21. Rasanen J, Heikkila J, Downs J, Nikki P, Vaisanen I, Viitanen A (1985) Continuous positive airway pressure by face mask in acute cardiogenic pulmonary edema. Am J Cardiol 55:296–300
22. Vaisanen IT, Rasanen J (1987) Continuous positive airway pressure and supplemental oxygen in the treatment of cardiogenic pulmonary edema. Chest 92:481–485
23. Lin M, Chiang HT (1991) The efficacy of early continuous positive airway pressure therapy in patients with acute cardiogenic pulmonary edema. J Formos Med Assoc 90:736–743
24. Bersten AD, Holt AW, Vedig AE, Skowronski GA, Baggoley CJ (1991) Treatment of severe cardiogenic pulmonary edema with continuous positive airway pressure delivered by face mask. N Engl J Med 325:1825–1830
25. Lin M, Yang YF, Chiang HT, Chang MS, Chiang BN, Cheitlin MD (1995) Reappraisal of continuous positive airway pressure therapy in acute cardiogenic pulmonary edema. Short-term results and long-term follow-up. Chest 107:1379–1386
26. Meduri GU, Conoscenti CC, Menashe P, et al (1989) Noninvasive face mask ventilation in patients with acute respiratory failure. Chest 95:865–870
27. Meduri GU, Turner RE, Abou-Shala N, et al (1996) Noninvasive positive pressure ventilation via face mask. First-line intervention in patients with acute hypercapnic and hypoxemic respiratory failure. Chest 109:179–193
28. Lapinsky SE, Mount DB, Mackey D, Grossman RF (1994) Management of acute respiratory failure due to pulmonary edema with nasal positive pressure support. Chest 105:229–231
29. Hoffmann B, Welte T (1999) The use of noninvasive pressure support ventilation for severe respiratory insufficiency due to pulmonary oedema. Intensive Care Med 25:15–20
30. Rusterholtz T, Kempf J, Berton C, et al (1999) Noninvasive pressure support ventilation (NIPSV) with face mask in patients with acute cardiogenic pulmonary edema (ACPE). Intensive Care Med 25:21–28
31. Wysocki M (1999) Noninvasive ventilation in acute cardiogenic pulmonary edema: better than continuous positive airway pressure? Intensive Care Med 25:1–2
32. Masip J, Betbese AJ, Paez J, et al (2000) Non-invasive pressure support ventilation versus conventional oxygen therapy in acute cardiogenic pulmonary oedema: a randomised trial. Lancet 356:2126–2132
33. Sharon A, Shpirer I, Kaluski E, et al (2000) High-dose intravenous isosorbide-dinitrate is safer and better than Bi-PAP ventilation combined with conventional treatment for severe pulmonary edema. J Am Coll Cardiol 36:832–837
34. Mehta S, Jay GD, Woolard RH, et al (1997) Randomized, prospective trial of bilevel versus continuous positive airway pressure in acute pulmonary edema. Crit Care Med 25:620–628
35. Levitt MA (2001) Prospective, randomized trial of BiPAP in severe acute congestive heart failure. J Emerg Med 21:363–369
36. Pang D, Keenan SP, Cook DJ, Sibbald WJ (1998) The effect of positive pressure airway support on mortality and the need for intubation in cardiogenic pulmonary edema: a systematic review. Chest 114:1185–1192
37. Antonelli M, Conti G, Bufi M, et al (2000) Noninvasive ventilation for treatment of acute respiratory failure in patients undergoing solid organ transplantation: a randomized trial. JAMA 283:235–241
38. Hilbert G, Gruson D, Vargas F, et al (2001) Noninvasive ventilation in immunosuppressed patients with pulmonary infiltrates, fever, and acute respiratory failure. N Engl J Med 344:481–487
39. Estopa R, Torres Marti A, Kastanos N, Rives A, Agusti-Vidal A, Rozman C (1984) Acute respiratory failure in severe hematologic disorders. Crit Care Med 12:26–28
40. Price KJ, Thall PF, Kish SK, et al (1998) Prognostic indicators for blood and marrow transplant patients admitted to an intensive care unit. Am J Respir Crit Care Med 158:876–884
41. Ewig S, Torres A, Riquelme R, et al (1998) Pulmonary complications in patients with haematological malignancies treated at a respiratory ICU. Eur Respir J 12:116–122

42. Tognet E, Mercatello A, Polo P, et al (1994) Treatment of acute respiratory failure with non-invasive intermittent positive pressure ventilation in haematological patients. Clin Intensive Care 5:282–288

43. Ognibene FP, Martin SE, Parker MM, et al (1986) Adult respiratory distress syndrome in patients with severe neutropenia. N Engl J Med 315:547–551

44. Rubenfeld GD, Crawford SW (1996) Withdrawing life support from mechanically ventilated recipients of bone marrow transplants: a case for evidence-based guidelines. Ann Intern Med 125:625–633

45. Crawford SW, Schwartz DA, Petersen FB, et al (1988) Mechanical ventilation after marrow transplantation. Risk factors and clinical outcome. Am Rev Respir Dis 137:682–687

46. Meduri GU, Cook TR, Turner RE, Cohen M, Leeper KV (1996) Noninvasive positive pressure ventilation in status asthmaticus. Chest 110:767–774

47. Fernandez MM, Villagra A, Blanch L, et al (2001) Non-invasive mechanical ventilation in status asthmaticus. Intensive Care Med 27:486–492

48. Holley MT, Morrissey TK, Seaberg DC, et al (2001) Ethical dilemmas in a randomized trial of asthma treatment: can Bayesian statistical analysis explain the results? Acad Emerg Med 8:1128–1135

49. Pollack CV, Jr., Fleisch KB, Dowsey K (1995) Treatment of acute bronchospasm with beta-adrenergic agonist aerosols delivered by a nasal bilevel positive airway pressure circuit. Ann Emerg Med 26:552–557

50. Hodson ME, Madden BP, Steven MH, et al (1991) Non-invasive mechanical ventilation for cystic fibrosis patients-a potential bridge to transplantation. Eur Respir J 4:524–527

51. Madden BP, Kariyawasam H, Siddiqi AJ, et al (2002) Noninvasive ventilation in cystic fibrosis patients with acute or chronic respiratory failure. Eur Respir J 19:310–313

52. Ambrosino N, Foglio K, Rubini F, Clini E, Nava S, Vitacca M (1995) Non-invasive mechanical ventilation in acute respiratory failure due to chronic obstructive pulmonary disease: correlates for success. Thorax 1995; 50:755–757

53. Confalonieri M, Potena A, Carbone G, et al (1999) Acute respiratory failure in patients with severe community-acquired pneumonia. A prospective randomized evaluation of noninvasive ventilation. Am J Respir Crit Care Med 160:1585–1591

54. Jolliet P, Abajo B, Pasquina P, et al (2001) Non-invasive pressure support ventilation in severe community-acquired pneumonia. Intensive Care Med 27:812–821

55. Nava S, Ambrosino N, Clini E, et al (1998) Noninvasive mechanical ventilation in the weaning of patients with respiratory failure due to chronic obstructive pulmonary disease. A randomized, controlled trial. Ann Intern Med 128:721–728

56. Girault C, Daudenthun I, Chevron V, Tamion F, Leroy J, Bonmarchand G (1999) Noninvasive ventilation as a systematic extubation and weaning technique in acute-on-chronic respiratory failure: a prospective, randomized controlled study. Am J Respir Crit Care Med 160:86–92

57. Hill N, Lin D, Levy M, et al (2000) Noninvasive positive pressure ventilation (NPPV) to facilitate extubation after acute respiratory failure: a feasibility study. Am J Respir Crit Care Med 161:A263 (abst)

58. Epstein SK, Ciubotaru RL, Wong JB (1997) Effect of failed extubation on the outcome of mechanical ventilation. Chest 112:186–192

59. Chevron V, Menard JF, Richard JC, et al (1998) Unplanned extubation: risk factors of development and predictive criteria for reintubation. Crit Care Med 26:1049–1053

60. Meduri GU, Abou-Shala N, Fox RC, Jones CB, Leeper KV, Wunderink RG (1991) Noninvasive face mask mechanical ventilation in patients with acute hypercapnic respiratory failure. Chest 100:445–454

61. Restrick LJ, Scott AD, Ward EM, et al (1993) Nasal intermittent positive-pressure ventilation in weaning intubated patients with chronic respiratory disease from assisted intermittent, positive-pressure ventilation. Respir Med 87:199–204

62. Hilbert G, Gruson D, Gbikpi-Benissan G, et al (1997) Sequential use of noninvasive pressure support ventilation for acute exacerbations of COPD. Intensive Care Med 23:955–961

63. Keenan SP, Powers C, McCormack DG, Block G (2002) Noninvasive positive-pressure ventilation for postextubation respiratory distress. JAMA 287:3238–3244
64. Jiang JS, Kao SJ, Wang SN (1999) Effect of early application of biphasic positive airway pressure on the outcome of extubation in ventilator weaning. Respirology 4:161–165
65. Pennock BE, Kaplan PD, Carlin BW, Sabangan JS, Magovern JA (1991) Pressure support ventilation with a simplified ventilatory support system administered with a nasal mask in patients with respiratory failure. Chest 100:1371–1376
66. Pennock BE, Crawshaw L, Kaplan PD (1994) Noninvasive nasal mask ventilation for acute respiratory failure. Institution of a new therapeutic technology for routine use. Chest 105:441–444
67. Gust R, Gottschalk A, Schmidt H, et al (1996) Effects of continuous (CPAP) and bi-level positive airway pressure (BiPAP) on extravascular lung water after extubation of the trachea in patients following coronary artery bypass grafting. Intensive Care Med 22:1345–1350
68. Matte P, Jacquet L, Van Dyck M, et al (2000) Effects of conventional physiotherapy, continuous positive airway pressure and non-invasive ventilatory support with bilevel positive airway pressure after coronary artery bypass grafting. Acta Anaesthesiol Scand 44:75–81
69. Aguilo R, Togores B, Pons S, Rubi M, Barbe F, Agusti AG (1997) Noninvasive ventilatory support after lung resectional surgery. Chest 112:117–121
70. Joris JL, Sottiaux TM, Chiche JD, et al (1997) Effect of bi-level positive airway pressure (BiPAP) nasal ventilation on the postoperative pulmonary restrictive syndrome in obese patients undergoing gastroplasty. Chest 111:665–670
71. Auriant I, Jallot A, Herve P, et al (2001) Noninvasive ventilation reduces mortality in acute respiratory failure following lung resection. Am J Respir Crit Care Med 164:1231–1235
72. Nelson D, et al. SK, Vespia J, et al. (2000) Outcomes of do-not-intubate patients treated with noninvasive bilevel positive pressure ventilation. Crit Care Med 29 (abst)
73. Freichels T (1994) Palliative ventilatory support: use of noninvasive positive pressure ventilation in terminal respiratory insufficiency. Am J Crit Care 3:6–10
74. Clarke DE, Vaughan L, Raffin TA (1994) Noninvasive positive pressure ventilation for patients with terminal respiratory failure: the ethical and economic costs of delaying the inevitable are too great. Am J Crit Care 3:4–5
75. Benhamou D, Girault C, Faure C, Portier F, Muir JF (1992) Nasal mask ventilation in acute respiratory failure. Experience in elderly patients. Chest 102:912–917
76. Meduri GU, Fox RC, Abou-Shala N, et al (1994) Noninvasive mechanical ventilation via face mask in patients with acute respiratory failure who refused endotracheal intubation. Crit Care Med 22:1584–1590
77. Sturani C, Galavotti V, Scarduelli C, et al (1994) Acute respiratory failure, due to severe obstructive sleep apnoea syndrome, managed with nasal positive pressure ventilation. Monaldi Arch Chest Dis 49:558–560
78. Wysocki M, Tric L, Wolff MA, et al (1993) Noninvasive pressure support ventilation in patients with acute respiratory failure. Chest 103:907–913
79. Antonelli M, Conti G, Rocco M, et al (1998) A comparison of noninvasive positive-pressure ventilation and conventional mechanical ventilation in patients with acute respiratory failure. N Engl J Med 339:429–435
80. Martin TJ, Hovis JD, Costantino JP, et al (2000) A randomized, prospective evaluation of noninvasive ventilation for acute respiratory failure. Am J Respir Crit Care Med 161:807–813
81. Rocker GM, Mackenzie MG, Williams B, et al (1999) Noninvasive positive pressure ventilation: successful outcome in patients with acute lung injury/ARDS. Chest 115:173–177
82. Beltrame F, Lucangelo U, Gregori D, Gregoretti C (1999) Noninvasive positive pressure ventilation in trauma patients with acute respiratory failure. Monaldi Arch Chest Dis 54:109–114
83. Anonymous (1999) Clinical indications for noninvasive positive pressure ventilation in chronic respiratory failure due to restrictive lung disease, COPD, and nocturnal hypoventilation – a consensus conference report. Chest 116:521–534

84. Bach JR (1996) Conventional approaches to managing neuromuscular ventilatory failure. In: Baxh JR (ed) Pulmonary Rehabilitation: The obstructive and Paralytic-Restrictive Syndromes. Henley & Belfus, Philadelphia, pp: 283–301
85. Finlay G, Concannon D, McDonnell TJ (1995) Treatment of respiratory failure due to kypho-scoliosis with nasal intermittent positive pressure ventilation (NIPPV). Ir J Med Sci 164:28–30
86. Bach JR, Ishikawa Y, Kim H (1997) Prevention of pulmonary morbidity for patients with Duchenne muscular dystrophy. Chest 112:1024–1028
87. Soo Hoo GW, Santiago S, Williams AJ (1994) Nasal mechanical ventilation for hypercapnic respiratory failure in chronic obstructive pulmonary disease: determinants of success and failure. Crit Care Med 22:1253–1261
88. Poponick JM, Renston JP, Bennett RP, et al (1999) Use of a ventilatory support system (BiPAP) for acute respiratory failure in the emergency department. Chest 116:166–171
89. Anton A, Guell R, Gomez J, et al (2000) Predicting the result of noninvasive ventilation in severe acute exacerbations of patients with chronic airflow limitation. Chest 117:828–833
90. Liesching T. Kwok HK, Hill NS, et al (2003) Acute application of non-invasive positive plessure ventilation. Chest (in press)

Non-invasive Ventilation:
Causes of Success or Failure

S. Nava and P. Ceriana

Introduction

Until fifteen years ago, mechanical ventilation was limited to the intensive care unit (ICU) because patients needed to be paralyzed and sedated. Over the last decade the great interest in non-invasive mechanical ventilation (NIV) has opened new horizons in the field of mechanical ventilation and the ways in which it can be applied. Indeed, as a result of various clinical and physiological evidence, NIV has become a first-line intervention in the management of severe exacerbations of chronic obstructive pulmonary disease (COPD) [1]. A recent International Consensus Conference in Intensive Care Medicine [2] concerning the use of noninvasive positive pressure ventilation (NPPV) in acute respiratory failure stated that "the addition of noninvasive positive pressure to standard medical treatment of patients with acute respiratory failure may prevent the need of intubation, and reduce the rate of complications and mortality in patients with hypercapnic respiratory failure". Moreover, it has been shown that NIV can be applied at an earlier stage in the evolution of ventilatory failure than would be usual when a patient is intubated and that the NIV can be administered even outside the ICU. The literature about NIV in the treatment of 'pure hypoxic' acute respiratory failure is also abundant, but conclusive results have been reached only in acute respiratory failure due to exacerbation of COPD. A meta-analysis by Keenan and co-workers [3] showed that NIV can reduce the need for endotracheal intubation with survival benefits in this population. Unfortunately, a meta-analysis cannot focus on what is the ideal setting in which to apply NIV or the best population to receive it. Nonetheless, it should be emphasized that the positive results reported NPPV were observed only in selected COPD patients with the majority excluded. Patients with COPD needing immediate intubation have regularly been excluded from all studies published to date [4]. This means that wherever NIV is performed, facilities for prompt endotracheal intubation should be readily available. Indeed, major problems regarding the use of NIV out of an ICU are the possible need for quick intubation and ways to provide sufficient assistance during NIV. Absolute contraindications to NIV have been clearly recognized as:

- Cardiac or respiratory arrest
- Non respiratory organ failure (i.e., severe encephalopathy, severe gastrointestinal bleeding and hemodynamic instability with or without unstable cardiac angina)

- Facial surgery or trauma
- Upper airway obstruction
- Inability to protect the airway and/or high risk of aspiration
- Inability to clear secretions.

Apart from these contraindications, several studies have indirectly suggested or directly investigated the possible indicators of NIV success or failure. The recognition of these parameters may be very important especially in environments outside the ICU, where it is mandatory to identify some 'quick' indicators of failure of NIV to avoid any undue delay in the time to intubation. In this chapter, we will discuss the utility of some predictors of NIV success or conversely of failure, depending on how you approach the problem (i.e, the glass may be half empty or half full), in both the situations of acute hypercapnic and 'pure hypoxemic' respiratory failure.

Acute Hypercapnic Respiratory Failure

In order to achieve the highest success rate during the application of NIV, an appropriate selection of patients who will benefit from this ventilatory technique must be made. The first step is to identify the patient in respiratory distress for whom ventilatory assistance is needed: clinical criteria include the presence of tachypnea, dyspnea, paradoxical abdominal breathing and accessory muscle activation while further indications can be given by the presence of respiratory acidosis ($PaCO_2 > 55$ mmHg and pH < 7.35). The second step is the identification of patients needing immediate intubation for whom NIV is not the technique of choice (see the above listed contraindications to NIV).

The reported rates of NIV failure in most important clinical trials range from 5 to 40% [4–7], hence it is likely that the early recognition of a subset of 'responders' could be helpful to avoid the delayed application of invasive ventilation in those patients who need endotracheal intubation.

Arterial blood gases

Respiratory acidosis is probably one of the most valuable indicators of the severity of COPD decompensation and all clinical studies report both pH and $PaCO_2$ values sampled always at baseline and after a certain time lag (generally one or a few hours) after the application of NIV. Ambrosino et al. [8] observed that, in a group of 47 patients with decompensated COPD, lower baseline values of pH and $PaCO_2$ were predictive of NIV failure; in those patients who were more acidemic before starting ventilation (pH 7.22 versus 7.28) NIV subsequently failed. pH values recorded 1 hour after the initial trial of NIV also accurately identified those patients who could be successfully ventilated. Furthermore, using a logistic regression analysis, baseline pH and pH after 1 hr of NIV maintained a valuable predictive power with a high degree of sensitivity (87–93%, respectively) and specificity (54% and 82%).

Similar results have been obtained by Meduri et al. [9] in a group of 158 patients with acute respiratory failure sustained by different causes. In a subgroup of 74 patients with hypercapnic ventilatory failure, NIV failed in patients with higher baseline $PaCO_2$ values and improvement of acidosis after a 2-hour NIV trial predicted a successful response to NIV.

Plant et al. [10] carried out a prospective multicenter randomized trial of NIV versus standard medical treatment on a population of 236 patients with an acute exacerbation of COPD and mild to moderate respiratory acidosis (pH range 7.25 7.35). They observed that a high degree of acidemia at study entry (pH<7.30) was associated with treatment failure and that improvement of pH after 4 hours of NIV was predictive of success. On the other hand, in a multicenter epidemiologic survey, Carlucci et al. [7] showed, in a group of 108 patients treated with NIV, most of them affected by COPD, that changes in arterial blood gases after 1 day of NIV could not discriminate responders and non-responders (7.37 versus 7.34) but that pH on admission was significantly higher in favorable cases (7.36 versus 7.30).

In a small group of twelve decompensated COPD patients treated with NIV plus medical therapy, Soo Hoo et al. [11] had a 50% rate of successful cases and observed no difference in baseline pH and $PaCO_2$ between failed and favorable cases. Yet, they were able to demonstrate that successful cases displayed a quicker correction of acidosis.

Anton et al. [12] applied NIV to 36 hypercapnic COPD patients with a success rate of 77%; in order to find predictive criteria for NIV failure they devised a multiple regression model and concluded that improvement in $PaCO_2$ and pH after one hour of NIV was a highly predictive index that enabled them to accurately predict NIV success in about 95% of cases.

While most authors have addressed the issue of 'early' NIV failure, Moretti et al. [13] tried to analyze predictors of 'late' failures, i.e., cases in which NIV failed a few days after its initial application, despite an initial improvement in clinical conditions and blood gas values. In a population of 134 patients with COPD exacerbation in whom NIMV was applied for > 24 hours, a subgroup of 31 patients did worse about 8 days after NIV application; a thorough evaluation of patient characteristics at study entry and at the moment of failure identified that a lower pH at admission, among with other variables, was predictive of late failure.

Table 1 summarizes the results regarding the achievement or not of statistical significance in predicting NIV success, for baseline pH and pH changes after a NIV trial.

Severity of Disease

The most commonly used indexes of severity of illness are APACHE II [14] and SAPS II [15] while other indexes, e.g., activities of daily living (ADL) [16] are specifically designed to indicate the degree of a patient's functional limitation. The association between indexes of severity of illness and NIV failure have been sought on the assumption that patients suffering from respiratory failure frequently have co-morbidities (malnutrition, cardiopathy, diabetes etc) and episodes of exacerbation are frequently associated with organ failures. Since during an episode of acute hypercapnic respiratory failure, the ventilator works mainly as an accessory muscle up to the resolution of the underlying decompensation, the greater the degree of

Table 1. The achievement (YES) or not (NOT) of statistical significance in predicting NIV success, for baseline pH or a change in pH during NIV

	Baseline pH	pH change after a NIV trial
Soo Hoo [11]	No	Yes
Moretti [13]	Yes	No
Anton [12]	No	Yes
Ambrosino [8]	Yes	Yes
Plant [10]	Yes	Yes
Carlucci [7]	Yes	No
Meduri [9]	Yes	Yes

organ failure, the slower will be the recovery process and the less likely will be the success of NIV.

A positive correlation between severity of underlying disease and NIV failure has been demonstrated by some authors. Moretti et al. [13] found that the presence of one or more complications at admission (i.e., severe hyperglycemia) together with marked functional disability (low ADL scale) were strong predictors of late NIV failure. A significantly greater severity of illness among patients who failed to improve with NIV was found by Ambrosino et al. [8] (mean APACHE II 24 versus 18 in successful cases) and by Soo Hoo et al. [11] who reported a mean APACHE II score of 21 in NIV failures and of 15 in successful cases. In the previously quoted epidemiologic survey [7], Carlucci et al., applying a multiple regression analysis, showed that SAPS II was an independent predictive factor of NIV failure. In another randomized prospective study in a general ICU, Conti et al. [17] treated 49 decompensated COPD patients (mean pH 7.2) with invasive (26 pts) or non-invasive (23 pts) ventilation after failure of medical treatment performed in the emergency department. The failure rate in the NIV group was 52% and patients who needed endotracheal intubation after a trial of NIV had a significantly higher SAPS II score (mean value=39) compared to patients who avoided intubation (mean value=35). However, using APACHE II, Anton et al. [12] and Meduri et al. [9] did not find any correlation between severity score and NIV failure. Similarly, Benhamou et al. [18], using SAPS II, was unable to find a link between patients' clinical status and NIV failure.

Table 2 summarizes the results concerning the achievement or not of statistical significance in predicting NIV success, for various indices of disease's severity.

Table 2. The achievement (YES) or not (NOT) of statistical significance in predicting NIV success, for various indices of disease's severity. ADL: activities of daily living scale

	SAPS II	APACHE II	ADL
Carlucci [7]	YES		
Meduri [9]		NO	
Ambrosino [8]		YES	
Moretti [13]			YES
Anton [12]		NO	
Soo Hoo [11]		YES	
Conti [17]	YES		
Benhamou [18]	NO		

Cooperation and Encephalopathy

Absence of encephalopathy, compliance and tolerance to NIV are important issues and essential requirements for effective ventilation. In case of respiratory distress, in fact, a tightly fitting mask is sometime poorly tolerated and if the patient is not cooperative, frequent movements and attempts to displace the mask and to loose the head straps cause large air leaks and ineffective triggering. Furthermore, a deteriorating mental status during NIV can indicate a worsening hypercarbia that requires immediate endotracheal intubation.

Some investigators have observed a positive correlation between baseline low mental status scored according to Kelly and Matthay [19] and NIV failure [8, 12, 17]. The problem of NIV tolerance and acceptance has been separately addressed using an arbitrary score: several groups [7, 8, 18] found that poor clinical tolerance to NIV was highly predictive of NIV failure. Interestingly, Soo Hoo et al. [11] observed that patients successfully treated with NIV were able to tolerate the mask for a longer period of time compared to unsuccessful cases.

'Mixed' Indices

Other indexes have been considered 'possible' predictors, although their statistical power has never been systematically addressed due to difficulties in finding homogeneous and objective systems of classification: for example, the degree of mask leak is closely connected to the team skill, to the patient's physical conformation, and to the availability of proper material [7, 11].

With respect to the ability to clear secretions, judgement can be highly subjective and variable among different operators. One of the few studies in which this issue has been addressed is that conducted by Carlucci et al. [7], who evaluated the ability to mobilize secretions using a simple binary scoring system (yes/no) and found more patients able to effectively clear sputum in the successfully treated group.

Training and Equipment

As stated before, the success of NIV largely depends on the acceptance and compliance of the patient, and these are likely to be associated with the way that this method of ventilation is applied by the operator. The learning and training process that a hospital team gains throughout the years may be important in this respect. Literature data indirectly raise this suspicion. For example, in 1992, Foglio et al. [20] concluded, from a retrospective study, that the use of NIV was not more effective than standard medical treatment alone in an acute respiratory failure due to COPD, but the same group later showed contrasting results [21], so that in an accompanying editorial [22] Brochard stated that "it was possible that some learning effects explained part of the improvement in the success rate".

It is, therefore, possible that progressively increasing experience of medical and paramedical personnel, derived from the systematic use of NIV over the years, may modify clinical practice (i.e., the severity of patients treated) and patient outcome. Several studies have demonstrated that NIV is no more demanding for the personnel than standard medical therapy or invasive ventilation, but interestingly enough Chevrolet et al. [23] demonstrated that NIV may be a very time-consuming procedure for nurses and so may be very difficult to apply; 10 years later they concluded that this technique, in experienced hands, appears not to influence the nurses' workload in the ICU significantly. Very recently, Carlucci et al. [24] have shown that the clinical practice of applying NIV for an acute exacerbation of COPD may change over time, so that with increased staff training, more severely ill patients may be treated with a reduced risk of failure. In the meantime, increased confidence with the technique may allow the same team to treat less severely ill patients outside the ICU, so that the total NIV costs per year decrease significantly. The severity of the episodes of acute respiratory failure, defined by pH and APACHE II score at admission, worsened significantly during the study period. In particular the change point statistical test showed a significant decrease in pH at admission after about 5 years of training (year 1997), thus allowing the authors to identify two different periods: 1992–1996 (first period) in which the mean pH at admission was 7.25 ± 0.07 and 1997–1999 (second period) during which the mean pH at admission was significantly lower (7.20 ± 0.08, p < 0.0001). As illustrated in Table 3, in the first period (1992–1996) among the variables recorded at admission, the severity of acidosis (pH and $PaCO_2$) and of illness (APACHE II), were significantly worse in the patients who failed NIV. In the second period (1997–1999), NIV failures differed only for a higher APACHE II (p<0.006). After one hour of treatment, two additional variables were associated with success of treatment, irrespective of the study period: an improvement in pH and $PaCO_2$ value (either in terms of absolute value or as change from admission time). Interestingly, failures of the first period had the same pH at admission as the successes in the second period (7.21 ± 0.06 vs 7.21 ± 0.08, respectively).

Table 3. Comparison of patients treated with non-invasive ventilation during 2 time periods. Modified from [24]

	Years 92–96 (n = 145)			Years 97–99 (n= 63)		
	Success (n = 119)	Failure (n = 26)	p value	Success (n = 53)	Failure (n = 10)	p value
APACHE II	21 ± 6	25 ± 6	0.005	24 ± 5	29 ± 7	0.006
pH adm	7.26 ± 0.07	7.21 ± 0.06	0.003	7.21 ± 0.08	7.18 ± 0.10	0.24
pH 1hr	7.31 ± 0.06	7.20 ± 0.09	< 0.0001	7.30 ± 0.06	7.18 ± 0.08	< 0.001
Δ pH	0.06 ± 0.03	– 0.01 ± 0.04	< 0.0001	0.09 ± 0.04	0.002 ± 0.06	< 0.0001
PCO$_2$ adm	83 ± 17	91 ± 14	0.03	88 ± 16	99 ± 22	0.06
PCO$_2$ 1hr	75 ± 14	95 ± 18	< 0.0001	77 ± 13	100 ± 22	< 0.0001
Δ PCO$_2$	– 8.3 ± 8	4.3 ± 6.2	< 0.0001	– 9.7 ± 7.4	1.9 ± 9.3	< 0.0001

The relative risk of failure of patients treated by NIV according to the severity of the respiratory failure at admission, was calculated for a pH of 7.30 and of 7.25. Compared with a patient with a pH of 7.30 treated in the second period, a patient with a pH of 7.25 had a 1.5-fold (95% CI 1 – 3.8) higher risk of failure if treated in the years 1997–1999 vs a 3.3-fold (95% CI 2.25.1) higher when treated in the years 92–96 (p = 0.03).

Equipment and in particular ventilators and monitoring systems also may be important in determining the success of NIV; the technology used in NIV has altered in the last decade and may have influenced the type of patient treated, since the success of NIV may depend on its acceptance. In particular, home care ventilators are now equipped with software developed to compensate for air-leaks, with new non-rebreathing devices and systems of triggering, so that the patient-ventilator interaction and CO$_2$ clearance may be better. The materials and the shapes of facial masks used for NIV have also dramatically improved over time so that the newer and more sophisticated interfaces may influence the tolerance of NIV and therefore the possibility to treat more severely ill patients with the same good outcomes.

Environment

The large majority of studies on NIV were performed in general ICUs [4–6], respiratory intermediate ICUs [8], and in pneumology wards [12], while only one study was performed directly in the emergency room [25]. No authors have compared outcomes of patients treated in different settings, but this would in any

Table 4. A schematic recommendation of where COPD patients should be treated in the case of an episode of acute hypercapnic respiratory failure, according to their baseline pH and clinical conditions.

Medical Ward
   To prevent 'overt' acute respiratory failure (pH from 7.30 to 7.35)

Respiratory ICU
   To treat severe acute respiratory failure (pH$\leq$7.30) but only if:

   1. Hemodynamic stability
   2. $PaO_2/FiO_2 \geq 1.5$
   3. No sepsis
   4. Minimal spontaneous capacity
   5. Normal sensorium
   6. No multiple organ failure

ICU
   To treat severe acute respiratory failure (pH<7.30)
   and in presence of one of the following contraindications
   for high dependency unit:

   1. $PaO_2/FiO_2 < 1.5$
   2. No spontaneous activity
   3. >1 organ failure

In All Other Conditions:
   Intubation

case be difficult because the severity of respiratory impairment of the patients in the studies differed greatly. In fact, all the studies performed in a general ward concerned patients with a mean pH >7.29, whilst patients admitted to ICU or respiratory intermediate ICU had more severe respiratory acidosis (pH <7.29). This pH value can reasonably be considered as a cut-off point for deciding whether a patient should be admitted to an ICU/respiratory intermediate ICU for NIV or whether they can stay in a general ward. This has been recently demonstrated in a large number of patients in the 'Yorkshire study' [26]. The severity of illness and the presence of co-morbid conditions must also be taken in account when deciding the optimal location for treatment. These two factors have been reported to be correlated with failure of NIV in acute respiratory failure [13]. Yet other factors must be considered before admitting a patient to an ICU, e.g., prior quality of life, functional status and central nervous system impairment. Table 4 is a schematic recommendation of where COPD patients should be treated in the case of an episode of acute hypercapnic respiratory failure, according to their baseline pH and clinical conditions.

Acute Hypoxic Respiratory Failure

Since the large majority of studies dealing with NIV were performed in patients with acute hypercapnic respiratory failure, it is not surprising that most of the literature dealing with predictors of success or failure is also concentrated in this field, so that there are scanty data about predictors of failure in 'pure' hypoxemic respiratory failure. The definition and severity of an episode of hypoxemic respiratory failure still relies on the PaO_2/FiO_2 ratio, thus including a variety of conditions of different etiologies and causes under the same umbrella. Most of the studies performed in 'pure' hypoxemic respiratory failure were focused particularly on a single pathology such as cardiogenic pulmonary edema [27], acute respiratory distress syndrome (ARDS), acute lung injury (ALI) [28] or community-acquired pneumonia [29, 30], so that a generalized recommendation on when NPPV should be avoided was difficult to make. Antonelli et al. [31] showed that application of the two different ventilatory techniques in hypoxemic respiratory failure resulted in similar short-term improvements in arterial blood gases, while non-invasive pressure support ventilation was associated with fewer serious complications and a shorter stay in the ICU stay when compared with conventional mechanical ventilation. Unfortunately, although the two groups of patients were apparently homogeneously composed, the small sample size did not allow the authors to perform a subgroup analysis according to the underlying diseases, so that it is possible that their results may have been influenced by a subgroup having a particularly better response to non-invasive pressure support ventilation. As a matter of fact, experience gained from other studies suggests, even though it has not clearly been demonstrated, that for a similar PaO_2/FiO_2 ratio the success or failure of NIV and therefore the patients' outcome depends predominantly on the underlying pathology, rather than on 'simple' indices. Confalonieri et al. [29] showed that in selected patients with acute respiratory failure caused by severe community-acquired pneumonia, NIV could significantly reduce the need for intubation when compared with medical treatment. But the subgroup analysis compels us to temper any excessive optimism since this clearly showed that only hypercapnic patients really benefited from the treatment, while in non-hypercapnic patients the rate of failure did not differ from that of the standard treatment. This was confirmed by Jolliet et al. [30], who in an uncontrolled study performed in non-COPD patients with community-acquired pneumonia showed an even higher rate of NIV failure than in the Italian study (66% vs 38%).

We know that hypercapnic respiratory failure is a direct consequence of alveolar hypoventilation whatever the cause leading to the impairment of the respiratory pump. In this condition, application of an artificial muscle, i.e., the ventilator, takes on the work of breathing entirely or in part, giving time to bronchodilator therapy to decrease airway obstruction and hyperinflation. On the other hand, hypoxemic respiratory failure can be the 'end-point' of several pathologies, each acting through different physiopathological mechanisms (shunt, ventilation/perfusion mismatch, impairment of alveolar-capillary diffusion). Providing adequate oxygenation is, therefore, the life-saving procedure. The addition of continuous positive airway pressure (CPAP) may be helpful in many ways, depending on the underlying pathologies, because it can increase functional residual capacity (FRC), improve respiratory mechanics and, therefore, oxygenation and, in certain instances such as cardiogenic pulmonary edema, decrease the left ventricular afterload. On the other hand, in most of these conditions, the inspiratory aid given by the ventilator may, theoretically, not be needed if hypercapnia, as a direct sign of respiratory pump failure, is not present. Once satisfactory oxygenation is reached, through one or more of the above mentioned mechanisms, the major determinant of the outcome remains the response to medical therapy.

Interestingly enough, Domenighetti et al. [32] published recently the first attempt to study whether similar degrees of hypoxia (PaO_2/FiO_2 ratio) with two different causes, have different outcomes. They showed that despite initial improvements being similar in terms of PaO_2/FiO_2 in the first hour of treatment, the outcome of patients affected by pneumonia was much worse than that of patients with cardiogenic pulmonary edema. Pneumonia has a relatively slow onset and time is also needed for conventional therapy to show its effects, conversely the onset of cardiogenic pulmonary edema is very rapid, but its resolution is similarly quick if the appropriate medical therapy works. Providing good oxygenation and ventilatory assistance, through an oxygen mask, NIV or invasive ventilation, may therefore not be enough in terms of outcomes when an inflammatory disease of any nature is healing too slowly. Interestingly in Domenighetti's study the only parameter recorded in the community-acquired pneumonia group after 60 minutes of NIV that resulted in statistically significant differences between success and failure was the respiratory rate, that tended to increase in the intubated patients and to significantly decreased in the successfully ventilated patients.

The only study that has addressed the presence of predictors of failure in patients with acute hypoxic respiratory failure was conducted prospectively on 354 patients with a PaO_2/FiO_2 at admission $\leq$ 200 mmHg [33]. The multivariate analysis identified the following as factors independently associated with failure:

- Age >40 years
- SAPS II $\geq$35
- Presence of ARDS and community-acquired pneumonia
- PaO_2/FiO_2 $\leq$146 mmHg after 1 hr of NIV

In this study the authors found, different to what is usually reported for hypercapnic respiratory failure, that the arterial blood gases at study entry had no predictive value, and that most of the failures were related to the inability to correct gas exchange after 1 hour. This may again reflect the importance of the individual response, depending on the different underlying pathologies, to the acute application of NIV.

Conclusion

In conclusion, NIV should be considered the first line treatment of mild to severe acute hypercapnic respiratory failure, while during an episode of 'pure' hypoxic respiratory failure the outcome seems to be related to the underlying disease, rather than to the degree of hypoxia.

Concerning hypercapnic respiratory failure, some indices such as admission pH and its changes after 1 hour of NIV, have been shown to be strong predictors of success or failure, while other possible indicators of success may be the integrity of the sensorium and the absence of co-morbidities and therefore the overall severity of illness of the patients. Great care should be taken to identify the subset of patients at risk of late NIV failure, since they have been shown to have a bad prognosis.

Concerning hypoxic respiratory failure, the presence of ARDS and community-acquired pneumonia seem to be high risk factors of failure, together with a lack of improvement in oxygenation after the first NIV attempt.

The inferences from all the indices proposed in everyday clinical practice should be made cautiously and specific studies validated on a large scale are needed. Indeed some of the 'cut-off' limits that have been shown to separate success from failure, may vary according to the specific training and familiarity of the staff with NIV, and according to the different environments and equipment, that may in fact modify the clinical approach to the patients.

References

1. Eliott MW (2002) Non-invasive ventilation in acute exacerbations of chronic obstructive pulmonary disease: a new gold standard? Intensive Care Med 28:1691–1694
2. Anonymous (2001) International Consensus Conference in Intensive Care Medicine: Noninvasive positive pressure ventilation in acute respiratory failure Am J Respir Crit Care Med 163:283–291
3. Keenan SP, Gregor J, Sibbald WJ, Cook DJ, Gafni A (2000) Noninvasive positive pressure ventilation in the setting of severe, acute exacerbations of chronic obstructive pulmonary disease: more effective and less expensive. Crit Care Med 28:2094–2102
4. Brochard L, Mancebo J, Wysocki M, et al (1995) Noninvasive ventilation for acute exacerbations of chronic obstructive pulmonary disease. N Engl J Med 333:817–822
5. Bott J, Carroll TH (1993) Randomized controlled trial of nasal ventilation in acute ventilatory failure due to chronic obstructive airway disease. Lancet 341:1555–1557
6. Celikel T, Sungur M, Ceyhan B, et al (1998) Comparison of noninvasive positive ventilation with standard medical therapy in hypercapnic acute respiratory failure. Chest 114:1636–1642
7. Carlucci A, Richard JC, Wisocki M, Lepage E, Brochard L (2001) Noninvasive versus conventional mechanical ventilation. An epidemiologic survey. Am J Respir Crit Care Med 163:874–880
8. Ambrosino N, Foglio K, Rubini F, Clini E, Nava S, Vitacca M (1995) Non-invasive mechanical ventilation in acute respiratory failure due to chronic obstructive pulmonary disease: correlates for success. Thorax 50:755–757
9. Meduri GU, Turner RE, Abou-Shala N, Wunderink R, Tolley E (1996) Noninvasive positive pressure ventilation via face mask. First-line intervention in patients with acute hypercapnic and hypoxemic respiratory failure. Chest 109:179–193
10. Plant PK, Owen JL, Eliott MW (2001) Non-invasive ventilation in acute exacerbations of chronic obstructive pulmonary disease: long term survival and predictors of in-hospital outcome. Thorax 56:708–712
11. Soo Hoo GW, Santiago S, Williams AJ (1994) Nasal mechanical ventilation for hypercapnic respiratory failure in chronic obstructive pulmonary disease: determinants of success and failure. Crit Care Med 22:1253–1261
12. Anton A, Güell R, Gomez J, et al (2000) Predicting the results of noninvasive ventilation in severe acute exacerbations of patients with chronic airflow limitation. Chest 117:828–833

13. Moretti M, Cilione C, Tampieri A, Fracchia C, Marchioni A, Nava S (2000) Incidence and causes of non-invasive mechanical ventilation failure after initial success. Thorax 55:819–825
14. Knaus WA, Draper EA, Wagner DP, et al (1985) APACHE II: a severity of disease classification system. Crit Care Med 13:818–829
15. Le Gall JR, Lemeshow S, Saulnier F (1993) A new simplified acute physiology score (SAPS II) based on a European/North american multicenter study. JAMA 270:2957–2963
16. Seneff MG, Wagner DP, Wagner RP, et al (1995) Hospital and 1-year survival of patients admitted to intensive care units with acute exacerbation of chronic obstructive pulmonary disease. JAMA 274:1852–1857
17. Conti G, Antonelli M, Navalesi P, et al (2002) Noninvasive vs. conventional mechanical ventilation in patients with chronic obstructive pulmonary disease after failure of medical treatment in the ward: a randomized trial. Intensive care Med 28:1701–1707
18. Benhamou D, Girault C, Faure C, et al (1992) Nasal mask ventilation in acute respiratory failure. Chest 102:912–917
19. Kelly BJ, Matthay MA (1993) Prevalence and severity of neurologic dysfunction in critically ill patients. Influence on need for continued mechanical ventilation. Chest 104:1818–1824
20. Foglio K, Vitacca M, Quadri A, Scalvini S, Marangoni S, Ambrosino N (1992) Acute exacerbations in severe COLD patients. Treatment using positive pressure ventilation by nasal mask. Chest 101:1533–1538
21. Vitacca M, Rubini F, Foglio K, Scalvini S, Nava S, Ambrosino N (1993) Non-invasive modalities of positive pressure ventilation improve the outcome of acute exacerbations in COLD patients. Intensive Care Med 19:450–455
22. Brochard L (1993) Non-invasive ventilation: practical issues. Intensive Care Med 19:431–432
23. Chevrolet JC, Jolliet P, Abajo B, Toussi A, Louis M (1991) Nasal positive pressure ventilation in patients with acute respiratory failure. Difficult and time-consuming procedure for nurses. Chest 100:775–782
24. Carlucci A, Delmastro M, Rubini F, Fracchia C, Nava S (2003) Changes in the practice of non-invasive ventilation in treating COPD patients over 8 years. Intensive Care Med 29:419–425
25. Wood KA, Lewis L, Von Harz B, Kollef MH (1998) The use of positive pressure ventilation in the emergency department. Chest 113:1339–1346
26. Plant PK, Owen JL, Eliott MW (2000) Early use of non-invasive ventilation for acute exacerbations of chronic obstructive pulmonary disease on general respiratory wards: a multicentre randomized controlled trial. Lancet 355:1931–1935
27. Pang D, Keenan SP, Cook DJ, Sibbald WJ (1998) The effect of positive pressure airway support on mortality and need for intubation in cardiogenic pulmonary edema: a systematic review. Chest 114:1185–1192
28. Rocker GM, Mackenzie MG, Williams B, Logan PM (1999) Noninvasive positive pressure ventilation. Successful outcome in patients with acute lung injury/ARDS. Chest 115:173–177
29. Confalonieri M, Potena A, Carbine G, Della Porta R, Tolley EA, Meduri U (1999) Acute respiratory failure in patients with severe community-acquired pneumonia. Am J Respir Crit Care Med 160:1585–1591
30. Jolliet P, Abajo B, Pasquina P, Chevrolet JC (2001) Non-invasive pressure support ventilation in severe community-acquired pneumonia. Intensive Care Med 27:812–821
31. Antonelli M, Conti G, Rocco M, et al (1998) A comparison of noninvasive positive-pressure ventilation and conventional mechanical ventilation in patients with acute respiratory failure. N Engl J Med 339:429–435
32. Domenighetti G, Gayer R, Gentilini R (2002) Noninvasive pressure support ventilation in non-COPD patients with acute cardiogenic pulmonary edema and severe community-acquired pneumonia: acute effects and outcome. Intensive Care Med 28:1226–1232
33. Antonelli M, Conti G, Moro ML, et al (2001) Predictors of failure of noninvasive positive pressure ventilation in patients with acute hypoxemic respiratory failure: a multi-center study. Intensive Care Med 27:1718–1728

Non-invasive Ventilation in Immunocompromised Patients

M. Antonelli, M. A. Pennisi, and G. Conti

Introduction

During the last two decades, the dramatic evolution of surgical techniques and the use of innovative immunosuppressive strategies has extended the applicability of solid organ transplantation to an increased number of patients suffering from end-stage failure of various organs. As a direct consequence, the survival rates after solid organ transplantation have dramatically improved. Despite this increase in the post-transplantation survival rate, respiratory complications are the principal cause of morbidity, together with acute organ rejection, and one of the main causes of mortality [1]. Approximately 5% of patients undergoing renal, hepatic, cardiac or pulmonary transplantation develop pneumonia after transplantation, with an attributable mortality of 37% [1].

Immunosuppressive treatments have produced an increase in the survival rates, but at the price of an increased susceptibility to severe infection, often caused by opportunistic agents (Table 1). The lung is the most commonly involved organ in the infectious processes.

During the immediate postoperative period, pneumonia is generally caused by Gram negative germs, that often colonize patients in the intensive care unit (ICU). In the late postoperative phase, Cytomegalovirus (CMV) is one of the most common causes of pneumonia [2, 4]. CMV infection can be primary or can be caused by the reactivation of a previous infection. *Pneumocystis carinii* is also a relatively common ethiologic agent for pneumonia occurring at least three months following transplantation.

Many immunosuppressed patients with hypoxemic acute respiratory failure develop acute lung injury (ALI) or acute respiratory distress syndrome (ARDS). In this situation, early application of optimal values of positive pressure ventilation is aimed for, to restore the decreased lung volume and increase oxygenation, reducing both the work of breathing and respiratory drive. Mechanical ventilation re-establishes patient equilibrium and buys time to allow the etiological treatment to be effective.

Endotracheal intubation is the conventional and accepted route to administer positive pressure ventilation. However the presence of an endotracheal tube represents the main risk factor for the development of nosocomial pneumonia and associated infectious complications [5]. In immunocompetent patients, endotracheal intubation induces a 1% increased risk for pneumonia per day of mechanical

Table 1. Common causes for respiratory infectious complications, in relation to the specific pattern of immunity alteration.

Cellular immunity alterations:	– intracellular bacteria (mycobacteria, atypic mycobacteria) – fungal infections (Pneumocystis carinii) – viral infections (CMV; Herpes virus)
Humoral immunity alterations:	– bacterial infections (mainly capsulated germs) – viral infections (syncitial respiratory virus, influenza virus, and parainfluenza virus)
Neutropenia:	– bacteria (Gram + and Gram -) – fungal infections (Candida, Aspergillus) – viral infections (herpes, syncitial respiratory virus)

ventilation [6]. This risk is likely to be largely increased in immunocompromised critically ill patients, but specific data are lacking.

These aspects have augmented the interest in non-invasive ventilation (NIV) techniques, which improve gas exchange with good patient tolerance and can decrease the rate of nosocomial infections.

Non-invasive Ventilation in Solid Organ Transplanted Patients and Acute Lung Injury

Over the last ten years several prospective non-randomized and randomized studies [7-15] have demonstrated the successful application of NIV in immuno-competent patients with hypoxemic acute respiratory failure of varied etiologies. In one observational trial [9] in patients with cystic fibrosis, NIV was used as a bridge to lung transplant.

Wysocki et al [14] randomized 41 patients with acute respiratory failure to receive NIV via face mask plus conventional medical treatment versus conventional medical therapy and oxygen supplementation via a Venturi mask. NIV reduced the need for endotracheal intubation (36 vs 100%, p = 0.02), the duration of ICU stay (13 ± 15 vs 32 ± 30 days, p = 0.04) and mortality rate (9 vs 66 %, p = 0.06) in the subgroup of patients with hypercapnia ($PaCO_2$ > 45 mmHg), but had no clear advantage in the hypoxemic patients with normocapnia.

Antonelli and colleagues [15] recently conducted a prospective, randomized study comparing NIV via a face mask to endotracheal intubation with conventional mechanical ventilation, in patients with hypoxemic acute respiratory failure who met predefined criteria for mechanical ventilation, after failure to improve with aggressive medical therapy. Sixty-four consecutive patients (32 in each arm) were enrolled. After 1 h of mechanical ventilation, both groups had a significant (p < 0.05) improvement in PaO_2/FiO_2. Ten (31%) patients randomized to NIV required endotracheal intubation. Patients randomized to conventional ventilation developed more frequent and serious complications (38 vs 66%, p = 0.02), and infectious complications (pneumonia or sinusitis) related to the endotracheal tube

(3 vs 31%; p = 0.004). Among survivors, patients randomized to NIV had a lower duration of mechanical ventilation (p = 0.006) and a shorter ICU stay (p = 0.002).

In conclusion, NIV was found to be as effective as conventional ventilation with endotracheal intubation in improving gas exchange. In the subgroup of patients successfully treated with NIV and who avoided endotracheal intubation the development of ventilator-associated pneumonia (VAP) was unlikely [15]

A recent prospective epidemiological survey of 320 consecutive immunocompetent patients with acute respiratory failure reported a lower rate of VAP in patients supported with NIV in comparison with those on conventional ventilation (0.16 per 100 days of NIV vs 0.85 per 100 days of tracheal intubation, p=0.004) [16].

For its positive effects on gas exchange, good tolerability and reduction in the incidence of nosocomial infections, NIV should be considered with interest also in the treatment of immunosuppressed patients. Small non-controlled studies in patients receiving lung transplantation have reported the efficacy of NIV in preventing endotracheal intubation, and treating acute respiratory failure [17-19]. In 1995, Kilger and colleagues described the successful application of NIV in a group of 6 patients who developed hypoxemic acute respiratory failure after bilateral lung transplantation. The authors administered pressure support ventilation-continuous positive airway pressure (PSV-CPAP) through a facial mask without side effects [17]. Two case reports described similar results in patients with single lung transplantation [18, 19].

We recently conducted a prospective randomized study to compare NIV delivered through a face mask to standard treatment with supplemental oxygen administration as a modality to avoid endotracheal intubation in 40 solid organ transplant recipients with acute hypoxemic respiratory failure [20]. Twenty patients were randomized to receive NIV and 20 to receive standard treatment with supplemental oxygen administration. Within the first hour of treatment, 14 (70%) patients in the NIV group, and 5 (25%) in the standard treatment group improved their PaO_2/FiO_2. Over time, a sustained improvement in PaO_2/FiO_2 was noted in 12 (60%) patients in the NIV group, but only in 5 patients (25%) randomized to standard treatment (p=0.03). The use of NIV was associated with a significant reduction in the rate of endotracheal intubation (20 vs 70%; p = 0.002), rate of fatal complications (20 vs 50%; p = 0.05), length of ICU stay (5.5 ± 3 vs 9 ± 4 days; p = 0.03) and ICU mortality (20 vs 50%; p = 0.05).

Rocco et al. [21], in a prospective non-randomized study, evaluated the application of NIV in a group of 21 patients developing postoperative acute respiratory failure after bilateral lung transplantation: the technique was well tolerated, improved gas exchange, and avoided endotracheal intubation in 86% of cases.

These data suggest that transplantation programs should consider the inclusion of NIV among the clinical tools for the treatment of transplant recipients with acute respiratory failure, especially if this approach can be used in an early phase of the respiratory failure, to prevent endotracheal intubation and its associated complications.

Practical Aspects of NIV Administration

As in immunocompetent patients with hypoxemic acute respiratory failure, in immunocompromised patients NIV should be administered preferably through a facial mask, which is generally well tolerated. A nasal mask can be used in a later phase, in selected and stabilized patients, for continuing the treatment. Mechanical ventilation is usually delivered in PSV mode, with variable levels of positive end-expiratory pressure (PEEP, usually within a range between 5 and 10 cmH_2O), according to the level of hypoxemia and clinical tolerance.

In our experience the continuous application of NIV is crucial, at least for the first 24 hours of treatment [15, 20], as these patients show a rapid deterioration of gas exchange if NIV is discontinued during the early phases of the disease. The ventilator is generally connected with conventional tubing to a clear, full face mask provided with an inflatable soft cushion seal. The mask is gently fitted to the patient's face, and secured with head straps. For patients with a nasogastric tube, a specific seal connector in the dome of the mask should be used to minimize air-leaks, especially if using ICU machines without leak compensation. After the mask is secured, the level of pressure support can be progressively increased to obtain an exhaled tidal volume (V_T) of 8-10 ml/kg with a respiratory rate less than 25 breaths/min and no accessory muscle contraction or paradoxical abdominal movements. Ventilator settings are then adjusted according to continuous pulse-oximetry and arterial blood gas data.

Contraindications to NIV application in immunosuppressed patients are generally similar to those described in patients with acute respiratory failure and are not specific (Table 2).

Table 2. Main contraindications to NIV in immunocompromised patients with acute respiratory failure.

- Hemodynamic and/or rhythm instability
- Neurologic alterations
- Uncooperative patients
- Facial deformitiy
- More than two organ failures
- Claustrophobia
- Recent acute myocardial infarction
- Severe anxiety

Non-invasive Ventilation in Immunocompromised Patients

Acute respiratory failure due to pulmonary infections represents a relatively common complication of hematological malignancies and their treatment. In the last twenty years, several investigators have underlined the negative prognosis for granulocytopenic patients with acute respiratory failure requiring endotracheal intubation and conventional mechanical ventilation [22-27]. This dramatically increased risk of death [25, 26] results from the combination of the damage induced by opportunistic infections, the direct toxicity of chemotherapy on pulmonary interstitial structures, and the complications directly related to endotracheal intubation.

Despite the fact that NIV could reduce the number of endotracheal intubations and the associated infection rate in these patients, the number of published studies on this topic is still very limited [27, 28]. Tognet and colleagues first reported good clinical results with the intermittent application of NIV in patients with hematological malignancies; 6 out of 11 patients with acute respiratory failure were successfully treated with NIV through a face-mask, using different levels of pressure support and PEEP [28]. Conti et al. evaluated the effects of NIV delivered via nasal mask utilizing a BiPAP®. ventilator (Respironics, USA) in 16 consecutive patients with hematological malignancies and acute respiratory failure [29]. Fifteen out of 16 individuals had an early and sustained improvement in gas exchange: PaO_2/FiO_2 after 1 h of treatment increased from 87 ± 22 to 175 ± 64 mmHg, and continued to improve in the following 24 h ($p < 0.01$). One patient failed to improve and another become intolerant to NIV, both were intubated and died from sepsis. Three other patients died from complications unrelated to respiratory failure. Eleven patients were successfully discharged from the ICU after 4.3 ± 2.4 days.

A recent randomized trial evaluated NIV as a means to avoid intubation and associated complications in immunocompromised patients admitted to the ICU for hypoxemic acute respiratory failure (PaO_2/FiO_2 below 200 mmHg), fever and lung infiltrates [30]. Fifty-two patients were enrolled in this study (30 patients with hematological malignancies and neutropenia,18 who received immunosuppressive treatment to prevent rejection after solid organ transplantation, bone marrow transplantation, or for other reasons, and four with acquired immunodeficiency syndrome [AIDS]) and were randomized to receive conventional treatment (O_2 plus aggressive medical therapy) or NIV plus conventional treatment [30]. NIV was intermittently administered with a face mask in PSV-CPAP. The two groups were comparable at study inclusion. NIV significantly reduced the rate of intubation (46 vs 77%, p=0.003) and serious complications (50 vs 81%, p=0.02). Both ICU (38 vs 69%, p=0.03) and hospital (50 vs 81%, p=0.02) mortality were significantly reduced. The authors concluded that the early intermittent application of NIV ameliorates the prognosis of immunocompromised patients admitted to the ICU. In this randomized study on immunocompromised patients treated with NIV, the results obtained in the subgroup of patients with hematologic malignancies and neutropenia were highly significant, suggesting an extended clinical role for the application of NIV to these conditions.

Table 3 summarizes the main studies on immunocompromised pantients.

Table 3. Main characteristics of the studies dedicated to the use of NIV in hypoxic acute respiratory failure in immunosuppressed and immunocompromised patients.

Author [ref]	Study	No of patients	Disease	Pts on NIV	Mask	PEEP	Modes of ventilation	Success rate (%)	Mortality
Kilger [18]	NR	30	Lung transplant	6	Facial	NE	PSV/CPAP	NE	NE
Varon [34]	NR	60	Solid cancer	60	Facial	NE	BiPAP	70 %	0%
Tognet [28]	NR	11	Hematologic malignancy	11	Facial	5	PSV/CPAP	55%	45%
Conti [29]	NR	16	Hematologic malignancy	16	Nasal	5	BiPAP	62%	38%
Antonelli [20]	R	40	Organ transplant	20	Facial	6	PSV/CPAP	80%	20%
Hilbert [30]	R	52	Mixed immuno-compromised	26	Facial	6	PSV-CPAP	50%	38%
Rocco [21]	NR	21	Lung transplant	21	Facial	6	PSV-CPAP	86%	9%

R = randomized; NR = non randomized; PEEP = positive end expiratory pressure; PSV = pressure support ventilation; CPAP = continous positive airways pressure; BiPAP = bilevel positive airways pressure; NE = not evaluated

NIV in Patients with Human Immunodeficiency Virus (HIV) Infection

Despite the dramatic improvement in the prognosis of HIV-infected patients due to the new anti-retroviral drugs, acute respiratory failure due to *P. carinii* and other opportunistic agents remains the main cause for ICU admission and mortality among patients with AIDS. These patients are generally treated with face-mask CPAP. Two groups have reported the use of non-invasive positive pressure ventilation (NPPV, CPAP + PSV) in patients with AIDS and hypoxemic acute respiratory failure [31-32].

In the first paper, 12 patients were treated with NPPV, 10 of them improved gas exchange and avoided intubation. PaO_2/FiO_2 increased from a baseline of 132 ± 71 to 222 ± 116 mmHg at 1 h and 285 ± 80 mmHg at 2-6 h. One of three patients failing to improve refused intubation and died. Overall, ICU survival was 67% (8 of 12), and hospital survival was 58%. Duration of NPPV was longer (39 ± 28 h) than in other conditions causing hypoxemic acute respiratory failure, but was safe (only two cases of facial skin necrosis) and well tolerated [31].

Rabbat et al. [32] reported on 18 patients suffering from acute respiratory failure complicating AIDS, treated with face-mask PSV-CPAP; NIV was successful and avoided endotracheal intubation in 13 patients, while five individuals failed and required endotracheal intubation (four of these patients died).

A recent case-control study by Confalonieri and colleagues [33] compared the results obtained with early NIV in 24 patients with AIDS and *P. carinii* pneumonia with those obtained in 24 matched controls treated with conventional ventilation for the same disease. NIV was successful and avoided endotracheal intubation in 67% of cases. Patients treated with NIV had a lower mortality rate not only in the ICU and in the hospital, but also at the two month follow up after the study entry.

Despite the relatively small amount of published data, it is reasonable to consider NIV as a useful therapeutic tool to avoid endotracheal intubation and associated infectious complications also when treating AIDS patients with acute respiratory failure.

Conclusion

The application of NIV to patients with immunological deficiencies is still considered a new approach that needs further clinical validation. A restricted number of studies focusing on the clinical use of NIV in immunocompromised and immunosuppressed patients have been published so far, but some evidence support a careful consideration of this approach when facing early respiratory decompensation.

NIV must be considered as a first-line treatment in patients who refuse sedation and endotracheal intubation, but agree to receive mechanical ventilatory support.

References

1. Mermel LA, Maki DG (1990) Bacterial pneumonia in solid organ transplantation. Semin Respir Infect 5:10-29
2. Schulman LL, Smith CR, Drusin R (1988) Respiratory complications after cardiac transplantation. Am J Med Sci 296:1-10
3. Velasco N, Catto GRD, Engeset NEJ, Moffat MAJ (1984) The effect of the dosage of steroids on the incidence of cytomegalovirus infection in renal transplant recipients. J Infect Dis 9:69-78
4. Pass RF, Whitley RJ, Diethelem AG, Whelchel JD, Reynolds DW, Alford CA (1980) Cytomegalovirus infection in patients with renal transplant: Potentiation by antithymocyte globulin and an incompatible graft. J Infect Dis 142:9-17
5. Meduri GU, Mauldin GL, Wunderink RG, Leeper KV, Jones C, Tolley E (1994). Causes of fever and pulmonary densities in patients with clinical manifestations of ventilator-associated pneumonia. Chest 106:221-235
6. Fagon JY, Chastre J, Domart Y (1989) Nosocomial pneumonia in patients receiving continuous mechanical ventilation : prospective analysis of 52 episodes with use of a protected specimen brush and quantitative culture techniques. Am Rev Respir Dis 139:877-884
7. Meduri GU, Conoscenti CC, Menashe P, Nair S (1989) Noninvasive face mask ventilation in patients with acute respiratory failure. Chest 95:865-870

8. Pennock BE, Kaplan PD, Carlin BW, Sabangan JS, Magovern JA (1991) Pressure support ventilation with a simplified ventilatory support system administered with a nasal mask in patients with respiratory failure. Chest 100:1371-1376

9. Hodson ME, Madden BP, Steven MH, Tsang VT, Yacoub MH (1991) Non-invasive mechanical ventilation for cystic fibrosis patients - a potential bridge to transplantation. Eur Respir J 4:524-527

10. Benhamou D, Girault C, Faure C, Portier F, Muir JF (1992) Nasal mask ventilation in acute respiratory failure. Experience in elderly patients. Chest 102:912-917

11. Wysocki M, Tric L, Wolff MA, Gertner J, Millet H, Herman B (1993) Noninvasive pressure support ventilation in patients with acute respiratory failure. Chest 103:907-913

12. Pennock BE, Crawshaw L, Kaplan PD (1994) Noninvasive nasal mask ventilation for acute respiratory failure. Chest 105:441-444

13. Meduri GU, Fox RC, Abou-Shala N, Leeper KV, Wunderink RG (1994) Noninvasive mechanical ventilation via face mask in patients with acute respiratory failure who refused endotracheal intubation. Crit Care Med 22:1584-1590

14. Wysocki M, Tric L, Wolff MA, Millet H, Herman B (1995) Noninvasive pressure support ventilation in patients wtih acute respiratory failure. A randomized comparison with conventional therapy. Chest 107:761-768

15. Antonelli M, Conti G, Rocco M, et al (1998) A comparison of noninvasive positive-pressure ventilation and conventional mechanical ventilation in patients with acute respiratory failure. N Engl J Med 339:429-435

16. Guerin C, Girard R, Chemorin C, De Varax R, Fournier G (1997) Facial mask noninvasive mechanical ventilation reduces the incidence of nosocomial pneumonia. A prospective epidemiological survey from a single ICU. Intensive Care Med 23:1024-1032

17. Ambrosino N, Rubini F, Callegari G, Nava S, Fracchia C, Rampulla C (1994) Non invasive mechanical ventilation in the treatment of acute respiratory failure due to infectious complication of lung transplantation. Monaldi Arch Chest Dis 49:311-314

18. Kilger E, Briegel J, Haller M (1995) Non invasive ventilation after lung transplantation. Med Klin 90:26-28

19. Rubini F, Nava S, Callegari G, Fracchia C, Ambrosino N (1994) Nasal pressure ventilation (NPSV) in a case of pneumocystis carinii pneimonia in single lung transplantation. Minerva Anestesiol 60:139-142

20. Antonelli M, Conti G, Bufi M, et al (2000) Noninvasive ventilation for treatment of acute respiratory failure in patients undergoing solid organ transplantation. JAMA 283:235-241

21. Rocco M, Conti G, Antonelli M, Bufi M, Costa MG (2001) Noninvasive pressure support ventilation in patients with acute respiratory failure after bilateral lung transplantation. Intensive Care Med; 27:1622-1626

22. Gachot B, Clair K, Wolff M, Reigner B, Vachon F (1992) Contonuous positive airway pressure by face-mask or mechanical ventilation in patients with HIV infection and Pneumocystis carinii pneumonie. Intensive Care Med 18:155-159

23 Lloyd -Thomas AR, Dhaliwal HS, Lister TA, Hindus CJ (1986) Intensive therapy for life-threatening medical complications of hematologic malignancy. Intensive Care Med 12:317-324

24. Denardo SJ, Oye RK, Bellamy PE (1989) Efficacy of intensive care for bone marrow transplant patients with respiratory failure. Crit Care Med 17:4-6

25. Crowford W, Schwartz DA, Petersen FB, Clark JG (1988) Mechanical ventilation after bone marrow transplantation. Risk factors and clinical outcome. Am J Respir Crit Care Med 137:682-687

26. Blot F, Guignet M, Nitenberg G, Leclercq B, Gachot B, Escudier B (1997) Prognostic factors for neutropenic patients in an intensive care unit. Respective roles of underlying malignancies and acute organ failures. Eur J Cancer 33:1031-1037

27. Ewig S, Torres A, Riquelme R (1998) Pulmonary complications in patients with haematological malignancies treated at a respiratory intensive care unit. Eur Respir J 12:116-122

28. Tognet E, Mercatello A, Polo P, et al (1994) Treatment of acute respiratory failure with non-invasive intermittent positive pressure ventilation in hematological patients. Clin Intensive Care 5:282-288
29. Conti G, Marino P, Cogliati A, et al (1998) Noninvasive ventilation for the treatment of acute respiratory failure in patients with hematologic malignancies: a pilot study. Intensive Care Med 24:1283-1288
30. Hilbert J, Grusìion D, Vargas F, Valentino R, Gbikpi-Benissan G, Cardinaud JP (2001) Noninvasive ventilation in immunosuppressed patients with pulmonary infiltrates, fever and acute respiratory failure. N Engl J Med 344:481-487
31. Meduri GU, Turner RE, Abou-Shala N, Wunderink R, Tolley E (1996) Non invasive positive pressure ventilation via face mask. First line intervention in patients with acute hypercapnic and hypoxemic respiratory failure. Chest 109:179-193
32. Rabbat A, Lelen G, Bekka F, Leroy F, Schelemmer B, Rochemaure J (1995) NIV in HIV patients with severe pneumocystis carinii pneumonia. Am J Respir Crit Care Med 151: 427 (abst)
33. Confalonieri M, Calderini E, Terraciano S, et al (2002) Noninvasive ventilation for treating acute respiratory failure in AIDS patients with PCP. Intensive Care Med 28:1233-1238
34. Varon J, Walsh GL, Fromm RE Jr (1998) Feasibility of noninvasive mechanical ventilation in the treatment of acute respiratory failure in postoperative cancer patients. J Crit Care 13:55-75

ARDS/VILI: Mechanisms

Biophysical Factors Leading to VILI

N. Vlahakis, J. C. Berrios, and R. D. Hubmayr

Introduction

In the past decade, the ventilatory management of patients with injured lungs has undergone a major paradigm shift. Whereas the old paradigm considered the sole goal of mechanical ventilation to be the correction of gas exchange failure, the new paradigm seeks to provide 'physical therapy' to an injured lung. This new paradigm embraces the hypothesis that both rate and amplitude of lung deformation affect numerous lung cell metabolic functions and consequently modulate transcellular as well as intercellular fluid transport, mechanisms of inflammation, host defense, and wound repair. These insights have profoundly altered the ventilator management of patients with injured lungs [1]. Although it is often difficult to assess the contribution of mechanical lung injury at the bedside relative to other disease mechanisms, a wealth of experimental and clinical data indicates that ventilator associated lung injury indeed exists [2, 3] and that it contributes to the mortality of patients [1].

Deformation of the Lung during Breathing

Micro-mechanics of the Normal Lung

It is remarkable that in 2003 there is still considerable uncertainty about the stresses and strains (a measure of deformation) of lung cells and connective tissue elements during breathing. It has been appreciated for more than 50 years that the topographical distributions of transpulmonary pressure and volume are non-uniform and the cause of this non-uniformity is generally understood (reviewed recently in [4]). Accordingly, the lungs and the boundary structures to which they must conform (ribcage, diaphragm abdomen, heart and mediastinum) are considered gravitationally deformed elastic solids. The shape matching of lung and boundary structures imposes a non-uniform strain field. Contrary to initial hypotheses the effects of gravity on the lungs themselves is only a minor determinant of non-uniform strain. The gravitational deformations of heart and diaphragm/abdomen turn out to be much more important determinants of regional volume and ventilation. However, with increasing precision of methods for measuring regional lung function it has become clear that there is considerable small scale heterogeneity in lung parenchymal strain that cannot be explained by a gravitational mechanism [5].

Measurements of regional lung expansion in dogs suggested that the linear dimensions of the lung increase by as much as 40% during an inspiratory capacity maneuver [6]. However, considering lung architecture this is a gross overestimate of lung cell and tissue strain. The lung parenchyma is a cell and connective tissue network that is distorted by surface tension. Embedded in this network are airways and blood vessels, which resist deformation to a greater extent than the surrounding parenchyma. This difference in mechanical properties is an important source of interdependence [7]. Models of lung micro-mechanics that are based on morphometric analyses of perfusion fixed tissue specimens consider the helical network of elastic and collagen fibers that form the alveolar ducts as the primary tissue stress bearing elements [8, 9]. The alveolar walls are largely supported by surface tension and simply unfold as lung volume increases [10]. This explains why macroscopic strains computed from lung regions >1 cm^3 may grossly overestimate the stretch experienced by lung cells during breathing. Aware of this limitation, Tschumperlin and Margulies traced the lengths of alveolar basement membranes in electron microscopic images of alveolar walls and estimated that their area changed by no more than 35% during an inspiratory capacity maneuver [11]. This corresponds to a linear strain of ~15%. These investigators also suggested that most of the stretch experienced by alveolar lining cells occurs at high lung volumes, i.e., after the alveolar wall has fully unfolded. It should be noted that the need for tissue fixation and the associated changes in hydration and surface tension leave lingering questions about the validity of all current alveolar micro-strain estimates. Alternative imaging approaches that enable morphometric measurements on live specimens ought to eliminate remaining uncertainties in this field.

Micro-mechanics of the Injured Lung

Data on the micro-mechanics of injured lungs are few and their interpretation is controversial [12, 13]. The long held view that the heavy injured lung collapses under its own weight has been challenged [4, 14]. The challenge rests on the assertion that fluid accumulates in small airways and distal airspaces which prevents rather promotes the collapse of dependent lung tissue. The effects on gas exchange, i.e., shunt and low ventilation/perfusion ratio (V/Q), are similar, regardless of whether one views the dependent lung as atelectatic (the alveoli are airless and collapsed) or expanded by edema. However, the stresses to which airway and alveolar lining cells are exposed during breathing could be quite different.

Two attributes of the injured lungs dominate injury mechanisms: 1) the number of alveoli capable of expanding during inspiration is decreased; 2) the distribution of liquid and surface tension in distal airspaces and hence the local impedances to lung expansion are heterogeneous. The first attribute was identified by Gattinoni's group and was characterized as "baby lung" [15]. It explains the increased risk of lung injury from regional overexpansion. The second attribute, namely heterogeneity in regional impedances to lung expansion, has several consequences. One is the shear stress between neighboring, interdependent units that operate at different volumes. The other consequence is injury to small airways and alveolar ducts caused by their repeated opening and collapse, by energy dissipation during liquid bridge fracture or resulting from the stress that is imposed on lining cells by the movement of air-liquid interfaces with respiration [16]. The relative contributions of these interrelated injury mechanisms in different syndromes and disease models is simply not known. Inferences from animal experiments with short term physiologic endpoints are at best hypothesis generating, but have yet to demonstrate the circumstance under which any one of these mechanisms prevails. Modeling approaches to bubble and liquid flow in tubes while constrained by simplifying assumptions, (e.g., rigid tube of uniform diameter, smooth surface) are beginning to shed some light on more quantitative aspects of this problem [17, 18].

Cellular Pathology of Ventilator Injured Lungs

Ventilator-induced lung injury (VILI) is characterized by a mechanical failure of the blood-gas barrier (Fig.1). As shown with electron microscopy more than 20 years ago, widespread endothelial and epithelial cell injury is one of the hallmarks of the entity and accounts at least in part for the increased microvascular permeability of ventilator-injured lungs [19–21]. Plasmamembrane blebs and cytoskeletal disruptions occur in association with intercellular and intracellular gaps exposing basement membrane. Based on studies on frog mesentery vessels Neal and Michel have argued that intra and intercellular gap formation is an adaptive cellular stress response rather than the consequence of a basement membrane break [22]. Whereas electron microscopy defines cellular ultrastructure in intricate detail, the technique is limited by finite sampling and is therefore not well suited for quantifying injury on the scale of whole lungs. Light microscopy, on the other hand, does not have sufficient spatial resolution to define lesions in individual cells. Therefore,

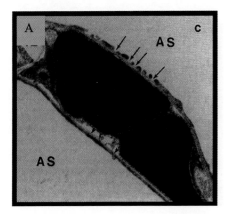 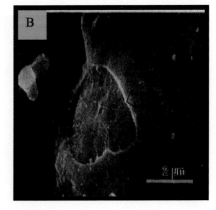

Fig. 1. Transmission (**A**) and scanning (**B**) electron microscopy images of alveolar pneumocytes that were injured by large volume ventilation (**A**) or capillary hypertension (**B**). AS: alveolar space. From [2, 19] with permission.

much VILI research has focused on the consequences of cellular injury such as edema, inflammation, and tissue remodeling rather than on the determinants of the cellular stress failure itself.

Gajic et al. have recently provided direct evidence that the VILI lesion is associated with a transient loss of endothelial and/or epithelial plasma membrane integrity [23]. Mechanically ventilated lungs were perfused with the membrane impermeable label propidium iodide (PI, Molecular Probe, Eugene, Oregon) and subpleural airspaces subsequently imaged with confocal microscopy. When PI enters a cell through a membrane defect it intercalates with DNA and emits a red fluorescence upon excitation with blue light. The number of cells with red fluorescence, therefore, identifies all subpleural cells that have suffered a transient or a permanent PM wound during the experiment.

Figure 2 shows the light microscopic characteristics of normal and injured lungs and the corresponding confocal images of sub-pleural lung regions. The image on

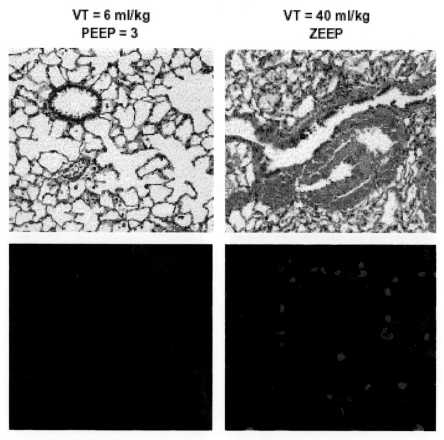

Fig. 2. Light microscopic (upper panel) and confocal images (lower panel) of a normal (left) and a ventilator injured lung (right). In the confocal images, blue fluorescence appears as dark gray, white red fluorescence appears as light gray. Adapted from [23] with permission

the left is from a lung which had been mechanically ventilated for 30 minutes at non-injurious settings (tidal volume, V_T = 6 ml/kg, positive end-expiratory pressure, PEEP = 3 cm H_2O). The blue autofluorescence outlines parenchyma and air spaces. No PI labeling (red fluorescence) is detected. In contrast, the image on the right outlines subpleural regions of a lung that had been mechanically ventilated for 30 minutes with high V_T (40 cc/kg), and zero end-expiratory pressure (ZEEP). There are a large number of red nuclei indicating that at some point during the experiment the PM of every one of these cells had become permeable, i.e., had been wounded. The fact that red fluorescence appears clustered near corners is suggestive of injury to endothelial cells in alveolar corner vessels or interstitial capillaries and/or of injury to type II pneumocytes.

Figure 3 shows a comparison of the PI based injury index between lungs that were labeled *during* injurious mechanical ventilation (left) and lungs that were subjected to the same injurious stress, but only labeled 2 minutes *after* its removal (right). Significantly fewer PI positive cells are identified when labeling is deferred to the post injury state. In the former instance all cells that acquire a membrane defect during injurious ventilation are labeled irrespective of their subsequent fate. In the latter instance only necrotic cells which have failed to reseal their membrane defects will be PI labeled. A comparison of the two cell populations suggests that normally over 60% of ventilator injured cells survive the insult. These observations are in keeping with data suggesting that removal of mechanical stress causes a rapid restoration of vascular barrier function [24–26].

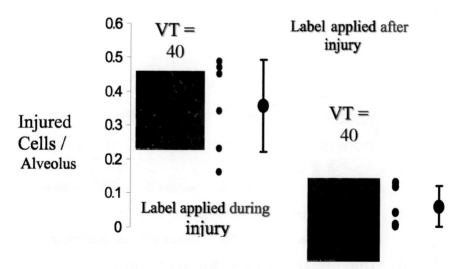

Fig. 3. Plasma membrane repair after removal of injurious stress. Adapted from [23] with permission

Effects of Deforming Stress on Cellular Structure and Function

Cell-matrix Interactions

Cells interact with their surroundings through adhesion receptors such as integrins which provide dynamic bidirectional links between the cytoskeleton and the extracellular matrix. [27, 28]. The extracellular matrix provides the scaffold in which cells live and to which they must conform. In the lung, an increase in basement membrane surface area that accompanies a large tidal breath imposes a shape change on adherent alveolar epithelial and microvascular endothelial cells. This shape change mandates that cell surface to volume ratio increase and hence requires a reorganization of the cell's stress bearing elements. If rate and amplitude of the deformation exceed the cell's capacity to remodel, structural failure occurs [29]. There is overwhelming experimental evidence that this reorganization involves active, energy dependent processes [30, 31], which challenges the validity of classic solid mechanics-based modeling approaches immeasurably.

Control of Plasma Membrane Tension

The plasma membrane carries a steady state tensile stress that is at least one order of magnitude lower than that born by fibrous actin. [32–34] Estimates of the tension at which the plasma membrane fractures range between 3 and 12 mN/m and vary with the composition and organization of the lipid bilayer [32, 33, 35]. Figure 4

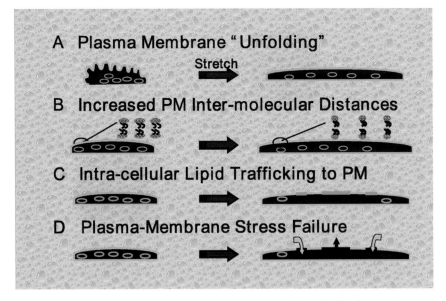

Fig. 4. The plasma membrane (PM) during cell stretch. Adapted from [31] with permission

summarizes the possible means by which a cell can accommodate increases in surface to volume ratio during an externally imposed shape change: a) unfolding of excess plasma membrane; b) elastic extension of the lipid bilayer c) a net-trafficking of lipid from intracellular membrane or lipid stores to the plasma membrane d) plasma membrane stress failure followed by secondary membrane repair or cell death. While the four mechanisms are not mutually exclusive, elastic expansion of the plasma membrane is limited because the lipid bilayer experiences lytic tensions at strains between 1 and 3% [35].

The plasma membrane of most cells has undulations and surface projections that offer relatively little resistance to unfolding when the membrane is laterally stressed. The complex cell surface topology reflects adhesive interactions between lipids and subcortical proteins and the intricate regulation of local actin assembly by highly charged membrane phospholipids [33, 36, 37]. Indeed, the only time the plasma membrane appears to be smooth is when it is blebbed, i.e., when the membrane is stressed by cytoplasmic liquid pressure and has lost contact with the subcortical cytoskeleton. The relative contributions of membrane unfolding and active transport to the so-called 'recruitable plasma membrane reservoir' have been studied in different cell models using patch clamp approaches [38], fluorescent lipid analoges [29, 31] and optical tweezers [39]. The use of optical (laser) tweezers to measure the elastic recoil of plasma membrane lipid tethers was pioneered by Sheetz and colleagues [39] and has laid the foundation for current views on the biophysical determinants of endocytosis and plasma membrane remodeling [33]. Accordingly, the in plane membrane tension and the adhesion energy between the plasma membrane and the subcortical cytoskeleton are tightly regulated. A key second messenger in the regulation of adhesion energy is the plasma membrane phosphatidylinositol 4,5-bisphosphate (PIP2), which binds tightly to actin regulatory proteins such as profilin, gelsolin and cofilin and mediates actin crosslinking and focal adhesion contact assembly [36]. To the extent to which tether force is a readout of adhesion energy interventions that decrease plasma membrane PIP2 such as phospholipase Cδ (PLCδ) activation have been shown to lower tether force and promote endocytosis [37]. It is intriguing to consider that deforming stress, which in some systems has been shown to activate phospholipase dependent signaling pathways [40], could also promote endocytosis by this mechanism.

Deformation Induced Lipid Trafficking

Vlahakis et al. have shown that stretching of alveolar epithelial cells in culture triggers a vigorous exocytic lipid trafficking response [31]. This trafficking response is vesicular in nature, varies with strain rate and amplitude, is temperature and energy dependent is associated with an increase in cell surface area and cell volume and can be pharmacologically manipulated [31, 41]. Based on the exclusion of membrane impermeant labels such as PI and fluorescine labeled dextran (FDx), Vlahakis concluded that deformation-induced lipid trafficking (DILT) is distinct from membrane trafficking that effects plasma membrane wound resealing. Inhibition of DILT increases the risk of plasma membrane stress failure and lowers the likelihood of subsequent plasma membrane repair [29]. DILT requires an intact cytoskeleton, specifically intact microfilaments and microtubules, is sensitive to plasma membrane cholesterol and is essential for preventing plasma membrane stress failure. These observations suggest that DILT is integral to the maintenance of plasma membrane tension at sublytic levels. They also suggest a central role for DILT in the pathogenesis of VILI and make DILT an attractive pharmaco-protective treatment target.

In preliminary experiments, Berrios et al. showed that cell stretch promotes trafficking of glycosphingolipids (GSL) not only *to* but also *from* the plasma membrane. The plasma membrane of eukaryotic cells is enriched in cholesterol and in addition to phosphatidylcholine (PC) contains high levels of sphingomyelin (SM) and GSL. GSLs are a class of sphingolipids (SL) which play important roles in a wide variety of cell functions including mechano-transduction [42]. Their concentration in cell membranes is tightly regulated in close association with cholesterol with which they form membrane micro-domains [43]. These microdomains (rafts) are signaling platforms which by virtue of their biophysical properties attract specific receptors and membrane proteins. In the plasma membrane rafts appear to have a preferential association with 50–100 nm pits called caveolae as defined by the marker protein, caveolin [44]. These structures play an important role in non-clathrin dependent endocytosis [45].

Figure 5 shows a representative example of stretch induced endocytosis of the fluorescent GSL analog BODIPY SM in A549 cells. In contrast to amino-phospholipids, the GSLs such as SM are essentially restricted to the outer layer of the plasma membrane. The asymmetry in lipid composition is maintained by a family of membrane bound ATPases (so-called flippases), which facilitate the translocation of amino-phospholipids to the inner leaflet [46]. To date, no flippase mediating the translocation of GSL across the plasma membrane has been identified. Therefore, barring plasma membrane wounding or a yet to be described stretch effect on membrane thermodynamics, GSLs can only be internalized by vesicular transport (endocytosis), a process that is shut down at 4°C.

Figure 5 illustrates several important preliminary findings:
(1) The initial plasma membrane label distribution (recorded at 10°C) appears uniform (left hand insert);
(2) following back exchange with defatted bovine serum albumin (BSA, (removes label from the outer plasma membrane layer) and rewarming to 37°C for 1 minute one observes fluorescence in peripherally located punctate structures;
(3) a single 1 minute stretch greatly enhances the uptake of SM into punctate structures that are now located throughout the cell;
(4) SM uptake from the plasma membrane is blocked at 4°C.

These observations are consistent with the hypothesis that deforming stresses promote plasma membrane remodeling not only via secretory but also endocytic pathways.

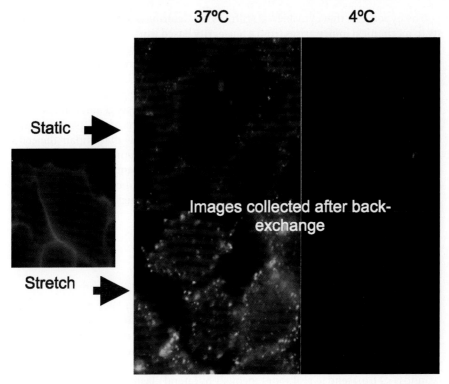

Fig. 5. Confocal images of BODIPY-SM labeled A549 cells (Berrios et al., unpublished observations)

Cytoskeletal Mechanics and the Probability of Deformation-Related Cell Wounding

Since it is known from work by Tschumperlin and Margulies [47], that primary rat type II alveolar pneumocytes (ATII) lose their susceptibility to deformation injury with time in liquid culture, Berrios et al. measured the apparent stiffness of primary rat ATIIs in various stages of differentiation using magnetic twisting cytometry (MTC) [30]. Indeed, ATIIs become more resistant to a shape change when they differentiate towards the ATI phenotype. However, Berrios's observations are insufficient to establish a cause and effect relationship between injury susceptibility and cell mechanical properties. MTC derived stiffness measurements are as much a readout of local cell adhesive properties as they are of global cell elastic moduli [48]. Berrios examined the number of RGD binding sites (an important integrin/matrix recognition sequence) on ATIIs and found them to increase greatly with time in culture. Therefore, it remains unclear if the increase in apparent cell stiffness is due to enhanced focal adhesion formation or a global change in cytoskeletal stiffness.

The hypothesis that cytoskeletal stiffness is a determinant of a cell's susceptibility to mechanical injury arises from a tensegrity based working model of cytoskeletal mechanics [28]. A tensegrity structure (such as a geodesic dome) is composed of a network of interconnected elements that are either compression or tension bearing. Based on this analogy, one may view the interconnected network of cytoskeletal biopolymers as loading the lipid envelope (the plasma membrane) of the cell. However, the usefulness of tensegrity as a hypothesis generating model is limited, because available data emphasize the importance of cell plasticity and structural remodeling over static mechanics. Interventions that impair the cell's ability to remodel make cells more susceptible to deformation injury, irrespective of their effects on apparent cell stiffness [29, 41]. In the absence of direct measurements of plasma membrane tension in externally deformed cells one should consider a deterministic relationship between cytoskelal stiffness and plasma membrane stress to be quite unlikely.

Mechanisms of Plasma Membrane Wound Repair

The cellular response to wounding has been investigated in many different systems [49]. Cardiologists and muscle physiologists, for example, have appreciated for some time that myocytes are subject to transient stress failure, that stress failure is an important stimulus for muscle remodeling, and that it need not be associated with significant loss of function [50]. The molecular mechanisms that drive plasma membrane resealing vary with cell type and lesion size. Small plasma membrane wounds (<1 μm) tend to seal spontaneously by lateral plasma membrane lipid flow. This is best demonstrated in red blood cells [51]. However most plasma membrane lesions, particularly if they are large, repair only if intracellular lipids are shuttled to the plasma membrane by an active, energy dependent and Ca^{++} regulated process [52]. The insertion of lipids to the plasma membrane causes a fall in plasma membrane tension, which in turn promotes 'self sealing' by lateral plasma membrane lipid flow [33, 53]. If the lesion is very large, extracellular Ca^{++} enters the cell and induces lipid vesicles to fuse and form a membrane patch [54]. Patch formation and the subsequent sealing of the surface break by site directed exocytosis requires the coordinated actions of vesicle fusion and docking proteins such as synaptotagmin, synaptobrevin, SNAP-25, and involves molecular motors of the kinesin family. In most cells the organelles that coalesce to form patches include lysosomes [55]. This has led to speculations that the process of patch resealing is a remnant of a primitive defense against invading microbes.

Effects of Mechanical Stress on Gene Expression

There are an exponentially increasing number of reports detailing the effects of deforming stress on gene expression in lung cells (recently reviewed in [3, 56]). It is known that deforming stress promotes the translocation of the nuclear transcription factor, nuclear factor-kappa B (NF-κB) and enhances inflammatory signaling by both macrophages and alveolar epithelial cells even in the absence of gross cell injury [57, 58]. Grembowicz et al. have shown that plasma membrane injury followed by membrane repair also leads to NF-κB translocation and upregulation of early stress-response genes [59]. As such, injured cells, despite having avoided the fate of necrosis, could serve as an important source of persistent pro-inflammatory and/or pro-fibrotic signals. This hypothesis raises several important questions: Is the pro-inflammatory signaling that accompanies most forms of VILI [60] the result of mechanical cell injury or the consequence of a regulated receptor mediated mechano-transduction event? Does plasma membrane wound resealing, which guarantees cell survival, generate more or less inflammation and tissue remodeling than cell necrosis, which invariably follows failure to reseal the plasma membrane wound? Considering that the probability of plasma membrane wound resealing can be experimentally manipulated [29] the second question is central to a cell resealing focused investigation of pharmacoprotection from VILI.

Conclusion

The clinical and experimental literature has unequivocally established that mechanical ventilation with large V_T is injurious to the lung. However, uncertainty about the micro-mechanics of injured lungs and the numerous degrees of freedom in ventilator settings leave many questions about the biophysical determinants of VILI unanswered. In this chapter, we have focused on the cell as opposed to the lung matrix as the primary injury target. We have emphasized the importance of deformation induced cell and plasma membrane remodeling and have reviewed the mechanisms cells use to maintain sublytic plasma membrane tensions in the face of deforming stresses. We have cited evidence that failure of remodeling, e.g., because of impaired DILT, predisposes the plasma membrane to mechanical stress failure. The demonstration of cell wounding and repair in intact ventilator injured lungs underscores the relevance of said mechanisms.

Acknowledgement: Supported by grants from the National Institutes of Health HL-63178, Glaxo-Smith-Kline and the Brewer Foundation.

References

1. The Acute Respiratory Distress Syndrome Network (2000) Ventilation with lower tidal volumes as compared with traditional tidal volumes for acute lung injury and the acute respiratory distress syndrome. N Engl J Med 342:1301–1308
2. Dreyfuss D, Saumon G (1998) Ventilator-induced lung injury: lessons from experimental studies. Am J Respir Crit Care Med 157:294–323
3. Uhlig S (2002) Mechanotransduction in the lung: Ventilation-induced lung injury and mechanotransduction: stretching it too far? Am J Physiol 282:L892–L896
4. Hubmayr RD (2002) Perspective on lung injury and recruitment: A skeptical look at the opening and collapse story. Am J Respir Crit Care Med 165:1647–1653
5. Chang H, Lai-Fook SJ, Domino KB, et al (2002) Spatial distribution of ventilation and perfusion in anesthetized dogs in lateral postures. J of Appl Physiol 92:745–762

6. Rodarte JF, Hubmayr RD, Stamenovic D, Walters BJ (1985) Regional lung strain in dogs during deflation from total lung capacity. J Appl Physiol 58:164–172
7. Lai-Fook SJ, Kallok MJ (1982) Bronchial-arterial interdependence in isolated dog lung. J Appl Physiol 52:1000–1007
8. Bachofen H, Schurch S, Urbinelli M, Weibel ER (1987) Relations among alveolar surface tension, surface area, volume, and recoil pressure. J Appl Physiol 62:1878–1887
9. Wilson TA, Bachofen H (1982) A model for mechanical structure of the alveolar duct. J Appl Physiol 52:1064–1070
10. Oldmixon EH, Hoppin FG Jr (1991) Alveolar septal folding and lung inflation history. J Appl Phys 71:2369–2379
11. Tschumperlin DJ, Margulies SS (1999) Alveolar epithelial surface area-volume relationship in isolated rat lungs. J Appl Physiol 86:2026–2033
12. McCann UG 2nd, Schiller HJ, Carney DE, Gatto LA, Steinberg JM, Nieman GF (2001) Visual validation of the mechanical stabilizing effects of positive end-expiratory pressure at the alveolar level. J Surg Res 99:335–442
13. Schiller HJ, McCann UG 2nd, Carney DE, Gatto LA, Steinberg JM, Nieman GF (2001) Altered alveolar mechanics in the acutely injured lung. Crit Care Med 29:1049–1055
14. Martynowicz MA, Minor TA, Walters BJ, Hubmayr RD (1999) Regional expansion of oleic acid-injured lungs. Am J Respir Crit Care Med 160:250–258
15. Gattinoni L, Pesenti A, Avalli L, Rossi F, Bombino M (1987) Pressure-volume curve of total respiratory system in acute respiratory failure: Computed tomographic scan study. Am Rev Respir Dis 136:730–736
16. Marini JJ (2001) Ventilator-induced airway dysfunction? Am J Respir Crit Care Med 163:806–807
17. Matthay MA, Bhattacharya S, Gaver D, et al (2002) Ventilator-induced lung injury: In vivo and in vitro mechanisms. Am J Physiol 283:L678–L682
18. Gaver DP III, Kute SM (1998) A theoretical model study of the influence of fluid stresses on a cell adhering to a microchannel wall. Biophys J 75:721–733
19. Costello ML, Mathieu-Costello O, West JB (1992) Stress failure of alveolar epithelial cells studied by scanning electron microscopy. Am Rev Respir Dis 145:1446–1455
20. Fu Z, Costello ML, Tsukimoto K, et al (1992) High lung volumes increases stress failure in pulmonary capillaries. J Appl Physiol 73:123–133
21. John E, McDevitt M, Wilborn W, Cassady G (1982) Ultrastructure of the lung after ventilation. Br J Exp Pathol 63:401–407
22. Savla U, Neal CR, Michel CC (2002) Openings in frog microvascular endothelium at different rates of increase in pressure and at different temperatures. J Physiol (Lond) 539:285–293
23. Gajic O, Lee J, Doerr CH, Berrios JC, Myers JL, Hubmayr RD (2003) Ventilator-induced cell wounding and repair in the intact lung. Am J Respir Crit Care Med 167:1057–1063
24. Neal CR, Michel CC (1996) Openings in frog microvascular endothelium induced by high intravascular pressures. J Appl Physiol 492:39–52
25. Dreyfuss D, Soler P, Saumon G (1992) Spontaneous resolution of pulmonary edema caused by short periods of cyclic overinflation J Appl Physiol 72:2081–2089
26. Elliott AR, Fu Z, Tsukimoto K, Prediletoo R, Mathieu-Costello O, West JB (1992) Short-term reversibility of ultrastructural changes in pulmonary capillaries caused by stress failure. J Appl Physiol 73:1150–1158
27. Geiger B, Bershadsky A, Pankov R, Yamada KM (2001) Transmembrane extracellular matrix-cytoskeleton crosstalk. Nat Rev Mol Cell Biol 2:793–805
28. Ingber DE (2000) Opposing views on tensegrity as a structural framework for understanding cell mechanics. J Appl Physiol 89:1663–1670
29. Vlahakis NE, Schroeder MA, Pagano RE, Hubmayr RD (2002) Role of deformation-induced lipid trafficking in the prevention of plasma membrane stress failure. Am J Respir Crit Care Med 166:1282–1289

30. Berrios JC, Schroeder MA, Hubmayr RD (2001) Mechanical properties of alveolar epithelial cells in culture. J Appl Physiol 91:65–73
31. Vlahakis NE, Schroeder MA, Pagano RE, Hubmayr RD (2001) Deformation-induced lipid trafficking in alveolar epithelial cells. Am J Physiol 280:L938–L946
32. Olbrich K, Rawicz W, Needham D, Evans E (2000) Water permeability and mechanical strength of polyunsaturated lipid bilayers. Biophys J 79:321–327
33. Sheetz MP (2001) Cell control by membrane-cytoskeleton adhesion. Nat Rev Mol Cell Biol 2:392–396
34. Wang N, Naruse K, Stamenovic D, et al (2001) Mechanical behavior in living cells consistent with the tensegrity model. Proc Natl Acad Sci USA 98:7765–7770
35. Waugh RE (1983) Effects of abnormal cytoskeletal structure on erythrocyte membrane mechanical properties. Cell Motil 3:609–622
36. Janmey PA (1995) Protein regulation by phosphatidylinositol lipids. Chem Biol 2:61–65
37. Raucher D, Stauffer T, Chen W et al (2000) Phosphatidylinositol 4,5-bisphosphate functions as a second messenger that regulates cytoskeleton-plasma membrane adhesion. Cell 100:221–228
38. Solsona C, Innocenti B, Fernandez JM (1998) Regulation of exocytotic fusion by cell inflation. Biophys J 74:1061–1073
39. Dai J, Sheetz MP (1999) Membrane tether formation from blebbing cells. Biophys J 77:3363–3370
40. Ruwhof C, van Wamel JET, Noordzij LAW, Aydin S. Harper JCR, van der Laarse A (2001) Mechanical stress stimulates phospholipase C activity and intracellular calcium ion levels in neonatal rat cardiomyocytes. Cell Calcium 29:73–83
41. Stroetz RW, Vlahakis NE, Walters BJ, et al (2001) Validation of a new live cell strain system: characterization of plasma membrane stress failure. J Appl Physiol 90:2361–2370
42. Park H, Go YM, Darji R, et al (2000) Caveolin-1 regulates sheer stress-dependent activation of extracellular signal-regulated kinase. Am J Physiol 278:H1285–H1293
43. Simons K, Toomre D (2000) Lipid rafts and signal transduction. Nat Rev Mol Cell Biol 1:31–39
44. Razani B, Woodman SE, Lisanti MP (2002) Caveolae: From cell biology to animal physiology. Pharmacol Rev 54:431–467
45. Puri V, Watanabe R, Singh RD, et al (2001) Clathrin-dependent and -independent internalization of plasma membrane sphingolipids initiates two Golgi targeting pathways. J Cell Biol 154:535–547
46. Devaux PF (1991) Static and dynamic lipid asymmetry in cell membranes. Biochemistry 30:1163–1173
47. Tschumperlin DJ, Margulies SS (1998) Equibiaxial deformation-induced injury of alveolar epithelial cells in vitro. Am J Physiol 275:L1173–1183
48. Hubmayr RD (2000) Biology lessons from oscillatory cell mechanics. J Appl Physiol 89:1617–1618
49. McNeil PL, Terasaki M (2001) Coping with the inevitable: how cells repair a torn surface membrane. Nat Cell Biol 3:E124–129
50. Fischer TA, McNeil PL, Khakee R, et al (1997) Cardiac myocyte membrant wounding in the abruptly pressure-overloaded rat heart under high wall stress. Hypertension 30:1041–1046
51. Benz R, Zimmermann U (1981) The resealing process of lipid bilayers after reversible electrical breakdown. Biochim Biophys Acta 640:169–178
52. Steinhardt RA, Bi G, Alderton JM (1994) Cell membrane resealing by a vesicular mechanism similar to neurotransmitter release. Science 263:390–393
53. Togo T, Krasieva TB, Steinhardt RA (2000) A decrease in membrane tension precedes successful cell-membrane repair. Mol Biol Cell 11:4339–4346
54. McNeil PL, Vogel SS, Miyake K, Terasaki M (2000) Patching plasma membrane disruptions with cytoplasmic membrane. J Cell Sci 113:1891–1902
55. Reddy A, Caler EV, Andrews NW (2001) Plasma membrane repair is mediated by Ca(2+)-regulated exocytosis of lysosomes. Cell 106:157–169

56. Liu, M., Tanswell AK, Post M (1999) Mechanical force-induced signal transduction in lung cells. Am J Physiol 277:L667–L683
57. Pugin J, Dunn I, Jolliet P, et al (1998) Activation of human macrophages by mechanical ventilation in vitro. Am J Physiol 275:L1040–L1050
58. Vlahakis NE, Schroeder MA, Limper AH, Hubmayr RD (1999) Stretch induces cytokine release by alveolar epithelial cells in vitro. Am J Physiol 277:L167–L173
59. Grembowicz KP, Sprague D, McNeil PL (1999) Temporary disruption of the plasma membrane is required for c-fos expression in response to mechanical stress. Mol Biol Cell 10:1247–1257
60. Tremblay L, Valenza F, Ribeiro SP, et al (1997) Injurious ventilatory strategies increase cytokines and c-fos m-RNA expression in an isolated rat lung model. J Clin Invest 99:944–952

Vascular Contribution to VILI

J. J. Marini, J. R. Hotchkiss, and A. F. Broccard

Introduction

Although ventilator-induced lung injury (VILI) is undoubtedly a complex process that is influenced by many factors, the great majority of investigative attention has been directed to airspace mechanics, as exemplified by tidal volume (V_T), plateau pressure, and positive end-expiratory pressure (PEEP). Yet, because the fragile alveolus serves as the interface between gas and blood, and because the intra-lumenal pressures applied to the airway epithelium and vascular endothelium are remarkably similar, the potential for *vascular* pressures and flows to impact the development or evolution of VILI also deserves close consideration. This chapter addresses the experimental evidence linking alveolar and vascular events in the generation of barrier breakdown.

Inflation and Pulmonary Vascular Pressure

The vascular pathway from pulmonary artery to left atrium can be considered as a series of three functional segments: arterial, 'intermediate' (which includes alveolar capillaries and contiguous microvessels), and venous [1]. Under normal condi-tions, arterial and venous segments – which are entirely extra-alveolar – contribute most to overall pulmonary vascular resistance. The compliant intermediate seg-ment however, is influenced primarily by alveolar pressures and as a consequence, influences the change in overall vascular resistance that occurs during ventilation.

The behavior of alveolar and extra-alveolar vessels during lung expansion is fundamentally different. The structural forces of interdependence cause interstitial pressures to fall during inflation, even during positive pressure ventilation [2]. This reduction of interstitial pressure increases the transmural pressure of the vessels in the immediate environment, tending to dilate them. Something quite different, however, happens at the alveolar level. During inflation of a normal, fully aerated ('open') lung, the majority of capillaries embedded within the alveolar wall are compressed by the expansion of adjoining alveoli, even as extra-alveolar vessels dilate and elongate (Fig. 1).

At all lung volumes above functional residual capacity (FRC), the effects of alveolar capillary compression and extra-alveolar vessel elongation outweigh the tendency for extra-alveolar vessels to dilate, so that pulmonary vascular resistance

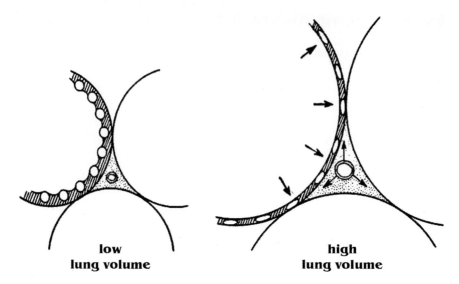

Fig. 1. Influence of lung expansion on alveolar and extra-alveolar vasculature. Inflation compresses wall-embedded capillaries but dilates extra-alveolar microvessels.

rises monotonically as a function of lung volume [3]. The so-called 'corner' vessels, which are located at the junctions of three or more alveolar septae, are simultaneously influenced by competing stresses arising from alveolar and interstitial pressures and do not behave as the wall-embedded capillaries do. Indeed, they may serve as a conduit for some blood to flow through the intermediate segment, even when alveolar pressure exceeds pulmonary arterial pressure [4]. With reference to the vascular contribution to VILI, it is important to consider that even for the normal lung, inflation imposes competing vascular stresses on different classes of microvessels. As discussed later, these competing forces are amplified by the heterogeneity of acute lung injury (ALI).

Interactions Between Airway and Pulmonary Vascular Pressures

The normal lung exhibits up to three perfusion zones, depending on the relationship between alveolar pressure and pulmonary arterial venous pressure. According to the familiar conceptual model popularized by West [5], gas pressures within aerated alveoli are everywhere equivalent under static conditions, whereas vascular pressures are influenced by gravity. Zone III conditions, under which both arterial and venous macrovascular pressures exceed alveolar pressure, allow flow to be governed by vascular pressure gradients and resistances. These conditions are most likely to be observed in dependent regions. When alveolar pressure exceeds both arterial and venous pressures, little blood flow occurs (except through corner vessels). Zone II exists where alveolar pressure exceeds pulmonary venous (but not arterial pressure), allowing flow to occur as regulated by the pressure gradient between arterial and alveolar pressures. These latter zones tend to develop in less dependent areas, where hydrostatic pressures are lower.

Unfortunately, the application of these useful concepts to the problem of the acutely injured lung is not straightforward. Indeed, their validity for this circumstance – in which collapsed, edematous, inflamed and even fibrotic lung units may coexist in the same micro-environment – can rightfully be questioned. In the setting of ALI, both alveolar and pulmonary arterial pressures are considerably greater than under normal conditions. Moreover, a variety of perfusion states is likely to exist, even along the same transverse plane. Filling of the small airways, alveolar, and interstitial spaces with cells and fluid alters the normal relationships among the pressures and flows of gases and blood. Independent of any variations of local pathology, increased lung tissue density and accentuated pleural pressure gradients tend to collapse dependent lung units, developing shunt and/or extending Zone II conditions to more caudal levels as the interstitial pressures surrounding the microvasculature rise.

Under the high permeability conditions of the first stage of ALI, even minor increases in pulmonary microvascular pressure will increase edema formation dramatically. Moreover, unlike healthy tissue whose blood-gas barrier is intact, there is no clear pressure threshold for edema formation [6]. The physiologic consequences of pulmonary edema are well known: alveolar edema compromises gas exchange, and edematous airways impede airflow and secretion clearance. From the standpoint of VILI, however, alveolar flooding may produce competing effects. A well known – if simplistic – model of interdependence proposed by Mead (see below) suggests that collapsed alveoli are subjected to shearing forces that are proportional to the disparity in alveolar dimensions between the collapsed alveolus and its distended neighbors [7]. Completely fluid-filled (flooded) alveoli, therefore, theoretically are subjected to lower shearing stresses than atelectatic units, as the gas-liquid interface is eliminated and alveolar dimensions increase. On the other hand, elimination of surface tension would cause capillaries that are fully embedded in the alveolar walls to bulge further into the interior, encouraging their rupture [8], and the increased weight of the edematous lung may encourage small airway compression and accentuate the tendency for tidal opening and closure to occur. Which of these competing effects predominates cannot be said with certainty. Thus, while the influence of pre-formed edema on lung mechanics and gas exchange is reasonably well described, the importance of the microvasculature to the generation of VILI is less understood. The remainder of this brief review will focus on what is currently known regarding the interactions between airway pressures and vascular pressures in the generation and maintenance of VILI.

What Disrupts the Blood Gas Barrier During VILI?

Clinicians have long been aware that certain inflammatory conditions of the lung produce tissue hemorrhage in the absence of ventilatory stress. These vessel-disrupting inflammatory injuries may originate from either the alveolar side (e.g., pneumonia, abscess) or from the vascular side of the blood-gas interface. Inflammatory conditions such as Wegener's granulomatosis, Goodpasture's syndrome, and pulmonary embolism are examples from the latter category, disrupting the delicate barrier between gas and blood and allowing erythrocytes to breech their vascular confines and migrate into the interstitium and air spaces.

Although inflammation is obviously of potential importance to the breakdown of the lung's structural architecture, simply elevating transmural pulmonary vascular pressure to high levels may cause vascular rents or tears. Perhaps the clearest example in this category occurs in severe mitral stenosis, a condition in which pulmonary venous and capillary pressures can exceed 35–40 mmHg. Acute edema that forms in this setting is typically blood-tinged, and the presence of hemosiderin-laden macrophages in expectorated or lavaged samples strongly suggests that this process originates at the alveolar level from the pulmonary (rather than the bronchial circulation). Another circumstance under which elevating transmural vascular pressures may cause hemoptysis in the absence of preexisting inflammation occurs during extreme exertion, when blood flows through the lung are extremely high and excursions of alveolar pressure are unusually large. Post-exertional lung hemorrhage is a well-described occurrence in racehorses [9], and hemoptysis has been reported after heavy exertion in elite human athletes as well [10]. Finally, forceful inspiratory efforts made during upper airway obstruction may produce transvascular pressures of sufficient magnitude to cause hemorrhagic pulmonary edema [11].

Elegant experiments undertaken in the laboratories of West and colleagues have used electron microscopy to demonstrate the potential for mechanical disruption of the microvasculature – 'capillary stress fracture' – to occur when microvascular pressures are elevated to very high levels relative to their usual operating conditions [12–15]. The pressures necessary to cause capillary stress fracture vary among species, with disruption being observed in healthy small animal lungs (e.g., rabbits), at pressures as low as 40 mmHg. Larger animals, such as dogs, withstand much higher microvascular pressures without losing the structural integrity of the capillary network [14]. Experimental studies reporting capillary stress fracture in animals have largely been undertaken in static preparations in which the airway pressure was held constant and the intralumenal vascular pressures upstream and downstream of the alveolus were equivalent. Under such conditions, structural breakdown is more likely to be seen at high lung volumes relative to resting conditions [15]. Although the range of microvascular pressure applied in these studies might seem to preclude their physiological relevance, much lower vascular pressures might be required if the framework of the lung were degraded by inflammation. Moreover, there is excellent reason to believe that regional transmural vascular forces may be dramatically different when mechanically heterogeneous lungs are ventilated with adverse ventilatory patterns.

Experimental Evidence Linking Vascular Pressure to VILI

Just as with inflammation, mechanical forces that tear the delicate alveolar-capillary membrane can originate on either side of the boundary. That the alveolar epithelium can be disrupted by sufficient airway pressure is evident when barotrauma develops. Clinicians recognize this damage radiographically as air that leaks into the interstitial spaces to cause intrapulmonary gas cysts, mediastinal emphysema, pneumothorax, and systemic gas embolism [16]. It is equally clear that the vasculature can lose its integrity in advance of epithelial fragmentation. Post-mortem examination of tissues from patients with ARDS often reveals areas of interstitial and alveolar hemorrhage, findings which generally have been attributed to the underlying inflammatory process. Yet, in both small and large animal models, the application of adverse ventilatory patterns to previously healthy lungs not only causes formation of proteinaceous edema, but also stimulates neutrophil aggregation and hemorrhage [17, 18]. Studies conducted in our laboratory strongly indicate that in the supine position, hemorrhagic edema forms preferentially in dependent areas [18, 19]. This proclivity is not subtle, and has been corroborated by the work of other investigators using different injury models [20]. It is worth emphasizing that our experiments have demonstrated that purely mechanical forces originating within the alveolus inflict hemorrhagic injury in the absence of pre-existing inflammation. It is somewhat counter-intuitive that tissue disruption should occur in areas in which transmural stretching forces (as defined by plateau pressure minus pleural pressure) are least. That is to say, 'alveolar stretch' is greatest in the *non*dependent regions, which are spared both the hemorrhagic infiltrate and most signs of inflammation. Why might this occur?

The tendency for hemorrhage to occur preferentially in the most dependent regions of the lung may have several explanations. One compelling reason to expect microvascular disruption to occur there is that the mechanical stresses applied by the tidal inflation cycle are greatly amplified at the interface of opened and closed lung tissues. More than three decades ago, Mead, Takashima, and Leith described a simplified model of alveolar mechanics in which they proposed that an alveolus attempting to close in an environment in which it was surrounded by inflated tissue would experience traction forces that are amplified in nonlinear proportion to the alveolar pressures existing in the open units [7]. By their reasoning, the co-efficient linking effective pressure (Peff) to that actually applied (Papp) is the ratio between the alveolar volume that corresponds to alveolar pressure (V) and the volume of the collapsed alveolus (V_0), raised to the 2/3 power: $Peff = Papp\ (V/V_0)^{2/3}$. Their admittedly oversimplified geometrical argument suggested that at 30 cmH2O alveolar pressure, for example, the effective stress applied at the junction of closed and open tissue might approximate a value 4.5 times as great as that experienced in the free walls of the open alveolus.

Whatever its quantitative accuracy, a similar line of reasoning might apply when tissues are already atelectatic and the lung is exposed to high ventilating pressures, as in ARDS. Extrapolating from the Mead equation, the traction forces applied to junctional tissues when alveolar pressure is 30 cmH2O could approximate 140 cmH2O, or ~100 mmHg. Thus, transvascular microvascular forces during tidal ventilation could be in the range that West and colleagues suggested necessary for a stress fracture to occur in large animals (dogs)[14]. Clearly, such theoretical arguments are widely open to criticism. However, it does seem reasonable to assume that mechanical shearing forces experienced in 'junctional' tissues are likely to exceed those elsewhere in the lung. Moreover, even within fully inflated regions, the competing forces of capillary compression and extra-alveolar vessel dilation/elongation would be expected to be amplified when both lung volumes and vascular pressures are high. These stresses would tug at the microvascular conduit that links the alveolar and extra-alveolar vessels with potentially damaging force. It is not difficult, therefore, to envision vascular rupture from ventilatory pressure under the pathological conditions of ALI. Although unstudied, surfactant depletion and inflammatory weakening of the interstitial structure could amplify the impact of such forces, whereas other changes of the microenvironment (e.g., flooding by edema) could abrogate the mechanical stresses experienced in distal lung units.

Another intriguing possibility to explain disproportionate vascular disruption in dependent lung regions is that dorsally situated tissues receive a majority of the lung's total blood flow and are subjected to greater hydrostatic pressures in the supine position. These higher intralumenal vascular pressures or flows might amplify tensile forces external to the microvessels or give rise to shearing stresses within the vascular endothelium that initiate inflammation-mediated tissue breakdown. There are hints in the early experimental literature of VILI that vascular pressure could play an important – if not a pivotal – role in VILI development or expression. Dreyfuss and Saumon, for example, found that ventilation with negative pressure caused damage more severe than that caused by positive pressure, implicating the role of increased blood flow to ventilation related damage [21]. These same investigators provided further support for this hypothesis in showing that rats given dopamine to increase cardiac output suffered increased albumin leak when ventilated with high pressure, and ascribed a major portion of PEEP's protective effect in the setting of high pressure ventilation to its reduction of pulmonary perfusion [22].

Our group has also explored the vascular contribution to VILI in a series of experiments using isolated ventilated and perfused (IVP) rodent lungs [23–26]. The IVP system offers numerous advantages for the investigation of the interactions between alveolar and vascular pressures:

1. The progress of edema formation can be monitored by continuously weighing the heart/lung block suspended from a strain gauge.
2. Breakdown of the alveolar capillary barrier can be inferred from the filtration constant (K_F) derived from the weight-time relationship.
3. In-flow and out-flow vascular pressures and perfusion rate can be precisely measured and/or regulated.
4. The composition and physical properties of the perfusate can be adjusted.

In the experiments described below, each heart-lung block was perfused with Krebs-Henseleit solution, doped with a small quantity of autologous blood to provide a histologically visible marker of overt vascular rupture. Sufficient albumin was added to achieve physiologic tonicity. The cumulative results of this work demonstrate unequivocally that variations of vascular pressure and flow have the potential to modulate the nature and severity of VILI.

Fig. 2. Effect of perfusion on VILI, as indexed by peri-vascular hemorrhage.
Although control, high (150% control) and low (50% control) perfusion groups of rabbit lungs were exposed for equal time periods to identical ventilatory conditions, damage was greater in the high perfusion group.
* $p < 0.05$ versus control;
** $p < 0.05$ versus control and low flow.
(Modified from [23] with permission)

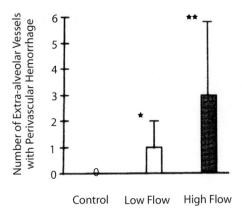

Pressure or Flow: Which is the Key Variable?

In our first experiment, we exposed isolated rabbit lungs to perfusion levels that were equivalent to, and ~ 50% greater or less than the normal resting blood flow of that animal species [23]. All lungs were ventilated identically with airway pressures that proved damaging *in vivo*. In this model of VILI, we demonstrated that perfusion amplitude contributed to the reduced lung compliance resulting from an adverse ventilatory pattern and promoted both lung edema and hemorrhage (Fig. 2).

We also found a strong correlation between indices of lung injury and the vascular pressure changes resulting from the interaction between ventilation and perfusion [23]. Although data from that experiment strongly suggested the primacy of perfusion pressure, it was not possible in that initial experiment to definitively determine which of those two variables was more important in modulating VILI, as vascular pressure increased in parallel with flow.

In a second isolated, ventilated perfused lung experiment designed to address that question, we varied airway pressure profiles to allow arterial pressure to vary while blood flow was held constant [24]. Our results indicated that mean airway pressure was a higher impact variable than tidal excursion amplitude in determining the severity of the lung hemorrhage and lung permeability alterations resulting from an adverse pattern of mechanical ventilation. Histologic injury scores were virtually identical for large and small V_T when high mean airway pressures were achieved, whether by lengthening inspiratory time or by increasing PEEP, respectively. A key difference between high mean airway pressure and low mean airway pressure preparations was the magnitude of the pulmonary arterial pressure and the length of time over which it was sustained. The results of those experiments emphasized the potential for deleterious interactions to occur between lung volumes and pulmonary hemodynamics. Taken together, our initial two studies demonstrated that modifications of vascular pressure within and upstream from the intermediate segment could influence the severity of VILI inflicted by an unchanging adverse pattern of ventilation.

How Does the Number of Ventilatory Cycles Influence the Expression of VILI?

Although ventilation is the product of V_T and frequency, surprisingly little attention has been directed to the role of the latter in the generation of VILI. Therefore, having concluded that upstream microvascular pressure might be an important co-factor in the development of VILI, we next addressed the question of how the number of ventilatory cycles occurring over a timed interval influences the rate of edema formation or severity of histologic alterations when maximum, minimum, and mean airway pressures are held identical.

Almost 15 years ago, Bshouty, and Younes reported that for the same minute ventilation target, raising V_T at a constant rate and raising frequency at a constant V_T produced similar degrees of edema in canine lobes perfused *in situ* at elevated hydrostatic pressures [27]. About the same time, Kolobow and colleagues demonstrated that sheep ventilated over many hours with high and moderate airway pressures sustained more lung injury than those sacrificed earlier, suggesting the potential for cumulative damage to occur under adverse ventilatory conditions [28, 29]. We used our isolated, ventilated and perfused model in experiments testing the hypothesis that cumulative damage occurs as a function of the number of stress cycles as well as stress magnitude. In these experiments, the pressure controlled mode with a peak pressure of 30 cmH$_2$O and a PEEP of 3 cmH$_2$O was used in each preparation [25]. Each experiment was conducted over 30 minutes. In one of three experimental groups of isolated and perfused rabbit lungs, a pulmonary artery peak pressure of 20 mmHg was matched to a ventilatory frequency of 20 cycles per minute to serve as our control. In a second set of perfused lungs, pulmonary artery pressure was allowed to rise to a maximum of 35 mmHg with each tidal cycle, at a frequency of 20 breaths per minute. In the third group, peak pulmonary artery pressure was again capped at 35 mmHg, but ventilator frequency was reduced to 3 cycles per minute with the same inspiratory time fraction as in the other two groups. Thus, mean airway pressure was identical for both high-pressure ventilatory patterns. The pH characteristics did not vary significantly among the groups. Our main findings were that lungs ventilated at low frequencies and high peak pulmonary artery pressures formed less edema and displayed markedly less perivascular hemorrhage than did those ventilated at higher frequencies but identical peak pulmonary artery pressures. In addition, lungs ventilated with high peak pulmonary artery pressures and flows demonstrated more extensive histologic alterations and edema formation than did those subjected to the same ventilatory pattern but at lower peak vascular pressures and flows [25] (Fig. 3).

Only a very small fraction of this difference was attributable to differences in mean hydraulic pressure. These data strongly indicated that not only are the characteristics of the tidal cycle and vascular pressures of fundamental importance to VILI, but also that minute ventilation, reflecting the number of stress cycles of a potentially damaging magnitude per unit time or their cumulative number, might be as well.

Whereas dependence of edema formation on minute-ventilation was previously noted in the aforementioned experimental study of isolated dog lobes by Bshouty and Younes [27], their experiments differed from ours in four notable ways. First,

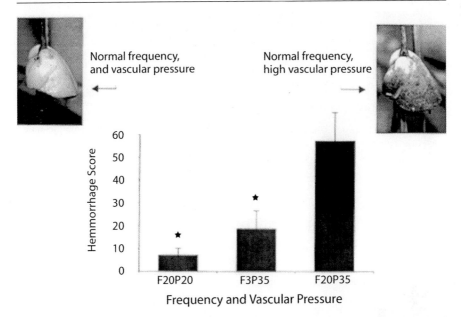

Fig. 3. Damaging effect of high vascular pressure and repeated cycling on isolated ventilated perfused rabbit lungs. For identical airway pressure profiles (plateau, mean, and end-expiratory pressures), higher peak inflow pressure (35 mmHg) was associated with greater damage, as compared to the control value of 20 mmHg. Reducing cycling frequency from 20 to 3 cycles per minute while holding airway and vascular pressures constant reduced injury severity. * p < 0.05 versus F20P35. (Modified from [25] with permission)

whereas their study was conducted with a physiological ventilatory pattern, we employed ventilatory patterns known to be potentially injurious. Second, vascular pressure in the Bshouty study was elevated by raising outflow (left atrial) pressure, thereby increasing pressure along the entire vascular tree (a simulation of left sided congestive heart failure). We held outflow pressure constant at a physiologically normal value while raising pressure selectively in those regions proximal to the intermediate vascular segment. Third, we used considerably higher vascular flows on a per gram of lung basis than did Bshouty and Younes [27]. Finally, we not only measured edema but also assessed histologic changes, as reflected by lung hemorrhage.

Several mechanisms come to mind to explain the diminution of lung edema formation and perivascular hemorrhage that we observed by decreasing respiratory frequency. A higher ventilatory frequency could have depleted surfactant more efficiently, thereby increasing alveolar surface tension and lowering end-expiratory extravascular pressure. The increased trans-vascular pressure gradient across extra-alveolar vessels would then favor fluid transudation, vessel disruption, and perivascular hemorrhage. Conceivably, the larger number of stress cycles imposed on the groups receiving 20 breaths per minute could have induced cumulative damage in a fashion similar to that experienced in a variety of bio-materials that

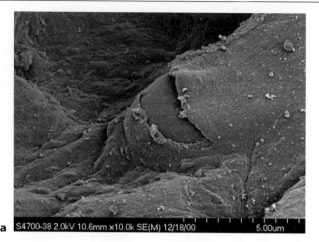

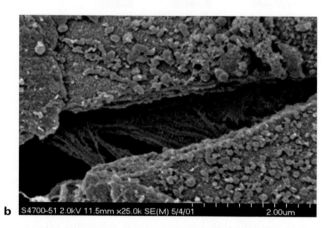

Fig. 4. Electron micrographs of rabbit lungs injured by high inflation pressures, low PEEP, and elevated vascular inflow pressure.
(**a**) Capillary stress fracture with incipient extravasation of an erythrocyte.
(**b**) Higher power view of stress fracture showing exposure of collagen filaments
(**c**) Peri-vascular hemorrhage.

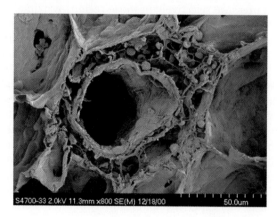

are subjected to sufficient repeated stress [30]. Overt stress fractures similar to those found by West and colleagues have been demonstrated by scanning electron microscopy in our laboratory (Fig. 4) and in a recently reported human patient [31]. A type of 'materials failure' of structural elements seems an attractive explanation, in that we found that both reducing stress application frequency (respiratory rate) and stress amplitude (pulmonary artery peak pressure) effectively limited VILI.

If cumulative damage is important, providing a lower frequency and/or lower pulmonary vascular pressure would be expected to reduce the tendency for material stress failure. Finally, it is interesting to consider that a low frequency may have allowed sufficient time between adjacent cycles for reparative processes to operate. Surprisingly little time appears to be needed to re-seal small disruptions in tissue barriers [32, 33].

What are the Relative Roles of Vascular and Airspace Pressures in VILI?

Because rigorous limitation of pulmonary vascular pressures significantly attenuated the damage in lungs exposed to a fixed ventilatory pattern, the work outlined above suggests that elevations of pulmonary vascular pressure arising from interactions between lung volume, pulmonary vascular resistance, and pulmonary vascular flow could worsen VILI. Our re-directed attention toward the vascular side of the alveolar capillary barrier stimulated us to ask the question: Does the mechanism by which pulmonary artery pressure is phasically increased influence the severity of lung damage during exposure to high alveolar pressure? In other words, is periodic inflation a necessary component of the vascular injury incurred during VILI?

Knowing that the frequency of ventilation was an important determinant of VILI, we reasoned that a lung exposed to pulsatile vascular pressure but not ventilated might experience significant injury, even without fluctuations of airway pressure. In an experiment designed to test this question, we applied a damaging pattern of airway pressure (plateau 30 cmH_2O, PEEP 5 cmH_2O) to one of three sets of lung preparations and allowed others to remain motionless [26]. In the ventilated group, peak pulmonary artery pressure was allowed to rise to 35 mmHg. Left atrial pressure was held at 10 mmHg and mean airway pressure at 17.5 cmH_2O. This set of ventilated preparations was compared to two unventilated groups held without tidal fluctuations of airway pressure (continuous positive airway pressure [CPAP]= 17.5 cmH_2O) in which in which all key hemodynamic pressures – peak, mean and nadir – were identical to their ventilated counterparts. In the latter two groups, a vascular pump applied pulsatile pulmonary artery pressure to the motionless lungs at frequencies of 3 or 20 pulses per minute. Each vascular stress cycle, whether generated by ventilation or by the vascular pump, was characterized by identical peak, mean, and nadir values. Our main findings were that lungs exposed to cyclic elevations of pulmonary artery pressure in the absence of ventilation formed less edema and displayed less perivascular and alveolar hemorrhage than ventilated lungs exposed to similar peak and mean pulmonary artery pressures and mean airway pressure [26]. Interestingly, under static CPAP conditions the higher pulsing frequency was associated with a greater degree of perivascular hemorrhage, indicating that the pulsatility of vascular pressure did contribute to VILI. Thus, the effects of respiratory frequency and vascular pressures on VILI are not mediated primarily by pulsatile vascular pressure *per se* but rather by a phenomenon related to cyclical modulation of the vascular microenvironment induced by ventilation. Because alveolar and extra-alveolar microvessels are stressed differently by lung expansion, these experiments focused our attention on the extra-alveolar microvasculature, suggesting the cyclic changes in perivascular pressure surrounding extra-alveolar, juxta-capillary microvessels might be important in the genesis of VILI.

Should Vascular Pressures be Lowered to Avert VILI?

Given that elevation of pulmonary vascular inflow pressure accentuated VILI, it seems logical that reduction of post-alveolar vascular pressure would also be protective. The merit of reducing left atrial pressure might be expected for at least two reasons. The edematous lungs tend to collapse under their own weight and to develop dependent atelectasis, which could lead to cyclic opening and collapse, intensified shear stresses, and a tendency for VILI in dependent areas. Moreover, exudation of protein-rich fluid has the potential to inactivate surfactant, further altering membrane permeability by increasing both surface tension and radial traction on pulmonary microvessels. On the other hand, increased left atrial pressure might help to limit VILI by flooding the alveoli of dependent regions, thereby reducing regional mechanical stresses. Moreover, reducing capillary pressure could promote cyclical vascular recruitment and derecruitment as the lungs transition from West's Zone III to Zone II condition during the course of the positive pressure inflation/deflation cycle. Hydrodynamic forces may well be accentuated by the higher velocities and surface shear stresses that occur along the vascular endothelium under such conditions. Moreover, reducing outflow pressure increases the gradient of pressure appearing across the alveoli, and consequently the energy dissipated across the intermediate segment. For these reasons, the impact of selectively reducing pulmonary venous pressure during ventilation with high airway pressure cannot be easily predicted.

A recently published comparison of lungs ventilated with moderately high peak alveolar pressures with normal and low left atrial pressures demonstrated a striking difference in favor of the normal vascular pressure subset [34] (Fig. 5).

This rather surprising result suggests that cyclical opening and closure of stressed microvessels could be important in the generation of VILI. Alternatively, decreasing outflow pressure might amplify microvascular stresses at or near the alveolar level, presumably acting through interdependence of the pulmonary vascular network. We speculate that direct mechanotransduction of inflammatory signals, increased transalveolar energy dissipation, or materials failure at the stressed boundary could be important linking mechanisms.

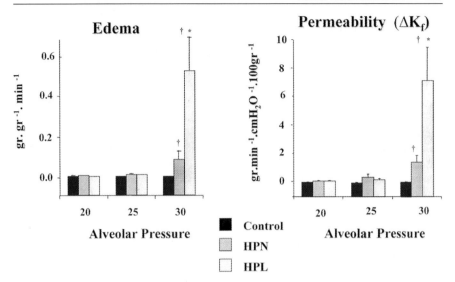

Fig. 5. Effect of reducing outflow pressure on edema formation and vascular permeability when ventilating isolated perfused rabbit lungs with high tidal inflation pressure and low PEEP. When peak alveolar pressure is 30 cmH$_2$O, lungs perfused with high inflow pressure and low outflow pressure sustain more edema and altered permeability than do lungs whose vascular outflow pressures are reduced. (Data from [34], with permission).

Potential Clinical Implications

Manipulation of cardiac output and vascular pressure is of vital importance in critical care management. The interactions between vascular pressure and ventilation outlined in this chapter suggest strongly that closer attention should be paid to interventions that impact vascular pressures, flows, and resistances when high inflation pressures are in use. Because microvascular stresses appear to be a potent cofactor in the development of pulmonary edema as well as lung damage resulting from an injurious pattern of ventilation, the clinician managing ALI must reconcile the competing objectives of ensuring adequate oxygen delivery and minimizing adverse effects. For example, an increase in cardiac output is generally held to be a beneficial consequence of management; however, increases in cardiac output are associated with an increased pre-alveolar microvascular pressure and a higher vascular pressure gradient across the lung. If increased pre-alveolar microvascular pressure accentuates a tendency for VILI, attempts to raise cardiac output may have unintended consequences. On the other hand, taking steps to reduce oxygen consumption demands could benefit the lung by reducing the pressure gradient developed across the microvasculature. Similarly, a reduction in left atrial pressure with maintained cardiac output is generally believed to benefit lung function, and this perception is almost certainly accurate with respect to hydrostatic edema formation. However, the results of the recent work already cited suggest that excessive reduction of left atrial pressure could amplify the tendency for VILI [34].

Because reducing ventilation frequency decreases the number of stress cycles, our work would suggest that a reduction in minute ventilation effected either by a decrease in V_T or a decrease in ventilatory frequency might have a salutary effect in reducing the tendency for VILI.

Reduced minute-ventilation is generally associated with increased CO_2 retention and hypercapnic acidosis, which until recently has been considered an undesirable but necessary consequence of a 'lung protective' ventilation strategy. However, when the lung's gas exchanging properties are not dramatically altered and CO_2 production remains unchanged, recently published experiments by Broccard, Sinclair and their respective colleagues strongly indicate that the generation of hypercapnic acidosis may exert a protective effect on the severity of VILI [35, 36]; this observation is consistent with elegant work that previously addressed ischemia/reperfusion injury [37].

Because interventions such as increasing PEEP or extending inspiratory time may redirect blood flow and radically alter the microvascular environment, it is conceivable that both benefit and harm could potentially result from these maneuvers. The body of investigative work just reviewed suggests that a reduction in the demands for cardiac output and ventilation could dramatically reduce the tendency for ventilator-induced lung injury even when using patterns that generate similar values for peak and end-expiratory alveolar pressures. Whether these intriguing possibilities are relevant to the clinical setting will require extensive and careful additional study.

References

1. Hakim TS, Michel RP, Chang HK (1982) Effect of lung inflation on pulmonary vascular resistance by arterial and venous occlusion. J Appl Physiol 53:1110–1115
2. Lai-Fook SJ (1982) Perivascular interstitial pressure measured by micro pipettes in isolated dog lung. J Appl Physiol 52:9–15
3. Fishman AP (1987) Pulmonary circulation. In: Fishman AP, Fisher AB, Geiger SR (eds) Handbook of Physiology-Section 3: The Respiratory System. Am Physiol Society, Bethesda, pp:93–97
4. Lamm WJ, Kirk KR, Hanson WL, Wagner WW Jr, Albert RK (1991) Flow through zone 1 lungs utilizes alveolar corner vessels. J Appl Physiol 70:1518–1523
5. West JB, Dollery CT, Naimark A (1964) Distribution of blood flow in isolated lung; relation to vascular and alveolar pressures. J Appl Physiol 19:713–724
6. Brigham KL, Woolverton WC, Blake LH, Staub NC (1974) Increased sheep lung vascular permeability caused by pseudomonas bacteremia. J Clin Invest 54:792–804
7. Mead J, Takishima T, Leith D (1970) Stress distribution in lungs: A model of pulmonary elasticity. J Appl Physiol 28:218–233
8. Namba Y, Kurdak SS, Fu Z, Mathieu-Costello O, West JB (1995) Effect of reducing alveolar surface tension on stress failure in pulmonary capillaries. J Appl Physiol 79:2114–2121
9. West JB, Mathieu-Costello O, Jones HJ, et al (1993) Stress failure of pulmonary capilaries in racehorses with exercise-induced pulmonary hemorrhage. J Appl Physiol 75:1097–1109
10. Hopkins SR, Schoene RB, Martin TR, Henderson WR, Spragg RG, West JB (1997) Intense exercise impairs the integrity of the pulmonary blood-gas barrier in elite athletes. Am J Respir Crit Care Med 155:1090–1094
11. Broccard AF, Liaudet L, Aubert JD, Schnyder P, Schaller MD (2001) Negative pressure post-tracheal extubation alveolar hemorrhage. Anesth Analg 92:273–275

12. Costello ML, Mathieu-Costello OM, West JB (1992) Stress failure of alveolar epithelial cells studied by scanning electron microscopy. Am Rev Respir Dis 145:1446–1455

13. West JB, Tsukimoto K, Mathieu-Costello O, Prediletto R (1991) Stress failure in pulmonary capillaries. J Appl Physiol 70:1731–1742

14. Mathieu-Costello O, Willford DC, Fu Z, Garden RM, West JB (1995) Pulmonary capillaries are more resistant to stress failure in dogs than in rabbits. J Appl Physiol 79:908–917

15. Fu Z, Costello ML, Tsukimoto K, et al (1992) High lung volume increases stress failure in pulmonary capillaries. J Appl Physiol 73:123–133

16. Amato MB, Marini JJ (1998) Barotrauma, volutrauma, and the ventilation of acute lung injury. In: Marini JJ, Slutsky AS (eds) Physiological Basis of Ventilatory Support. Marcel Dekker, New York, pp:1187–1245

17. Dreyfuss D, Saumon G (1998) Ventilator-induced lung injury: lessons from experimental studies. Am J Respir Crit Care Med 157:294–323

18. Broccard A, Shapiro R, Schmitz L, Adams AB, Nahum A, Marini JJ (2000) Prone positioning attenuates and redistributes ventilator-induced lung injury in dogs. Crit Care Med 28:295–303

19. Broccard AF, Shapiro RS, Schmitz LL, Ravenscraft SA, Marini JJ (1997) Influence of prone position on the extent and distribution of lung injury in a high tidal volume oleic acid model of acute respiratory distress syndrome. Crit Care Med 25:16–27

20. Hirschl RB, Tooley R, Parent A, Johnson K, Bartlett RH (1996) Evaluation of gas exchange, pulmonary compliance, and lung injury during total and partial liquid ventilation in the acute respiratory distress syndrome. Crit Care Med 24:1001–1008

21. Dreyfuss D, Saumon G (1993) Role of tidal volume, FRC, and end-inspiratory volume in the development of pulmonary edema following mechanical ventilation. Am Rev Respir Dis 148:1194–1203

22. Dreyfuss D, Soler P, Basset G, Saumon G (1988) High inflation pressure pulmonary edema. Respective effects of high airway pressure, high tidal volume, and positive end-expiratory pressure. Am Rev Respir Dis 137:1159–1164

23. Broccard AF, Hothchkiss JR, Kuwayama N, et al (1998) Consequences of vascular flow on lung injury induced by mechanical ventilation. Am J Respir Crit Care Med 157:1935–1942

24. Broccard AF, Hotchkiss JR, Suzuki S, Olson D, Marini JJ (1999) Effects of mean airway pressure and tidal excursion on lung injury induced by mechanical ventilation in an isolated perfused rabbit lung model. Crit Care Med 27:1533–1541

25. Hotchkiss JR, Blanch LL, Murias G, et al (2000) Effects of decreased respiratory frequency on ventilator induced lung injury. Am J Respir Crit Care Med 161:463–468

26. Hotchkiss JR, Blanch LL, Naviera A, Adams AB, Olson D, Marini JJ (2001) Relative roles of vascular and airspace pressures in ventilator induced lung injury. Crit Care Med 29:1593–1598

27. Bshouty Z, Younes M (1992) Effect of breathing pattern and level of ventilation on pulmonary fluid filtration in dog lung. Am Rev Respir Dis 145:3672–3676

28. Kolobow T, Moretti MP, Fumagalli R, et al (1987) Severe impairment in lung function induced by high peak airway pressuring during mechanical ventilation. An experimental study. Am Rev Respir Dis 135:312–315

29. Tsuno K, Miura K, Takeya M, Kolobow T, Morioka T (1991) Histopathologic pulmonary changes from mechanical ventilation at high peak airway pressures. Am Rev Respir Dis 143:1115–1120

30. Hashin Z, Rotem A (1978) A cumulative damage theory of fatigue failure. Mater Sci Eng 34:147–160

31. Hotchkiss JR, Simonson DA, Marek DJ, Marini JJ, Dries DJ (2002) Pulmonary microvascular fracture in a patient with acute respiratory distress syndrome. Crit Care Med 30:2368–2370

32. Dreyfuss D, Soler P, Saumon G (1992) Spontaneous resolution of pulmonary edema caused by short periods of cyclic overinflation. J Appl Physiol 72:2081–2089

33. Vlahakis NE, Hubmayr RD (2000) Invited review: Plasma membrane stress failure in alveolar epithelial cells. J Appl Physiol 89:2490–2496

34. Broccard A, Vannay C, Feihl F, Schaller MD (2002) Impact of low pulmonary vascular pressure on ventilator-induced lung injury. Crit Care Med 30:2183–2190
35. Sinclair SE, Kregenow DA, Lamm WJ, Starr IR, Chi EY, Hlastala MP (2002) Hypercapnic acidosis is protective in an in vivo model of ventilator-induced lung injury. Am J Respir Crit Care Med 166:403–408
36. Broccard AF, Hotchkiss JR, Vannay C, et al (2001) Protective effects of hypercapnic acidosis on ventilator-induced lung injury. Am J Respir Crit Care Med 164:802–806
37. Laffey JG, Tanaka M, Engelberts D, et al (2000) Therapeutic hypercapnia reduces pulmonary and systemic injury following in vivo lung reperfusion. Am J Respir Crit Care Med 162:2021–2022

VILI: Physiological Evidence

J. D. Ricard, D. Dreyfuss, and G. Saumon

Introduction

Mechanical ventilation has been part of basic life support for several decades. Several potential drawbacks and complications were identified early in the use of mechanical ventilation [1]. Of these, ventilator-induced lung injury (VILI) has recently received much attention in both the experimental [2] and the clinical field [3-7]. The purpose of this chapter is to review the physiological evidence for VILI based on animal studies and to place these results into a clinical perspective of ventilatory management of acute respiratory distress syndrome (ARDS).

Evidence for VILI

Ventilation of Intact Lungs

High lung volume VILI

Webb and Tierney were the first to demonstrate that mechanical ventilation could cause pulmonary edema in intact animals [8]. They were able to show in rats subjected to positive airway pressure ventilation that pulmonary edema was more severe and occurred more rapidly when the animals were ventilated with 45 cmH$_2$O than with 30 cmH$_2$O peak airway pressure. Animals ventilated for 1 hour with 14 cmH$_2$O peak airway pressure did not develop edema. It was later confirmed that ventilation with high airway pressure produces capillary permeability alterations, non-hydrostatic pulmonary edema and tissue damage resembling that observed during ARDS [9]. Further studies demonstrated that VILI depended mainly on lung volume and especially on the end-inspiratory volume [10]. The corresponding pressure is termed 'plateau' pressure and its clinical importance has been empha-sized in a Consensus Conference on mechanical ventilation [11]. The respective roles of increased airway pressure and increased lung volume on the development of VILI were clarified by showing that mechanical ventilation of intact rats with large or low tidal volume (V$_T$), but with identical peak airway pressures (45 cmH$_2$O) [10] did not result in the same lung alterations. Pulmonary edema and cellular ultrastructural abnormalities were encountered only in rats subjected to high V$_T$ and not in those in which lung distention was limited by thoraco-abdominal strapping [10]. Furthermore, animals ventilated with large V$_T$ but negative airway pressure (by means of an iron lung) still developed pulmonary edema thus demonstrating that airway pressure is not a determinant for pulmonary edema [10]. Consequently, it was suggested that the term 'volutrauma' would be more appropriate than barotrauma in this situation [12, 13]. Other investigators have reached the same conclusions with different protocols and species. Hernandez and coworkers compared the capillary filtration coefficient (a measure of capillary permeability) of the lungs of rabbits ventilated with 15, 30 and 45 cmH_2O peak airway pressures with that of animals ventilated with the same airway pressures but with limitation of thoraco-abdominal excursions by plaster casts placed around the chest and the abdomen [14]. The capillary filtration coefficient of the lungs removed after ventilation was normal in animals ventilated at 15 cmH_2O peak pressure, increased by 31% at 30 cmH_2O peak pressure and by 430% at 45 cmH_2O peak pressure in animals without restriction of lung distention. In striking contrast, limiting lung inflation prevented the increase of the capillary filtration coefficient [14]. Carlton and coworkers confirmed this observation in lambs [15]. Besides the lung distention that occurs during mechanical ventilation, the rate at which lung volume varies may also affect microvascular permeability. Peevy and coworkers [16] used isolated perfused rabbit lungs to determine the capillary filtration coefficient of lungs ventilated with various V_T and inspiratory flow rates. They found that small V_T with a high flow rate increased the filtration coefficient to the same extent (approximately 6 times baseline value) as ventilation with a markedly higher V_T but a lower inspiratory flow rate for the same peak airway pressure [16].

Taken together, these experimental studies have demonstrated that large volume rather than high intrathoracic pressures *per se* results in ventilator-induced lung edema in intact animals.

Low lung volume VILI

Unlike high volume lung injury (which can be observed in non-injured animals), low lung volume injury is not seen in healthy lungs, which can tolerate mechanical ventilation with physiologic V_T and low levels of positive end-expiratory pressure (PEEP) for prolonged periods of time without any apparent damage. Taskar and colleagues [17] have shown that the repetitive collapse and reopening of terminal units during 1 h does not seem to damage healthy lungs (although it does alter gas exchange and reduces compliance).

Ventilation of Damaged Lungs

High-volume lung injury

Several investigators have evaluated the effect of mechanical ventilation with overdistension on damaged lungs. Results from these studies consistently stress the increased susceptibility of diseased lungs to the detrimental effects of mechanical ventilation.

The first studies were performed on isolated lungs. Bowton and Kong [18] showed that isolated perfused rabbit lungs injured by oleic acid gained significantly more weight when ventilated with 18 ml/kg bw than when ventilated with 6 ml/kg bw V_T. Hernandez and colleagues [19] compared the effects of oleic acid alone, mechanical ventilation alone, and a combination, on the capillary filtration coefficient and wet-to-dry weight ratio of isolated perfused lungs from young rabbits. These measurements were not significantly affected by low doses of oleic acid, or mechanical ventilation with a peak inspiratory pressure of 25 cmH$_2$O for 15 min. However, the filtration coefficient increased significantly when oleic acid injury was followed by mechanical ventilation. The wet-to-dry weight ratio (a marker of edema severity) of these lungs was significantly higher than that of the lungs subjected to oleic acid injury or ventilation alone. The same workers also showed that the increased filtration coefficient produced by ventilating isolated blood-perfused rabbit lungs with 30–45 cmH$_2$O peak pressure was greater when surfactant was inactivated by instilling dioctyl-succinate [20]. Whereas light microscope examination showed only minor abnormalities (minimal hemorrhage and vascular congestion) in the lungs of animals subjected to ventilation alone, or surfactant inactivation alone, the combination of the two caused severe damage (edema and flooding, hyaline membranes and extensive alveolar hemorrhage).

These results on isolated lungs suggested that VILI might develop at lower airway pressure in abnormal isolated lungs. Whether this could also be the case in whole animals with 'pre-injured lungs' was investigated by comparing the effects of different degrees of lung distention during mechanical ventilation in rats whose lungs had been injured by α-naphtylthiourea (ANTU) [21]. ANTU infusion alone caused moderate interstitial pulmonary edema of the permeability type. Mechanical ventilation of intact rats for 2 min resulted in a permeability edema whose severity depended on the V$_T$ amplitude. It was possible to calculate how much mechanical ventilation would theoretically injure lungs diseased by ANTU by summing up the separate effect of mechanical ventilation alone or ANTU alone on edema severity. The results showed that the lungs of the animals injured by ANTU ventilated at high volume (45 ml/kg bw) had more severe permeability edema than predicted, indicating synergism between the two insults rather than addition. Even minor alterations, such as those produced by spontaneous ventilation during prolonged anesthesia (which degrades surfactant activity and promotes focal atelectasis [22, 23]), are sufficient to synergistically increase the harmful effects of high volume ventilation [21]. The extent to which lung mechanical properties have deteriorated prior to ventilation is a key factor in this synergy. The amount of edema produced by high volume mechanical ventilation in the lungs of animals given ANTU, or that had undergone prolonged anesthesia was inversely proportional to the respiratory system compliance measured at the very beginning of mechanical ventilation [21]. Thus, the more severe the existing lung abnormalities before ventilation, the more severe the VILI. The reason for this synergy requires clarification. The presence of local alveolar flooding in animals given the most harmful ventilation protocol was the most evident difference from those ventilated with lower, less harmful, V$_T$ [21]. It is conceivable that flooding reduced the number of alveoli that received the V$_T$, exposing them to overinflation and rendering them more susceptible to injury, further reducing the aerated lung volume and resulting in positive feed-back. The same reasoning applies to prolonged anesthesia, during which the aerated lung volume was probably gradually reduced by atelectasis [21]. Both flooding and atelectasis decrease compliance, likely to an extent that is correlated with their spreading. It is thus not surprising that the lower the lung distensibility before ventilation (as inversely reflected by quasi-static compliance, an index of the amount of lung that remains open), the more severe the alterations induced by high volume ventilation [21]. Thus, uneven distribution of ventilation that occurs during acute lung injury (ALI) [24] may render lungs more prone to regional overinflation and injury. To explore this possibility, alveolar flooding was produced by instilling 2 ml saline into the trachea. The rats were then immediately ventilated for 10 minutes with V_T of up to 33 ml/kg. Flooding with saline did not significantly affect microvascular permeability when V_T was low. As V_T was increased, capillary permeability alterations were larger in flooded than in intact animals, reflecting further impairment of their endothelial barrier. There was also a correlation between end-inspiratory airway pressure, the pressure at which was found the lower inflection point on the pressure-volume (PV) curve, and capillary permeability alterations in flooded animals ventilated with a high V_T [25]. Thus, the less compliant and recruitable the lung was after saline flooding, the more severe were the changes in permeability caused by lung distention.

Low lung-volume injury

There may be an increase in trapped gas volume during pulmonary edema and ALI, especially when surfactant properties are altered, because of terminal unit closure [26]. Under such conditions, the slope of the inspiratory PV curve of the respiratory system often displays an abrupt increase at low lung volume. This change reflects the massive opening of previously closed units and has been termed the 'lower inflection point'. Most clinicians are aware of the importance of this phenomenon in terms of arterial oxygenation, since setting PEEP above this inflection point usually results in a very abrupt decrease in shunt and increase in PaO_2 [27–30].

Attention has focused only relatively recently on the possibility that pulmonary lesions may be aggravated if this inflection point lies within the V_T. Experimental evidence for this was initially provided by studies comparing conventional mechanical ventilation with high frequency oscillatory ventilation (HFOV) in premature or surfactant-depleted lungs. More recently, studies performed during conventional mechanical ventilation of surfactant-depleted lungs with various levels of PEEP also support the possibility that the repeated opening and closing of terminal units cause additional injury [31–33]. Sykes and coworkers [31, 32] studied this issue by ventilating rabbits whose lungs were depleted of surfactant by lavage. Peak inspiratory pressure was 15 mmHg at the beginning of the experiment and 25 mmHg at the end (5 hours later), because lung compliance decreased (V_T was set but not stated). PEEP was adjusted so that functional residual capacity (FRC) was either above or below the lower inflection point on the inspiratory limb of the PV curve. This resulted in PEEP levels of about 1–2 mmHg (below inflection) and 8–12 mmHg (above inflection). The mortality rates in the two groups were identical, but the arterial PaO_2 was better preserved and there was less hyaline membrane formation in the high PEEP group [31, 32]. This lessening of pathological alterations occurred even when the mean airway pressures in the low and high PEEP groups were kept at the same level by adjusting the inspiratory/expiratory time ratio [32]. Muscedere and colleagues [33] recently reported similar results for isolated, unperfused, lavaged rabbit lungs ventilated with a low (5–6 ml/kg bw) V_T and with a PEEP set below or above the inflection point. However, Sohma and colleagues could not replicate these findings in rabbits with hydrochloric acid-injured lungs using the same ventilation settings [34]. The reality of the repetitive opening and closure of terminal units and the significance of the lower inflection point on the PV curve have been recently challenged by Martynowicz and coworkers [35]. They studied the regional expansion of oleic acid-injured lungs using the parenchymal marker technique. They found that the gravitational distribution of volume at the FRC was not affected by oleic acid injury and that the injury was not associated with decreased parenchymal volume of dependent regions. In addition, they found that the temporal inhomogeneity of regional tidal expansion did not increase with oleic acid injury. Their findings are, therefore, in contradiction with the hypothesis that a gravitational gradient in superimposed pressure during VILI produces compression atelectasis of dependent lung that in turn produces shear injury from cyclic recruitment and collapse [35]. They propose a different explanation for the occurrence of a lower inflection point on the PV curve, namely the displacement of air-liquid interfaces along the tracheo-bronchial tree rather than alveolar recruitment and derecruitment and thus a different mechanism by which PEEP restores the regional tidal expansion of dependent regions and conclude that the knee in the P-V curve is the result of the mechanics of parenchyma with constant surface tension and partially fluid-filled alveoli, not the result of abrupt opening of airways or atelectatic parenchyma [36]. It, therefore, remains unsettled whether injury caused by the repetitive reopening of collapsed terminal units and the protective effect of PEEP is restricted to the peculiar situation of surfactant depletion. In the clinical field, the recent negative results of the ALVEOLI trial (http://hedwig.mgh.harvard.edu/ardsnet/ards04.html) cast doubt on the clinical existence of repetitive opening and closing lung injury [37].

Roles of V_T, PEEP, and Overall Lung Distention

The influence of PEEP on ALI (and more specifically on ventilator-induced pulmonary edema) must be studied with respect to the level of V_T used. Indeed, PEEP increases FRC and opens the lung but also displaces end-inspiratory volume towards total lung capacity when V_T is kept constant possibly thus favoring overinflation. PEEP may also affect hemodynamics and lung fluid balance. Therefore, close analysis of the numerous studies which have been done to clarify the relationships between PEEP, oxygenation, and the accumulation of extravascular lung water during hydrostatic or permeability type edema must take into account the experimental approach used, i.e., intact animals or isolated lungs (for which lung water content will differ) and whether or not V_T is reduced (thus increasing or not end-inspiratory lung volume).

Effects of PEEP when V_T is kept constant

Application of PEEP may result in lung overinflation if it is followed by a significant change in FRC owing to the increase in end-inspiratory volume. Depending on the homogeneity of ventilation distribution, this overinflation will affect preferentially the more distensible areas, thus accounting for the usual lack of reduction or even the worsening of edema reported with PEEP during most experiments [38]. In intact animals, application of PEEP does not counteract the accumulation of edema fluid during hydrostatic type edema [39] or permeability type edema [39, 40], though it improves oxygenation [39] because of the reopening of flooded alveoli. In isolated ventilated-perfused lung, PEEP aggravates edema fluid accumulation [41]. Thus, for a given V_T, increasing FRC with PEEP has dissimilar effects on edema accumulation in isolated lungs and in intact animals. In the latter, the lack of effect of PEEP depends on the balance between PEEP-induced increase in end-inspiratory lung volume which decrease interstitial pressure and favors fluid filtration in extra-alveolar vessels and the hemodynamic depression due to elevated intrathoracic pressure that will decreases filtration pressure. In contrast, the preservation of perfusion-rate in isolated-perfused lungs favors the increase in edema [41].

Effects of PEEP when V_T is reduced

Edema is less severe when V_T is decreased and end-inspiratory lung volume is kept constant by increasing FRC with PEEP during high-volume ventilation [2]. Webb and Tierney showed that edema was lessened by 10 cmH$_2$O PEEP application during ventilation with 45 cmH$_2$O peak airway pressure [8]. The authors attributed this beneficial effect of PEEP to the preservation of surfactant activity. It was shown later that although PEEP decreased the amount of edema, it did not change the severity of the permeability alterations as assessed by the increase in dry lung weight [10]. However, no alveolar damage was observed in animals ventilated with PEEP in comparison with those ventilated in zero end-expiratory pressure (ZEEP). The only ultrastructural alterations observed with PEEP consisted of endothelial blebbing [10]. This preservation of the epithelial layer has received no satisfactory explanation. It may be that PEEP prevented repetitive opening and closing of terminal units, thereby decreasing shear stress at this level. Similar observations have been made by other investigators in intact animals [42, 43] and in perfused canine lobes [44]. The potential role of hemodynamic alterations induced by PEEP should be considered. For a given end-inspiratory airway pressure, application of PEEP produces an increase in intrathoracic pressure which adversely affects cardiac output [45, 46]. Indeed, rats submitted to high-peak airway pressure ventilation with 10 cmH$_2$O PEEP had more severe edema when the hemodynamic alterations induced by PEEP were corrected with dopamine [47]. The amount of edema was correlated with systemic blood pressure, suggesting that improvement in cardiac output and increased filtration were responsible for this aggravation. In conclusion, the reduction of edema and of the severity of cell damage by PEEP during ventilation-induced pulmonary edema may be linked to reduced tissue stress (by decreasing volume-pressure excursion) and capillary filtration, as well as to the preservation of surfactant activity.

Importance of overall lung distention

Lung volume at the end of inspiration (i.e., the overall degree of lung distention) is probably the main determinant of VILI severity. Rats ventilated with a low V_T and 15 cmH$_2$O PEEP developed pulmonary edema whereas rats ventilated with the same V_T but 10 cmH$_2$O PEEP did not [47]. Similarly, doubling V_T (which was not deleterious in animals ventilated in ZEEP) resulted in edema in the presence of 10 cmH$_2$O PEEP. Thus the safety of a given V$_T$ depends on how much FRC is increased.

In conclusion, VILI and edema occur when a certain degree of lung overinflation is reached. This situation is met when V$_T$ is increased at a given end-inspiratory pressure. By contrast, when PEEP is added to reach the same end-inspiratory pressure, it seems to slow the development of edema and diminish the severity of tissue injury, although the occurrence of microvascular permeability alterations is not prevented [10, 47]. Finally, when PEEP results in additional overinflation, there is greater edema [47].

Possible Mechanisms of VILI

It is now clear that ventilation-induced pulmonary edema is essentially the result of severe changes in the permeability of the alveolar-capillary barrier. Small increases in microvascular transmural pressure may add their effects to those of altered permeability to enhance edema severity.

Depending on the duration of the aggression, two different kinds of injury probably occur. Small animals very rapidly develop a severe permeability pulmonary edema as a consequence of acute extreme lung stretching. This edema probably does not involve inflammatory cell recruitment or secretion of mediators. Edema develops more slowly in larger animals, in particular in response to moderately high airway pressures, rendering the situation more complex. A low lung volume injury probably adds its own effects to the direct mechanical aggression at high end-inspiratory volume. Indeed, high V$_T$ mechanical ventilation without PEEP may reduce the aerated volume and gradually cause mechanical non-uniformity. This lung inhomogeneity will in turn promote overinflation of the more distensible and probably healthier zones, leading to positive feed-back aggravation. In addition, lung injury develops slowly enough in large animals for inflammatory pathways to become involved.

Mechanisms of Increased Vascular Transmural Pressure

Increased fluid filtration by this mechanism may occur at both extra-alveolar [48, 49] and alveolar [50–52] sites during mechanical ventilation. Increased transmural pressure in extra-alveolar vessels may result from the increase in lung volume, a consequence of lung interdependence [45, 53, 54], whereas increased filtration across alveolar microvessels may be the consequence of surfactant inactivation [8, 52].

Mechanisms of Altered Permeability

While permeability alterations are obvious and severe during ventilator-induced edema, the underlying mechanisms are not fully understood, and there are probably several. In particular, as previously stressed, the mechanisms of lung injury may well vary according to the extent and duration of lung overdistension.

Effects of surfactant inactivation

In addition to its effects on fluid filtration, surfactant inactivation and elevated alveolar surface tension may increase alveolar epithelial permeability to small solutes. DTPA clearance in rabbits [55] and dogs [56] was increased following surfactant inactivation by detergent aerosolization. This effect was ascribed to the uneven distribution of lung mechanical properties resulting in ventilation inhomogeneities and regional overexpansion, rather than to the elimination of peculiar barrier properties of surfactant [56]. The effects of surfactant inactivation and large V_T ventilation on alveolocapillar permeability (as assessed by pulmonary DTPA clearance) are additive [57]. Increased surface tension may also alter endothelial permeability as a result of increased radial traction on pulmonary microvessels [52].

Participation of inflammatory cells and mediators

Role of inflammatory cells: The endothelial cell disruptions that have been observed during overinflation edema in small animals may allow direct contact between polymorphonuclear cells and basement membrane. This contact may promote leukocyte activation. As previously mentioned, the short duration of experiments conducted in small animals did not allow massive leukocyte recruitment. A striking feature of the VILI that occurs after several hours in larger animals is the infiltration of inflammatory cells into the interstitial and alveolar spaces. In one of the earliest studies on this subject, Woo and Hedley-White [58] observed that overinflation produced edema in open-chest dogs, and that leukocytes accumulated in the vasculature and macrophages in the alveoli. Further studies have confirmed these results [59] and shown that high transpulmonary pressure increased the transit time of leukocytes in the lungs of rabbits [60]. Conversely, when animals are depleted in neutrophils, high volume pulmonary edema is less severe than in non-depleted animals [61].

Role of inflammatory mediators: The participation of inflammatory cytokines in the course of VILI has been the subject of recent studies and is a matter of debate [62]. Tremblay and colleagues [63] examined the effects of different ventilatory strategies on the level of several cytokines in bronchoalveolar lavage (BAL) fluid of isolated rat lungs ventilated with different end-expiratory pressures and V_T. High V_T ventilation (40 ml/kg bw) with ZEEP resulted in considerable increases in tumor necrosis factor (TNF)-α, interleukin (IL)-1ß and IL-6 and in macrophage inhibitory protein (MIP)-2. Unfortunately, results from this study have not been replicated by another group using the same *ex vivo* lung model [64]. It is worth noting that stretching *in vitro* human alveolar macrophages [65] or A549 epithelial cells [66] led to no TNF-α release, but to IL-8 release. *In vivo* studies of intact animals show that high volume mechanical ventilation that produces a very severe pulmonary edema does not induce the release of TNF-α [64, 67]. Studies on TNF-α mRNA also yield conflicting results since Takata and coworkers [68] showed large increases in TNF-α mRNA in the intraalveolar cells of surfactant-depleted rabbits after one hour of conventional mechanical ventilation with peak inspiratory and end-expiratory pressures of 28 and 5 cmH$_2$0 (resulting in a mean airway pressure of 13 cmH$_2$O) whereas Imanaka and colleagues showed no increase in lung tissue TNF-α mRNA of rats ventilated by high pressure (45 cmH$_2$O of peak inspiratory pressure [69].

The only mediator which is constantly found in the different experimental studies is MIP-2 (or IL-8, pending on the experimental model). The presence of this neutrophil chemoattractant mediator in lungs subjected to high volume ventilation is in agreement with the well documented recruitment of neutrophils that occurs after long term ventilation [59, 70–72].

In addition to increasing the amount of cytokines in the lung, it has been suspected that overinflation during mechanical ventilation may promote the release of cytokines [73, 74] or bacteria [75, 76] into the blood, thus giving a causative role for mechanical ventilation in multiorgan dysfunction [77, 78]. However, this hypothesis remains to be proven [79].

New Insights into VILI

Cellular Response to Mechanical Strain

Growing interest has focused on the cellular response to mechanical strain, which has been comprehensively reviewed lately [80]. Parker and colleagues studied the different signal transduction pathways that may be involved in the microvascular permeability increases observed during experimental VILI [81]. They found that gadolinium (that blocks stretch-activated nonselective cation channels) annulled the increases in vascular permeability induced by high airway pressure [82]. Authors concluded that stretch-activated cation channels might initiate the increase in permeability induced by mechanical ventilation through increases in intracellular Ca^{2+} concentration. To further explore this hypothesis, the same team studied the effect of inhibitors of the Ca^{2+}/calmodulin – myosin light chain kinase pathway on vascular permeability [83]. Using an isolated perfused rat model, they showed that kinase inhibitors, which may prevent Ca^{2+} entry, contraction of the actin-myosin filaments or release of adhesion proteins, could significantly attenuate the vascular permeability increase induced by high pressure mechanical ventilation [83]. Taken together, these results suggest that the increase in microvascular permeability may not be a simply passive physical phenomenon (a "stress failure" [84, 85]), but the result of biochemical reactions. Maintenance of plasma membrane integrity is essential in response to mechanical stress. Recently, Vlahakis and colleagues reported a heretofore-undescribed response of alveolar epithelial cells to deformation [86]. They labeled membrane lipids to study deformation-induced lipid trafficking and observed in a direct manner (laser confocal microscopy) epithelial cells of the alveolar basement membrane response to deforming forces. A 25% stretch deformation resulted in lipid transport to the plasma membrane to ensure its integrity and an increase in epithelial cell surface area. This lipid trafficking occurred in all cells, in contrast with plasma breaks which were seen in only a small percentage of cells. Authors concluded that deformation-induced lipid trafficking serves, in part, to repair plasma breaks in order to maintain plasma membrane integrity and cell viability, and that this could be viewed as a cytoprotective mechanism against plasma membrane stress failure seen during VILI [10, 85]. Other investigators have focused on the relative importance of deformation frequency, duration, and amplitude in deformation-induced cell injury [87]. Exposing rat primary alveolar epithelial cells to cyclic deformation (25, 37 and 60% increase in membrane surface area [ΔSA]) led to significantly greater cell death in comparison with static deformation. To investigate the relative importance of peak deformation magnitude a cyclic deformation amplitude on deformation-induced injury, cells were submitted to cyclic deformation amplitudes of 12% and 25% ΔSA superimposed on a static deformation of 25% ΔSA, thus resulting in a peak deformation magnitude of 37 and 50% ΔSA, respectively. Interestingly, authors found that limiting the deformation amplitude resulted in significant reductions in cell death at identical peak deformations. From these results, an analogy can be drawn with experiments that showed a decrease in lung injury when V_T was reduced with a constant PEEP level, thus reducing end-inspiratory lung volume [47].

Influence of Capnia on VILI

Deleterious effects of hypocapnia have been extensively 287 reviewed recently [88] and are addressed in the chapter by Brian Kavanagh (page 287). However, it is important to note that in addition to detrimental effects of hypocapnia [89] or of hypercapnic acidosis buffering [90] on ischemia-reperfusion lung injury, experimental studies have shown that hypercapnic acidosis is protective of VILI [91, 92].

Strategies to Reduce VILI: Use of the PV Curve

The ARDS network trial [6] has undisputedly shown that reducing V_T from 12 ml/kg to 6 ml/kg resulted in a 22% reduction of mortality. Due to protocol, the same reduction of V_T was applied in all the patients allocated to the low V_T group. However, it has repeatedly been shown that the pressure and the volume that are considered safe for some ARDS patients may cause lung overdistension in others [93–96]. Conversely, arbitrary settings may result in an unnecessary reduction in V_T, which a recent meta-analysis has suggested as being potentially harmful [7]. It has been suggested that information from the inspiratory PV curve of the respiratory system could be used to tailor ventilator settings. For instance, the presence of an opening pressure (lower inflection point) could be used to adjust the PEEP [27–29]. In addition to improving oxygenation, PEEP reduces the severity of VILI [10] and may lessen the damage produced by the repeated opening and closing of lung units in surfactant-depleted lungs [31, 33]. However, PEEP may favor overinflation if V_T is not reduced [2, 97]. It has been proposed that the V_T be adjusted according to PV curve analysis by limiting end-inspiratory pressures to below the decrease in slope seen at high pressure/volume, called the upper inflection point (UIP) [3, 95, 96]. The UIP often seen in patients with ARDS has been ascribed to overinflation [95, 96], or to the end of recruitment [98, 99] during lung expansion. However, whether or not ventilator settings that would result in pressure/volume excursions above the UIP are deleterious remains unsettled, and has never been assessed experimentally. The impact of pulmonary edema and the resulting decrease in ventilatable lung volume on the inspiratory limb of the respiratory system PV curve has not yet been evaluated. A better understanding of its significance is required before the UIP can be used to set V_T in patients. A recent experimental study was designed to examine several hypotheses [100]. The first was that the reduction in ventilatable lung volume (the baby-lung effect) not only decreases the compliance of the lung [93, 101] but also affects the position of the UIP. The second was that the development of edema alters the PV curve essentially because of distal airway obstruction. And the third was that individual characteristics of the PV curve reflect the susceptibility of the lungs to the deleterious effects of high volume ventilation. The first two hypotheses were tested by obstructing the distal airways of rats by instilling a viscous liquid and by comparing the PV curves obtained to those obtained during hyperinflation ventilation of intact rats. Authors found that changes in the shape of the PV curve (gradual decrease in compliance and volume at which the UIP was seen, and progressive increase in end-inspiratory pressure) were very similar whether they were due to viscous instillation into the lungs or due to the development of overdistension pulmonary edema. To test the third hypothesis, PV curves prior to mechanical overinflation were examined with respect to the amount of pulmonary edema induced by overinflation in lungs injured by α-naphthylthiourea (ANTU). Authors found that the higher the compliance and the position of the UIP before overinflation, the less edema occurred after overinflation. Taken together, these results suggest that the position of the UIP is a marker of ventilatable lung volume and is both influenced by and predictive of the development of edema during mechanical ventilation.

Conclusion and Clinical Applications

The experimental concept of VILI has recently received a resounding clinical relevance [6]. However, what might have been seen as the final step in ARDS ventilatory strategy knowledge (i.e., unilateral drastic V_T reduction for every ARDS patient) has very recently been shaken [7]. For the time being and until further evidence, one may put forward the following conclusions :
- drastic V_T reduction may not be justified for every ARDS patient.
- reasoned V_T reduction, designed to avoid volutrauma, may be guided by the state of lung mechanical properties as can be provided by the respiratory system PV curve, in order to avoid excessive or insufficient V_T reduction.
- use of high levels of PEEP is not to date justified.
- Evidence-based ventilatory management of ARDS is a difficult art; luckily basic physiology is still there to help clinicians [37, 62, 102, 103].

counts, as well as reduced histological evidence of lung injury. Narimanbekov and colleagues [49] used an IL-1β receptor antagonist and found reduced lung lavage concentrations of a number of markers of lung injury (i.e., albumin, elastase, and neutrophils) in a saline-lavaged rabbit model.

Recently Held and colleagues [50] demonstrated in isolated perfused mouse lungs that both LPS and overventilation caused translocation of NF-κB to the nucleus, leading to release of MIP-2. However, there were major differences in response to the two different stimuli when they used LPS-resistant C3H/HeJ mice, which have abnormalities in Toll like receptor (TLR)-4. In LPS-resistant C3H/HeJ mice overventilation, but not LPS, caused translocation of NF-κB and release of MIP-2, suggesting that initial signaling steps between LPS and ventilation differ and that the NF-κB translocation elicited by overventilation is independent of TLR4.

Passage of Mediators from Lung to Bloodstream

One important question is where the increased systemic pro-inflammatory media-tors originate from. Loss of compartmentalization of local pulmonary inflamma-tory mediators due to mechanical ventilation has been recently proposed. The alveolar barrier restricts transport of macro-molecules of a size similar to that of cytokines (15–20 kDa). After secretion in the lung, cytokines such as TNF-α remain in the alveolar space and leak into the circulation only if there is injury of the alveolar barrier. Several investigators have shown that increased permeability of the alveolar-capillary interface, as a result of lung injury leads to the release of mediators into circulation that would normally have remained compartmentalized within the alveolar space [51, 52]. Tutor and colleagues [51] employed an isolated perfused rat lung model in which they injected TNF-α into the lung and measured its appearance in the perfusate. They found that the perfusate TNF-α concentra-tions were increased only when alveolar-capillary permeability was increased and not in normal lung, suggesting that loss of compartmentalization of alveolar TNF-α could occur, but only in the context of damage to the alveolar-capillary membrane. Von Bethman and colleagues [8] reported that in an isolated perfused murine lung model, ventilation with higher transpulmonary pressure (25 cmH2O) versus nor-mal pressure (10 cmH2O) led to a significant increase in concentration of both TNF-α and IL-6 in the perfusate. As compartmentalization of the local pulmonary response is lost, systemic release of inflammatory mediators may promote the massive inflammatory response that underlies MODS.

ARDS is characterized by a loss of integrity of the alveolar capillary barrier due to severe diffuse alveolar damage, leading to bidirectional protein flux. Therefore, not only pro-inflammatory cytokines but also locally secreted proteins, particularly the surfactant-associated protein (SP) may pass into the systemic circulation. SP-A, SP-B and SP-D, which have anti-inflammatory properties, have been detected in serum of ARDS patients, and have been associated with outcome of patients with ARDS [53, 54]. The balance between the pro- and anti-inflammatory cytokines passing from the lung to the bloodstream may be more important in determining the subsequent effect than the absolute values of any single mediators.

Bacterial Translocation in Mechanical Ventilation

Another mechanism whereby mechanical ventilation may contribute to the development of a systemic inflammatory response is by promoting bacterial translocation from the air spaces into the circulation. Two recent studies evaluated the influence of mechanical ventilatory strategy on the translocation of bacteria from the lung into the bloodstream in dogs and rats[55, 56]. After intratracheal instillation of bacteria, these animals were ventilated with a high transpulmonary pressure ($-30 \, cmH_2O$) and minimal (0 to 3 cmH_2O) or 10 cmH_2O PEEP. Bacteremia seldom occurred in control animals ventilated with low airway pressure, whereas it was found in nearly all animals ventilated with high V_T and a low PEEP. In contrast, ventilation with the same transpulmonary pressure but with 10 cmH_2O PEEP resulted in rates of bacteremia as low as in controls. In a saline-lavaged rabbit lung injury model, mechanical ventilation with a V_T of 12 ml/kg and without PEEP resulted in translocation of intratracheally instilled endotoxin into the systemic circulation, but ventilation with a V_T of 5 ml/kg and a PEEP of 10 cm H_2O did not. The appearance of endotoxin in the blood stream was associated with an increase in plasma TNF-α [57]. Since the gut could be a "motor" of MODS, bacterial and endotoxin translocation caused by mechanical ventilation may play a role in development of MODS [15].

Pulmonary and Systemic Inflammatory Mediators in VILI in Clinical Studies

Elevated levels of pro-inflammatory mediators have been measured in airspace lavage fluid and in the plasma of patients with ARDS. Ranieri and colleagues [11] measured BAL and plasma levels of several pro-inflammatory cytokines in 44 patients with ARDS. At study entry, patients were randomized to receive mechanical ventilation with a conventional strategy (mean V_T of 11.1 ml/kg, mean plateau airway pressure 31 cmH_2O, and mean PEEP of 6.5 cmH_2O), or a protective ventilatory strategy with V_T (7.6 ml/kg) and higher PEEP (14.8 cmH_2O) with a mean plateau airway pressure of 24.6 cmH_2O. PEEP in the latter group was set above the lower inflection point of the respiratory system pressure volume curve. Baseline measurements of cytokines were made at the time of admission (study entry), and were then measured serially for three days. By 36 hours, BAL fluid from patients in the protective ventilation group had significantly fewer polymorphonuclear cells and lower concentrations of TNF-α, IL-1β, IL-6, and IL-8. Plasma levels of IL-6 were also significantly lower in the patients receiving protective ventilation. The NIH ARDS Network study found lower levels of plasma IL-6 at three days in patients ventilated with low V_T compared with conventional V_T [12].

In patients with ARDS, concentration of TNF-α, IL-1β and IL-6 were higher in the arterialized blood (obtained via a wedged Swan-Ganz catheter), as compared with mixed venous blood, suggesting that the lungs in these patients were contributing cytokines to the systemic circulation [58]. Recently, Stuber and colleagues [59] studied patients with ALI and found that switching to conventional mechanical ventilation (V_T of 12 ml/kg, PEEP of 5 cmH_2O) from a lung protective strategy (V_T

of 5 ml/kg, PEEP of 15 cmH2O) was associated with a marked increase in plasma cytokine levels within 1 h, while plasma cytokine levels returned to baseline when lung protective settings was reestablished. In contrast, in 39 patients with normal lungs, without ARDS, Wrigge and colleagues [60] found that ventilation with a high V_T (15 ml/kg) and zero PEEP did not affect plasma levels of either IL-6, TNF-α, IL-1 receptor antagonist, or IL-10. These data suggest that if the lung is normal, mechanical ventilation, even with relatively large V_T, is unlikely to increase alveolar capillary permeability and augment the pulmonary inflammatory response, leading to increased production of inflammatory mediators.

Multiple Organ Dysfunction and VILI in Clinical Studies

There are now prospective data in the literature examining the hypothesis that a protective ventilatory strategy can have an impact on the development of MODS As previously mentioned, Ranieri and colleagues reported that the use of a lung-protective strategy in patients with ARDS attenuated an increase in pulmonary and systemic cytokine levels including TNF-α and IL-6 [11]. In a subsequent *post hoc* analysis (Fig. 2), they found a higher incidence of renal failure in ARDS patients ventilated with conventional ventilation compared with a lung protective strategy. Furthermore, they found a significant correlation between overall MODS score with changes in plasma concentration of a number of inflammatory mediators (IL6, TNF-α, IL-1β and IL-8), which are involved in MODS [13]. Similarly, the NIH ARDS Network reported the results of a randomized, clinical trial comparing a V_T of 12 ml/kg with 6 ml/kg (predicted body weight). They found lower levels of plasma IL-6 in the 6 ml/kg tidal volume group, associated with a greater number of organ failure-free days and a 22% reduction in mortality rate [12]. These data suggest that mechanical ventilation, which is invariably used in the care of patients with ARDS, can increase alveolar capillary permeability and augment the pulmonary inflammatory response, leading to increased production of inflammatory mediators. If these mediators (e.g., cytokines) enter the circulation, they could contribute to the development of MODS. It is important to emphasize that MODS is a complex syndrome, often precipitated and intensified by a series of events rather than a single event. A likely scenario is that there is an ongoing inflammatory response as a result of the persistence of the factors that either initiated or exacerbated the response, and/or failure of intrinsic regulatory mechanisms. Conversely, patients with normal lungs who receive prolonged ventilation (e.g., neuromuscular disease with respiratory failure) would not develop VILI nor MODS.

Implications

In this review, we have focused mainly on the effects of mechanical ventilation on hemodynamics and systemic inflammation, but how might these lead to end organ dysfunction? Recently, it has been shown that inflammatory cytokines/chemokines can modulate apoptosis in various cell types [61] and increased apoptosis has been detected in animal model of CLP [62, 63] as well as in patients dying of sepsis and

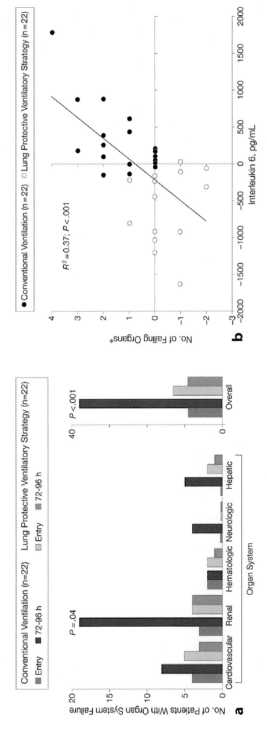

Fig. 2. a. Number of patients with organ system failure in the 2 groups of patients on entry and within 72 hours of mechanical ventilation. Patients may have failure of more than 1 organ system. **b.** Changes in total number of failing organs and in plasma concentration of interleukin 6. Asterisk indicates number of failing organ systems at 72 hours minus number on entry. Dagger indicates change in interleukin 6 derived from value at 36 hours minus entry value. From [13] with permission.

MODS [64]. Imai and colleagues have demonstrated increases in end organ epithelial cell apoptosis after injurious mechanical ventilation in an *in vivo* rabbit ARDS model [65]. Apoptosis might thus be an important down-stream effect in the development of systemic inflammatory response syndrome (SIRS)/MODS caused by VILI in ALI/ARDS, although there are insufficient data to confirm this hypothesis at present.

Conclusion

Based on the paradigm developed in this chapter, it is suggested that in patients with ARDS, VILI plays a crucial role in initiating and/or propagating a systemic inflammatory response leading to MODS. As such, protective ventilatory strategies in concert with other novel therapies could reduce the development of MODS and decrease mortality in mechanically ventilated patients. Furthermore, pharmacological modulation of cellular and molecular sequelae may reduce VILI and/or development of MODS.

References

1. Esteban A, Anzueto A, Frutos F, et al (2002) Characteristics and outcomes in adult patients receiving mechanical ventilation: a 28-day international study. JAMA 287:345–355
2. Slutsky AS, Tremblay LN (1998) Multiple system organ failure. Is mechanical ventilation a contributing factor? Am J Respir Crit Care Med 157:1721–1725
3. Grembowicz KP, Sprague D, McNeil PL (1999) Temporary disruption of the plasma membrane is required for c-fos expression in response to mechanical stress. Mol Biol Cell 10:1247–1257
4. Mourgeon E, Isowa N, Keshavjee S, Zhang X, Slutsky AS, Liu M (2000) Mechanical stretch stimulates macrophage inflammatory protein-2 secretion from fetal rat lung cells. Am J Physiol 279:L699–L706
5. Pugin J, Dunn I, Jolliet P, et al (1998) Activation of human macrophages by mechanical ventilation in vitro. Am J Physiol 275:L1040–L1050
6. Quinn D, Tager A, Joseph PM, Bonventre JV, Force T, Hales CA (1999) Stretch-induced mitogen-activated protein kinase activation and interleukin-8 production in type II alveolar cells. Chest 116:89S–90S
7. Vlahakis NE, Schroeder MA, Limper AH, Hubmayr RD (1999) Stretch induces cytokine release by alveolar epithelial cells in vitro. Am J Physiol 277:L167–L173
8. von Bethmann AN, Brasch F, Nusing R, et al (1998) Hyperventilation induces release of cytokines from perfused mouse lung. Am J Respir Crit Care Med 157:263–272
9. Tremblay L, Valenza F, Ribeiro SP, Li J, Slutsky AS (1997) Injurious ventilatory strategies increase cytokines and c-fos m-RNA expression in an isolated rat lung model. J Clin Invest 99:944–952
10. Chiumello D, Pristine G, Slutsky AS (1999) Mechanical ventilation affects local and systemic cytokines in an animal model of acute respiratory distress syndrome. Am J Respir Crit Care Med 160:109–116
11. Ranieri VM, Suter PM, Tortorella C, et al (1999) Effect of mechanical ventilation on inflammatory mediators in patients with acute respiratory distress syndrome: a randomized controlled trial. JAMA 282:54–61

12. The Acute Respiratory Distress Syndrome Network (2000) Ventilation with lower tidal volumes as compared with traditional tidal volumes for acute lung injury and the acute respiratory distress syndrome. N Engl J Med 342:1301–1308
13. Ranieri VM, Giunta F, Suter PM, Slutsky AS (2000) Mechanical ventilation as a mediator of multisystem organ failure in acute respiratory distress syndrome. JAMA 284:43–44
14. Amato MB, Barbas CS, Medeiros DM, et al (1998) Effect of a protective-ventilation strategy on mortality in the acute respiratory distress syndrome. N Engl J Med 338:347–354
15. Carrico CJ, Meakins JL, Marshall JC, Fry D, Maier RV (1986) Multiple-organ-failure syndrome. Arch Surg 121:196–208
16. Le Gall JR, Klar J, Lemeshow S, et al (1996) The Logistic Organ Dysfunction system. A new way to assess organ dysfunction in the intensive care unit. ICU Scoring Group. JAMA 276:802–810
17. De Backer D (2000) The effects of positive end-expiratory pressure on the splanchnic circulation. Intensive Care Med 26:361–363
18. Pinsky MR (2002) Recent advances in the clinical application of heart-lung interactions. Curr Opin Crit Care 8:26–31
19. Russell JA, Phang PT (1994) The oxygen delivery/consumption controversy. Approaches to management of the critically ill. Am J Respir Crit Care Med 149:533–537
20. Fessler HE, Brower RG, Wise RA, Permutt S (1991) Effects of positive end-expiratory pressure on the gradient for venous return. Am Rev Respir Dis 143:19–24
21. Jardin F, Farcot JC, Boisante L, Curien N, Margairaz A, Bourdarias JP (1981) Influence of positive end-expiratory pressure on left ventricular performance. N Engl J Med 304:387–392
22. Robotham JL, Lixfeld W, Holland L, et al (1980) The effects of positive end-expiratory pressure on right and left ventricular performance. Am Rev Respir Dis 121:677–683
23. Brienza N, Revelly JP, Ayuse T, Robotham JL (1995) Effects of PEEP on liver arterial and venous blood flows. Am J Respir Crit Care Med 152:504–510
24. Dorinsky PM, Hamlin RL, Gadek JE (1987) Alterations in regional blood flow during positive end-expiratory pressure ventilation. Crit Care Med 15:106–113
25. Matuschak GM, Pinsky MR, Rogers RM (1987) Effects of positive end-expiratory pressure on hepatic blood flow and performance. J Appl Physiol 62:1377–1383
26. Sha M, Saito Y, Yokoyama K, Sawa T, Amaha K (1987) Effects of continuous positive-pressure ventilation on hepatic blood flow and intrahepatic oxygen delivery in dogs. Crit Care Med 15:1040–1043
27. Aneman A, Eisenhofer G, Fandriks L, et al (1999) Splanchnic circulation and regional sympathetic outflow during peroperative PEEP ventilation in humans. Br J Anaesth 82:838–842
28. Trager K, Radermacher P, Georgieff M (1996) PEEP and hepatic metabolic performance in septic shock. Intensive Care Med 22:1274–1275
29. Kiefer P, Nunes S, Kosonen P, Takala J (2000) Effect of positive end-expiratory pressure on splanchnic perfusion in acute lung injury. Intensive Care Med 26:376–383
30. Fournell A, Scheeren TW, Schwarte LA (1997) Oxygenation of the intestinal mucosa in anaesthetized dogs is attenuated by intermittent positive pressure ventilation (IPPV) with positive end-expiratory pressure (PEEP). Adv Exp Med Biol 428:385–389
31. Seeman-Lodding H, Haggmark S, Jern C, et al (1999) Systemic levels and preportal organ release of tissue-type plasminogen activator are enhanced by PEEP in the pig. Acta Anaesthesiol Scand 43:623–633
32. Kiiski R, Takala J, Kari A, Milic-Emili J (1992) Effect of tidal volume on gas exchange and oxygen transport in the adult respiratory distress syndrome. Am Rev Respir Dis 146:1131–1135
33. Thorens JB, Jolliet P, Ritz M, Chevrolet JC (1996) Effects of rapid permissive hypercapnia on hemodynamics, gas exchange, and oxygen transport and consumption during mechanical ventilation for the acute respiratory distress syndrome. Intensive Care Med 22:182–191
34. Brofman JD, Leff AR, Munoz NM, Kirchhoff C, White SR (1990) Sympathetic secretory response to hypercapnic acidosis in swine. J Appl Physiol 69:710–717

35. Rose CE Jr, Althaus JA, Kaiser DL, Miller ED, Carey RM (1983) Acute hypoxemia and hypercapnia: increase in plasma catecholamines in conscious dogs. Am J Physiol 245:H924–H929

36. Cardenas VJ Jr, Zwischenberger JB, Tao W, et al (1996) Correction of blood pH attenuates changes in hemodynamics and organ blood flow during permissive hypercapnia. Crit Care Med 24:827–834

37. Sitbon P, Teboul JL, Duranteau J, Anguel N, Richard C, Samii K (2001) Effects of tidal volume reduction in acute respiratory distress syndrome on gastric mucosal perfusion. Intensive Care Med 27:911–915

38. Dos Santos CC, Slutsky AS (2000) Invited review: mechanisms of ventilator-induced lung injury: a perspective. J Appl Physiol 89:1645–1655

39. Fisher AB, Chien S, Barakat AI, Nerem RM (2001) Endothelial cellular response to altered shear stress. Am J Physiol 281:L529–L533

40. Liu M, Post M (2000) Invited review: mechanochemical signal transduction in the fetal lung. J Appl Physiol 89:2078–2084

41. Uhlig S (2002) Ventilation-induced lung injury and mechanotransduction: stretching it too far? Am J Physiol 282:L892–L896

42. Waters CM, Sporn PH, Liu M, Fredberg JJ (2002) Cellular biomechanics in the lung. Am J Physiol 283:L503–L509

43. Vlahakis NE, Hubmayr RD (2000) Invited review: plasma membrane stress failure in alveolar epithelial cells. J Appl Physiol 89:2490–2496

44. Dunn I, Pugin J (1999) Mechanical ventilation of various human lung cells in vitro: identification of the macrophage as the main producer of inflammatory mediators. Chest 116:95S–97S

45. Gan L, Doroudi R, Hagg U, Johansson A, Selin-Sjogren L, Jern S (2000) Differential immediate-early gene responses to shear stress and intraluminal pressure in intact human conduit vessels. FEBS Lett 477:89–94

46. Gan L, Miocic M, Doroudi R, Selin-Sjogren L, Jern S (2000) Distinct regulation of vascular endothelial growth factor in intact human conduit vessels exposed to laminar fluid shear stress and pressure. Biochem Biophys Res Commun 272:490–496

47. Haitsma JJ, Uhlig S, Goggel R, Verbrugge SJ, Lachmann U, Lachmann B (2000) Ventilator-induced lung injury leads to loss of alveolar and systemic compartmentalization of tumor necrosis factor-alpha. Intensive Care Med 26:1515–1522

48. Imai Y, Kawano T, Iwamoto S, Nakagawa S, Takata M, Miyasaka K (1999) Intratracheal anti-tumor necrosis factor-alpha antibody attenuates ventilator-induced lung injury in rabbits. J Appl Physiol 87:510–515

49. Narimanbekov IO, Rozycki HJ (1995) Effect of IL-1 blockade on inflammatory manifestations of acute ventilator-induced lung injury in a rabbit model. Exp Lung Res 21:239–254

50. Held HD, Boettcher S, Hamann L, Uhlig S (2001) Ventilation-induced chemokine and cytokine release is associated with activation of nuclear factor-kappa B and is blocked by steroids. Am J Respir Crit Care Med 163:711–716

51. Tutor JD, Mason CM, Dobard E, Beckerman RC, Summer WR, Nelson S (1994) Loss of compartmentalization of alveolar tumor necrosis factor after lung injury. Am J Respir Crit Care Med 149:1107–1111

52. Kurahashi K, Kajikawa O, Sawa T, et al (1999) Pathogenesis of septic shock in Pseudomonas aeruginosa pneumonia. J Clin Invest 104:743–750

53. Greene KE, Wright JR, Steinberg KP, et al (1999) Serial changes in surfactant-associated proteins in lung and serum before and after onset of ARDS. Am J Respir Crit Care Med 160:1843–1850

54. Doyle IR, Bersten AD, Nicholas TE (1997) Surfactant proteins-A and -B are elevated in plasma of patients with acute respiratory failure. Am J Respir Crit Care Med 156:1217–1229

55. Nahum A, Hoyt J, Schmitz L, Moody J, Shapiro R, Marini JJ (1997) Effect of mechanical ventilation strategy on dissemination of intratracheally instilled Escherichia coli in dogs. Crit Care Med 25:1733–1743

56. Verbrugge SJ, Sorm V, van't Vee A, Mouton JW, Gommers D, Lachmann B (1998) Lung overinflation without positive end-expiratory pressure promotes bacteremia after experimental Klebsiella pneumoniae inoculation. Intensive Care Med. 24:172–177.
57. Murphy DB, Cregg N, Tremblay L, et al (2000) Adverse ventilatory strategy causes pulmonary-to-systemic translocation of endotoxin. Am J Respir Crit Care Med 162:27–33
58. Douzinas EE, Tsidemiadou PD, Pitaridis MT, et al (1997) The regional production of cytokines and lactate in sepsis-related multiple organ failure. Am J Respir Crit Care Med 155:53–59
59. Stuber F, Wrigge H, Schroeder S, et al (2002) Kinetic and reversibility of mechanical ventilation-associated pulmonary and systemic inflammatory response in patients with acute lung injury. Intensive Care Med 28:834–841
60. Wrigge H, Zinserling J, Stuber F, et al (2000) Effects of mechanical ventilation on release of cytokines into systemic circulation in patients with normal pulmonary function. Anesthesiology 93:1413–1417
61. Papathanassoglou ED, Moynihan JA, Ackerman MH (2000) Does programmed cell death (apoptosis) play a role in the development of multiple organ dysfunction in critically ill patients? a review and a theoretical framework. Crit Care Med 28:537–549
62. Hiramatsu M, Hotchkiss RS, Karl IE, Buchman TG (1997) Cecal ligation and puncture (CLP) induces apoptosis in thymus, spleen, lung, and gut by an endotoxin and TNF-independent pathway. Shock 7:247–253
63. Hotchkiss RS, Swanson PE, Cobb JP, Jacobson A, Buchman TG, Karl IE (1997) Apoptosis in lymphoid and parenchymal cells during sepsis: findings in normal and T- and B-cel-deficient mice. Crit Care Med 25:1298–1307
64. Hotchkiss RS, Swanson PE, Freeman BD, et al (1999) Apoptotic cell death in patients with sepsis, shock, and multiple organ dysfunction. Crit Care Med 27:1230–1251
65. Imai Y, Parodo J, Kajikawa O, et al (2003) Injurious mechanical ventilation and end-organ epithelial cell apoptosis and organ dysfunction in an experimental model of ARDS. JAMA 289:2104–2112

ARDS/VILI: Assessment

Chest Wall Mechanics in ARDS

L. Gattinoni, D. Chiumello, and P. Pelosi

Introduction

The respiratory system is composed of the lung and the chest wall, and these two structures are mechanically in series. The chest wall is considered as any part of the body that surrounds the lung, and is composed by two structures in parallel: the rib cage and the abdomen [1]. The sum of the pressures used to inflate the lung and the chest wall represents the total pressure required to inflate the respiratory system. It is assumed that the changes in volume of lung and chest wall are equal to the change in volume of the respiratory system. In this way, any possible blood movement in/out of the chest wall is excluded [1].

In clinical practice, to study total respiratory mechanics and those of its compartments (lung and chest wall), we need to measure the airway, esophageal pressure, and the tidal volume (V_T) excursions. The method most commonly used to compute respiratory mechanics (in this chapter we only refer to the elastance) is the rapid occlusion technique during constant flow inflation [2]. Table 1 shows the most common formulas used to compute the total and the partitioned respiratory mechanics [3].

Table 1. Formulas used to compute total and partitioned elastance

$$E_{rs} = \frac{Paw - Pbs}{\Delta V}$$

$$E_l = \frac{Paw - Pes}{\Delta V}$$

$$E_{cw} = \frac{Pes - Pbs}{\Delta V}$$

$$E_{rc\_rs} = \frac{Paw - Pbs}{\Delta Vrc}$$

$$E_{ab\_rs} = \frac{Paw - Pbs}{\Delta V_{ab}}$$

Paw = Airway pressure; Pbs = Atmospheric pressure; Pes = Esophageal pressure; ΔV = Chest wall volume; ΔVrc = Rib cage volume; ΔVab = Abdominal volume

In this chapter, we will discuss the different types of acute respiratory distress syndrome (ARDS, pulmonary and extrapulmonary) and the consequences of an increase in the intraabdominal pressure (IAP) on the prone position, recruitment maneuver, and hemodynamics.

Pulmonary and Extrapulmonary ARDS

A few years ago, the consensus conference on ARDS stated that: "ARDS could be due to a direct insult (a direct injury on lung cells, ARDSp) or to an indirect insult (a systemic effect of the inflammatory response, ARDSexp)"[4]. At the present time, several studies have showed that ARDSp and ARDSexp have not only different pathogenic pathways but also different respiratory mechanics and morphological aspects.

Pathogenetic Pathways

Direct pulmonary insult has been studied in experimental models by using intra-tracheal instillation of endotoxin [5], complement [6], and tumor necrosis factor (TNF) [7]. After a direct insult, the primary lung structure to be injured is the alveolar epithelium. This damage causes activation of alveolar macrophages and of the inflammatory network, leading to intrapulmonary inflammation. The prevalence of the epithelial damage determines a localization of the pathological abnormality in the intra-alveolar space, with alveolar filling by edema, fibrin, collagen, neutrophilic aggregates, and/or blood, and is often described as pulmonary consolidation.

Indirect pulmonary insult has been studied in experimental models by intravenous [8] or intraperitoneal [9] toxic injection. After an indirect insult, the lung injury originates from the action of inflammatory mediators released from extrapulmonary foci into the systemic circulation. In this case, the first target of damage is the pulmonary vascular endothelial cell, with an increase in vascular permeability and recruitment of monocytes, polymorphonuclear leukocytes, platelets, and other cells. Thus, the pathological alteration due to an indirect insult is primarily microvascular congestion and interstitial edema, with relative sparing of the intra-alveolar spaces.

From these data, it is possible that different cytokine levels in the lung or in serum in ARDSp and ARDSexp will be involved. Chollet-Martin et al. found an increase in bronchoalveolar lavage (BAL) and serum interleukin (IL)-8 in ARDSexp [10] while Bauer et al. found increased levels of serum TNF- only in patients with ARDSexp compared to ARDSp [11].

However, it is worth noting the possible coexistence in the same patients of the two insults: one directly in the lung (as pneumonia) and the other indirectly (through mediator release from extrapulmonary foci) that may mix the model.

Respiratory Mechanics

It is well known that ARDS patients are usually characterized by an increase in respiratory system elastance mainly attributed to an alteration in the lung elastance [12]. However, there are several studies showing that the increase in respiratory system elastance could be due also to an increase in the chest wall elastance [13]. In 16 acute lung injury (ALI)/ARDS patients we found a significant increase in lung and chest wall elastance compared to normal anesthetized subjects. The increase in chest wall elastance could be due to several factors such as a decrease in functional residual capacity (FRC), pleural effusion, and abdominal distension (abdominal hemorrhage, intestinal obstruction, ileus, and ascites). Further, we found that although the respiratory system elastance was similarly increased in both types of ARDS, lung elastance was higher in the ARDSp compared to ARDSexp [14] (Fig 1.). On the contrary, only the ARDSexp patients presented a higher chest wall elastance. Increasing positive end-expiratory pressure (PEEP) in these ARDS patients differently affected the respiratory mechanics: in the ARDSp the respiratory system and lung elastance increased while in the ARDSexp the respiratory system, lung and chest wall elastance decreased. These data suggest that the ARDSp patients present a stiffer lung which does not improve with PEEP, while in ARDSexp the lung and chest wall elastance improve with PEEP. ARDSp is likely characterized by more consolidated areas (i.e., severe alveolar flooding) less responsive to PEEP compared to ARDSexp in which the atelectatic areas are predominant and more responsive to PEEP.

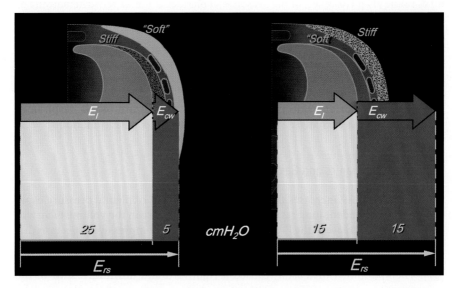

Fig. 1. An example of how pulmonary (left panel) and extrapulmonary (right panel) ARDS may affect the total, lung and chest wall elastance. Ers = total respiratory system elastance; El = lung elastance; Ecw = chest wall elastance.

Morphological Aspects

We retrospectively scored the chest x-rays, performed in a standardized way, in 21 ARDS patients (9 ARDSp and 12 ARDSexp), to identify the amount of 'hazy' and 'diffuse' lung densities – likely representing interstitial edema and compression atelectasis – and patchy densities-likely representing pulmonary consolidations [15]. Patients with ARDSp had an increased number of patchy densities compared to ARDSexp patients.

Goodman et al. studied the difference in morphological aspects at computed tomography (CT) between ARDSp and ARDSexp in the early phase of disease [16]. In ARDSexp the ground glass areas (expression of atelectasis or edema from the inflammatory systemic response) were more than twice as extensive as consolidation (expression of the initial insult inside the alveoli). On the contrary in ARDSp consolidation and ground glass opacification were similarly presented.

Intraabdominal Pressure

The IAP is the pressure generated inside the abdomen and depends on the status of diaphragm, the abdominal wall, and the viscera [17]. The abdomen and its contents should be considered as non-compressive and primarily fluid, that follow Pascal's law. The normal pressure in humans is between 5–15 cmH$_2$O. The two most common methods to measure the IAP are direct measurement of the gastric pressure and the measurement of bladder pressure [18]. The bladder pressure is usually measured by inflating the bladder through a bladder catheter with 50–200 ml of saline [17]. However, in the presence of bladder trauma, pelvic hematoma or in cases of low bladder compliance, the bladder pressure is not a reliable indicator of the IAP and the gastric pressure is better [19].

An increase in IAP can occur in the presence of hemorrhage, ascites, bowel edema, or external compression [17]. The incidence of an increase in the IAP (above 15 cmH$_2$O) varies according to the underlying diseases but seems to be around 30 % in the surgical intensive care population [20].

The most important side effects of an elevated IAP are on: 1) respiratory mechanics and gas exchange; 2) hemodynamics and; 3) edema formation

Respiratory Mechanics and Gas Exchange

The increase in IAP increases the gravitational gradient of pleural pressure especially in the dependent lung regions, inducing an increase in the volume of airway closure, and a decrease in the FRC, with possible risk of compressive atelectasis due to the upward push of the diaphragm to the lung. Mutho et al. evaluated the effect of abdominal distension on the lung and chest wall mechanics in anesthetized pigs [21]. The abdominal distension caused a rightward and downward shift of the pressure volume curve (PV curve) of the respiratory system and the chest wall by a stiffening of the diaphragm/abdomen and by a reduction in lung expansion. Similarly Ranieri et al. found that surgical ARDS patients presented a rightward shift of the thoracic and abdominal PV curves compared to medical ARDS patients, related to abdominal distension [22]. When these patients underwent abdominal decompression, the PV curve of the thorax and abdomen moved upward and leftward.

Our group showed that ARDSexp, due to intraabdominal pathologic conditions, presented a higher IAP compared to ARDSp [14]. We found a direct correlation between the IAP and the chest wall elastance, i.e., patients with a higher IAP have a higher chest wall elastance which reflected the increase stiffness of the thoracic rib cage.

We analyzed the sonographic findings of the abdomen in normal spontaneously breathing subjects, in patients with ARDSexp due to abdominal sepsis, and in patients with ARDSp due to community acquired pneumonia [23]. In the normal subjects it was difficult to recognize the abdominal wall and the gut anatomical structure. In the patients with ARDSexp and with related abdominal problems, the increased dimension and thickness of the gut due to intraluminal debris and fluid and also with reduced peristaltic movements were visible. In the patients with ARDSp, the dimensions of the gut were slightly increased while the gut wall thickness was not increased, without any consistent debris or fluid.

These findings, thus, suggest that in ARDS the increase in respiratory system elastance may be produced by two different mechanisms: in ARDSp a high lung elastance is the major component, whereas in ARDSexp the lung and the chest wall elastance equally contribute to the increase in the respiratory system elastance.

Abdominal distension can also impair gas exchange. Mure et al., evaluating the effects of abdominal distension in anesthetized pigs, found that animals with abdominal distension presented a lower arterial oxygenation, higher ventilation/perfusion (V/Q) heterogeneity and dead space compared to normal animals [24].

We performed a prospective observational multicenter Italian study on IAP in critically ill patients [17]. The IAP was significantly increased in intubated compared to non-intubated patients (14.6±6 vs 12.3±7 cmH$_2$O). Considering three ranges of IAP: patients with IAP < 10 cmH$_2$O, patients with IAP between 10 and 20 cmH$_2$O and patients > 20 cmH$_2$O, the PaO$_2$/FiO$_2$ significantly decreased from 322±138 to 286±126 to 235±136 mm Hg while the PaCO$_2$ did not change.

Hemodynamics

An elevated IAP may cause hypoperfusion, because the diaphragm is pushed upward transmitting the abdominal pressure to the heart and big vessels causing a decrease in cardiac output [17, 20, 24, 25]. Further, several studies have shown a reduction in renal blood flow with consequent increase in serum creatinine due to a direct compression of renal parenchyma or to a compression of renal veins when the IAP was increased [17, 20, 26, 27].

The intracardiac pressures (central venous or wedge pressure) used as an estimation of the preload, could be falsely elevated in the presence of an elevated IAP [17, 20]. Consequently, for a correct evaluation of the preload, the intracardiac pressures should be measured against the intrathoracic pressure and not, as is usually done, against the atmospheric pressure [17, 20]. In such situations the estimation of the preload by the volume indexes should be more accurate.

Edema Formation

Recently we investigated the impact of changes in IAP due to pneumoperitoneum, in healthy animals and in an oleic acid animal model by CT scan analysis (Luecke T, et al, unpublished data). In the healthy group, an IAP of 20 cmH_2O significantly decreased the gas volume compared to IAP of 0 cmH_2O. In the oleic acid group at IAP of 0 cmH_2O the gas volume was lower and despite the edema formation the total lung volume decreased compared to the healthy lung group. This may suggest that the edema increase did not fully compensate for the reduction in gas volume. On raising the IAP to 20 cmH_2O, the tissue increased by almost threefold. The edema formation at the highest IAP was due to concomitant effects: 1) an increase in the central venous pressure, 2) a blood shift from the abdomen to the thorax, and 3) a reduction of edema clearance due to the increase in the pleural pressure.

These data clearly stress the importance of measuring IAP at the bedside in critically ill patients as an invaluable tool to optimize the clinical management.

Prone Position

In clinical practice the prone position is commonly used to improve the arterial oxygenation in ARDS patients [28]. However, the positive effect on gas exchange is present in only 60–70 % of patients. From animal and human data several mechanisms have been proposed to explain how prone positioning may affect gas exchange. The first suggested mechanism was related to an increase in FRC passing from supine to prone position [29]. However, when the FRC was measured it was found not to change between supine and prone [30, 31]. Two human studies evaluated the effect of prone position on the partitioned respiratory mechanics and found an increase in the chest wall elastance [30, 31]. The increase of chest wall elastance was due to a greater rigidity of the rib cage component of the chest wall in prone position compared to the supine because the IAP did not change. The rib cage is constituted by a ventral part (sternal) with a large facility to move compared to the dorsal part (vertebral) [32]. In prone position, the stiffer component of the rib cage (dorsal part) is free to move, whereas the movement of the more complaint (ventral part) is reduced by the bed surface. This can explain the increase in the chest wall elastance. The prone position due to the modification of respiratory mechanics could induce a redistribution of ventilation towards the dependent ventral regions with an overall more homogeneous regional distribution compared to the supine position.

A significant correlation was found between the changes in chest wall elastance and arterial oxygenation between supine and prone position [31]. The greater the stiffness of the dorsal part of the rib cage, the greater the ventilation of the less inflated ventral regions, and the greater the improvement in arterial oxygenation.

Prone positioning may improve arterial oxygenation also by decreasing the V/Q heterogeneity [33]. An elevated IAP is usually present in ARDSexp. Mure et al. found a greater improvement in oxygenation and in V/Q heterogeneity in the presence of elevated IAP compared to a normal IAP [24]. The increase in IAP can increase the gravitational gradient of pleural pressure that became more positive in the dependent lung regions (see above). In the prone position, the pleural pressure in these regions is reduced and the gradient becomes flatter. An attenuation of the vertical gradient of pleural pressure in the prone position means an increase in the transpulmonary pressure (i.e., the real opening alveolar pressure) that might better reopen the atelectatic lung regions. Therefore a greater improvement in gas exchange could be expected especially in the presence of elevated IAP.

Recently, we performed a large prospective trial in 73 patients (51 ARDSp and 22 ARDSexp) with bilateral chest infiltrates, a PaO_2/FiO_2 ratio lower than 200 mmHg with PEEP higher or equal to 5 cmH_2O, and no evidence of cardiac problems [35]. Patients were evaluated daily for a 10-day period for the presence of respiratory failure criteria (the same as entry criteria). Patients who met these criteria were placed in a prone position for 6 hours once a day. The improvement in oxygenation was greater in ARDSexp compared with ARDSp, although the overall mortality was not different between the two groups.

Lim et al. showed that ARDSp and ARDSexp patients showed different time courses of arterial oxygenation during prone positioning [34]. The ARDSexp patients, with more prevalent compressive atelectasis lung regions presented a significant increase in the arterial oxygenation just after 0.5 hour, compared to ARDSp patients. The ARDSp patients, characterized by more prevalent consolidation lung regions were less affected by the increase in transpulmonary pressure obtained by the prone position.

The different time course of oxygenation according to the etiology of ARDS suggests that the mechanisms of oxygenation in the prone position may be multifactorial or time-dependent, or both. An attenuation of the vertical gradients of the pleural pressure, or an increased effective transpulmonary pressure in the dependent lung regions, is obtained immediately as the patients are turned to the prone position. This mechanical benefit could then result in the reversal of compressive atelectasis in ARDSexp, but would not bring about an immediate change in the consolidated lung units in ARDSp. The greater decrease in consolidation densities in the prone position of ARDSexp as compared with ARDSp suggests that the effects of position and the mechanism through which it may improve respiratory function can be different in ARDSp and ARDSexp. In ARDSexp, in which collapse and compression atelectasis together with an increase of intra-abdominal pressure play a major role in inducing hypoxia, the redistribution of atelectasis from dorsal to ventral and possibly the changes in regional transpulmonary pressure may induce an immediate improvement in oxygenation [35]. In ARDSp, in which collapse is likely less relevant, the same mechanism may operate to a lesser degree and possibly the redistribution of ventilation may play an additional role. These two studies reinforce the hypothesis that the mechanism by which prone position improves oxygenation may be different or may operate to different degrees in ARDSp and ARDSexp.

In anesthetized patients during general anesthesia when positioned in prone position, the arterial pressure and cardiac output decrease, raising concerns for ARDS patients. However, in ARDS patients the prone position has not been shown to alter cardiac output [35]. Despite no change in cardiac output during prone position, problems could arise from a possible decrease in splanchnic perfusion due to an increase in IAP. Hering et al. evaluating renal function and gastric to arterial PCO_2 differences in prone position did not find any adverse effects [36]. At the present time we do not know if the prone position can worsen splanchnic perfusion in patients with elevated IAP and cardiovascular instability.

Recruitment

The alveolar derecruitment during mechanical ventilation using a low V_T ventilation strategy can occur due to V/Q heterogeneity or an inadequate level of PEEP to counteract the superimposed pressure, or to the use of high FiO_2. Recruitment maneuvers have been introduced to recruit the lung in ARDS patients (i.e., try to reopen the closed not ventilated lung regions) [37]. However, we must keep in mind that the actual opening pressure is the transpulmonary pressure, which strictly depends on the elastance of the lung and chest wall.

In fact,

transpulmonary pressure = Paw*[El / (El + Ecw)]

in which Paw is the applied airway pressure, El is the lung elastance, and Ecw the chest wall elastance.

Grasso et al. found that responder patients (i.e., patients in which the PaO_2/FiO_2 increases more than 50 %) after application of a recruitment maneuver, applying a continuous positive pressure at 40 cmH_2O for 40 seconds, presented a relatively normal chest wall elastance compared to non-responders [38]. In the responders, the transpulmonary pressure reached was 28, compared to 18 cmH_2O in the non responders.

Our group found that in ARDS the introduction of 3 consecutive sighs per minute, as a recruitment maneuver, at 45 cmH_2O of airway plateau pressure, increased the arterial oxygenation and the end expiratory lung volume [37]. However, when considering ARDSp and ARDSexp, the recruitment maneuver was more effective in ARDSexp. Although the transpulmonary pressure was higher in ARDSp due to a relatively normal chest wall elastance compared to ARDSexp, the obtained lung recruitment was lower in ARDSp. This could be explained by the lower potential for lung recruitment in ARDSp due to a more prevalent alveolar consolidation compared to ARDSexp.

At the present time we do not know of any possible barotrauma induced by recruitment maneuvers. However, recruitment maneuvers are not always beneficial in ARDS patients. Villagrà et al. evaluated the effect of a recruitment maneuver (2 minutes of pressure controlled ventilation at a peak pressure of 50 cmH_2O and PEEP above the upper inflection point) in ARDS patients and found no improvement in gas exchange [39]. Although the recruitment maneuver improved the end expiratory lung volume in these patients, gas exchange did not improved suggesting an alveolar overdistension compared to a 'true recruitment'.

Two problems can arise during the application of a recruitment maneuver as a sustained inflation. The interruption of ventilation may cause hypercapnia with a reduction in the systemic vascular resistance and an increase in cardiac output. On the contrary, the increase in intrathoracic pressure due to the transmission of airway pressure could reduce the preload and/or the increase in the lung volume could increase the afterload with a reduction in the cardiac output. The final hemodynamic effect depends on the balance of these two phenomena. Consequently, in clinical practice in ARDSexp, obese or trauma patients or in all conditions where there is an increase in chest wall elastance, higher airway pressures (>60–70 cmH$_2$O) are necessary to reach an adequate transpulmonary pressure to open up the atelectatic lung regions.

Hemodynamic Interactions

The hemodynamic impact of a given applied airway pressure in ARDS patients depends on two factors: 1) the lung volume and 2) the venous return.

By increasing the lung volume during mechanical ventilation, the blood is squeezed out from the thorax to the periphery, causing a decrease in the preload and an increase in the afterload with a decrease in cardiac output [38].

The effect on venous return is mediated by the changes in the pleural pressure. The pleural pressure (Ppl) is usually estimated by measuring the esophageal pressure and results from the interaction of two structures (the lung and the chest wall). The changes in Ppl due to a given applied airway pressure depends not only on the absolute value of Paw but also on the chest wall and total respiratory system elastance according to the following formula:

$$\Delta Ppl = \Delta Paw * Ecw/Ers \text{ or } Pes/Paw$$

in which Ers is the respiratory system elastance, and Pes the esophageal pressure

To test this formula, we evaluated the volume shift in ARDS patients during a PV curve, as the difference between the gas volume insufflated and the chest wall volume at the same pressure points. The chest wall volume was measured by the optoelectronic plethysmography, a quite recent technique already validated in the ICU [40]. The volume shift varied widely among the patients, ranging from 44 to 133 ml [41]. A linear regression showed that the volume shift could be a function of two factors: 1) the area under the curve of the applied pressure airway pressure vs the inflation time (i.e., the lung volume reached), and 2) the ratio of ΔPes to ΔPaw, indicating that for a given applied pressure to the airways the greater is the increase of Pes and the greater is the absolute volume shift out of the chest wall.

Based on these formula and these data, in patients with a higher chest wall elastance the variations in pleural pressure will be higher compared to patients with normal chest wall elastance. So, the hemodynamic impact of the variations in airway pressure induced by PEEP, recruitment maneuver or V$_T$ will be different in ARDSp or ARDSexp based on the different mechanical characteristics.

Conclusion

In summary, whenever in clinical practice we are faced with a new ARDS patients we should try:
1) to understand which type of ARDS is present
2) to measure the IAP, lung and chest wall elastance
3) to maximize the lung recruitment with adequate airway pressure and also with the prone position, and
4) to apply adequate levels of PEEP to maintain the lung open.

Acknowledgements. The authors would like to thank Dr. M. Quintel, Dr. G. LiBassi and Dr. E. Storelli for their precious collaboration and suggestions.

References

1. Pelosi P, Aliverti A, Dellacà R (2000) Chest wall mechanics in normal subjects and in critically ill patients. Intensivmed 37:341–351
2. D'Angelo E, Robatto FM, Calderini E, Tavola M, Bono D, Milic-Emili J (1991) Pulmonary and chest wall mechanics in anesthetized and paralyzed humans. J Appl Physiol 70:2602–2610
3. Barnas GM, Green MD, Mackenzie CF, et al (1993) Effect of posture on lung and regional chest wall mechanics. Anesthesiology 78:251–259
4. Bernard GR, Artigas A, Brigham KL, et al (1994) The American-European consensus conference on ARDS. Am J Respir Crit Care Med 149:818–824
5. Terashima T, Kanazawa M, Sayama K (1994) Granulocyte colony-stimulating factor exacerbates acute lung injury induced by intratracheal endotoxin in guinea pigs. Am J Respir Crit Care Med 149:1295–1303
6. Shaw JO, Henson PM, Henson J, Webster RO (1980) Lung inflammation induced by complement derived chemotatic fragments in the alveolus. Lab Invest 42:547–558
7. Tutor JD, Mason CM, Dobard E, Beckerman C, Summer WR, Nelson S (1994) Loss of compartimentalization of alveolar tumor necrosis factor after lung unjury. Am J Respir Crit Care Med 149:1107–1111
8. Muller-Leisse C, Klosterhalfen B, Hauptmann S (1993) Computed tomography and histologic results in the early stages of endotoxin-injury lungs as a model for adult respiratory distress syndrome. Invest Radio 28:39–45
9. Seidenfeld JJ, Curtix Mullins R, Fowler SR, Johanson WG (1986) Bacterial infection and acute lung injury in amsters. Am Rev Respir Dis 134:22–26
10. Chollet-Martin S, Montravers P, Gilbert C, et al (1993) High levels of IL-8 in the blood and alveolar spaces in patients with pneumonia and ARDS. Infect Immun 61:4553–4559
11. Bauer TT, Monton C, Torres A, Cabello, et al (2000) Comparison of systemic cytokine levels in patients with acute respiratory distress syndrome, severe pneumonia and controls. Thorax 55:46–52
12. Polese G, Rossi A, Appendini L, Brandi G, Bates JH, Brabdolese (1991) Partitioning of respiratory mechanics in mechanically ventilated patients. J Appl Physiol 71:2425–2433
13. Pelosi P, Cereda M, Foti G, Giacomini M, Pesenti A (1995) Alteration of lung and chest wall mechanics in patients with acute lung injury: effects of positive end-expiratory pressure. Am J Respir Crit Care Med 152:531–537
14. Gattinoni L, Pelosi P, Suter PM, Pedoto A, Vercesi P, Lissoni A (1998) Acute respiratory distress syndrome caused by pulmonary and extrapulmonary disease. Am J Respir Crit Care Med 158:3–11

15. Pelosi P, Brazzi L, Gattinoni L (1999) Diagnostic imaging in acute respiratory distress sindrome. Curr Opin Crit Care 5:9–16
16. Goodman LR, Fumagalli R, Tagliabue P, et al (1999) Adult respiratory distress syndrome due to pulmonary and extrapulmonary causes: CT, clinical and functional correlations. Radiology 213: 545–552
17. Pelosi P, Aspesi M, Gamberoni C, et al (2002) Measuring intra-abdominal pressure in the intensive care setting. Intensivmed 39:509–519
18. Iberti TJ, Kelly KM, Gentili DR, Hirsch S, Benjamin E (1987) A simple technique to accurately determine intra-abdominal pressure. Crit Care Med 15:1140–1142
19. Collee GG, Lomax DM, Ferguson C, Hanson GC (1993) Bedside measurement of intraabdominal pressure (IAP) via an indwelling naso-gastric tube: clinical validation of the technique. Intensive Care Med 19:478–480
20. Malbrain MLNG (1999) Abdominal pressure in the critically ill: measurement and clinical relevance. Intensive Care Med 25:1453–1458
21. Mutoh T, Lamm WJ, Embree LJ, Hildebrandt J, Albert RK (1992) Volume infusion produces abdominal distension, lung compression, and chest wall stiffening in pigs. J Appl Physiol 72:575–582
22. Ranieri VM, Brienza N, Santostasi S, et al (1997) Impairment of lung and chest wall mechanics in patients with acute respiratory distress syndrome: Role of abdominal distension. Am J Respir Crit Care Med 156:1082–1091
23. Pelosi P, Caironi P, Gattinoni L (2001) Pulmonary and extrapulmonary forms of acute respiratory distress syndrome. Semin Respir Crit Care Med 22:254–268
24. Mure M, Glenny RW, Domino KB, Hlastala MP (1998) Pulmonary gas exchange improves in the prone position with abdominal distension. Am J Respir Crit Care 157:1785–1790
25. Cullen DJ, Coyle JP, Teplick R, Long M (1989) Cardiovascular, pulmonary and renal effects of massively increased intra-abdominal pressure in critically ill patients. Crit Care Med 17:118–121
26. Shenasky JH, Gillenwater JY (1972) The renal hemodynamic and functional effects of external counterpressure. Surg Gynecol Obstet 134:253–258
27. Bradley SE, Bradley GP (1947) The effect of increased intra-abdominal pressure on renal function in man. J Clin Invest 26:1010–1020
28. Gattinoni L, Tognoni G, Pesenti A, et al (2001) Effect of prone position on the survival of patients with acute respiratory failure. N Engl J Med 345: 568–573
29. Phiel MA, Brown RS (1976) Use of extreme position changes in acute respiratory failure. Crit Care Med 4:13–14
30. Guerin C, Badet M, Rosselli S, et al (1999) Effects of prone position on alveolar recruitment and oxygenation in acute lung injury. Intensive Care Med 25:1222–1230
31. Pelosi P, Tubiolo D, Mascheroni D, et al (1998) Effects of the prone position on respiratory mechanics and gas exchange during acute lung injury. Am J Respir Crit Care Med 157:1–7
32. Osmon GO. Functional anatomy of the chest wall. In Roussos (ed) The Thorax, 2nd ed. Marcel Dekker, New York, pp:413–443
33. Lamm WJ, Graham MM, Albert RK (1994) Mechanism by which the prone position improves oxygenation in acute lung injury. Am J Respir Crit Care Med 150:184–193
34. Lim CM, Koh Y, Chin JY, et al (1999) Respiratory and haemodynamic effects of the prone position at two different levels of PEEP in a canine acute lung injury model. Eur Respir J 13:163–168
35. Pelosi P, Brazzi L, Gattinoni L (2002) Prone position in acute respiratory distress syndrome. Eur Respir J 20:1017–1028
36. Hering R, Wrigge H, Vorwerk R, et al (2001) The effects of prone positioning on intraabdominal pressure and cardiovascular and renal function in patients with acute lung injury. Anesth Analg 92:1226–1231
37. Pelosi P, Cadringher P, Bottino N, et al (1999) Sigh in acute respiratory distress syndrome. Am J Respir Crit Care Med 159:872–880

38. Grasso S, Mascia L, Del Turco M, et al (2002) Effects of recruiting maneuvers in patients with acute respiratory ditstress syndrome ventilated with protective ventilatory strategy. Anesthesiology 96:795–802
39. Villagrà A, Ochagavia A, Vatua S, et al (2002) Recruitment maneuvers during lung protective ventilation in acute respiratory distress syndrome. Am J Respir Crit Care Med 165:165–170
40. Aliverti A, Dellaca R, Pelosi P, Chiumello D, Pedotti A, Gattinoni L (2000) Optoelectornic plethysmography in intensive care patients. Am J Respir Crit Care Med 161:1564–1552
41. Chiumello D, Aliverti A, Dellaca' R, Carlesso E, Gattinoni L (2002) The blood shift during the pressure volume curve. Crit Care 6 (suppl 1):P10 (abst)

Targets in Mechanical Ventilation for ARDS

B. P. Kavanagh

Introduction

The conventional aims of mechanical ventilation are to provide adequate oxygenation, carbon dioxide (CO_2) clearance and relieve work of breathing. An additional aim is the recruitment of lung tissue based on multiple animal experiments and some clinical experiments, although this could not be considered a conventional aim at present. A final aim is to prevent multiple organ failure and death, although the appropriate means or targets necessary to achieve this are not at this stage validated for use by the bedside physician. In addition to providing benefit, an aim must be to prevent harm. In this context, the clinician tries to avoid barotrauma, multiple organ dysfunction, atelectasis, hemodynamic impairment, and patient ventilator asynchrony. This chapter will review the key conventional targets and some potential future targets. The advantages of each target will be reviewed and finally the 'trade off' of competing ventilation targets will be discussed. Although critically important, titration towards ventilator-patient interactions and sedation are beyond the scope of this chapter.

Titration against Targets

Titrating towards a parameter in the ICU suggests that the parameter is valid (a worthy goal), and that the clinician balances the risks and benefits of such titration. In terms of oxygenation, ICU clinicians opt for similar qualitative targets; however the quantitative variability is large [1]. It is anticipated that among other – less 'established' – ventilatory targets, the variability may be greater.

Oxygenation as a Target

Adequacy of tissue oxygenation is a key aim in mechanical ventilation. However, although measurement of arterial oxygen tension is a valid, reproducible standard at the bedside, the overall aim, of course is adequacy of tissue oxygenation. Thus, arterial oxygenation should be viewed as an intermediate therapeutic target 10 [2], that is necessary – but not sufficient – as an end-point in targeting mechanical ventilation.

Measures of arterial oxygenation can be characterized by whether they take account of ventilatory parameters, oxygen delivery or tissue oxygen supply balance.

Measures Independent of Ventilatory Parameters

Arterial oxygen saturation is continuously available at the bedside and is a sensitive and robust parameter. An oxygen content measured with a co-oximeter is more meaningful when measuring venous oxygen levels, and is currently available as a continuous parameter. Although these measures provide a good idea of the oxygen content, once the number approaches 100% there can still be a profound intrapulmonary shunt that is detectable only by changes in arterial oxygen tension. Continuous PaO_2 is measurable with bedside arterial blood gas sampling, or by use of intra-arterial opthode devices. The latter technology, especially in small children or in adults with significant peripheral vascular disease, may be limited by the relative dimensions of the intra-arterial device, and the diameter of the artery. In terms of titrating, for example, inspired oxygen fraction (FiO_2) or positive end-expiratory pressure (PEEP), pulse oximetry oxygen saturation (SpO_2) is insensitive when above 94–96% because significant shunt can exist with PaO_2 values of 9–50 kPa (I kPa = 7.5 mmHg), all of which correspond to a SpO_2 of 100%. Therefore, when using SpO_2 for titration, the process must commence with SpO_2 in the range of 90–92%, so that increases in oxygen tension can be appreciated. PaO_2 can also be used, and is highly sensitive to improvements in oxygenation (calculation of the A-aO_2 differences might be more sensitive to reductions in ventilation/perfusion [V/Q] mismatch, although unless automated, it is somewhat cumbersome). The limitations, in the absence of an indwelling analyzer, are the times required for sampling and laboratory (or 'point of care') processing.

Markers Incorporating Ventilatory Parameters

The ratio of the partial pressure of arterial oxygen (PaO_2) to the fraction of inspired oxygen (FiO_2) was initially devised as an entry criteria definition for oxygenation impairment in ARDS by a Consensus Conference group10 [3]. This is extremely useful in the sense that when FiO_2 is altered, this alteration is factored into the picture. Thus PaO_2 has far more meaning with the physician knows the value of the FiO_2. In addition, although mean airway pressure is not incorporated into the PaO_2/FiO_2 quotient, alterations in PEEP or mean airway pressure will be reflected in a changed PaO_2/FiO_2 ratio. This translates into a useful index, because if the PEEP or mean airway pressure has been increased, and this increase is accompanied by a 'better', i.e., higher, PaO_2/FiO_2 ratio), this indicates a successful result of the pressure alteration (e.g., successful recruitment).

A potential advance on the PaO_2/FiO_2 ratio is the oxygenation index. This was initially developed for pediatrics, and is a composite quotient taking account of three parameters (FiO_2, mean airway pressure, and PaO_2), and thus provides – in theory – a more robust sense of the gas exchange efficiency of the lung. It is expressed as:

$$\text{Oxygenation index} = \frac{(FiO_2 \times \text{mean airway pressure} \times 100)}{PaO_2}$$

There are several important differences between the PaO_2/FiO_2 ratio and the oxygenation index. First, an increased PaO_2/FiO_2 ratio indicates 'better' oxygenation, whereas an increase in the oxygenation index indicates a *worsening* of the oxygenation status. Second, where the oxygenation index is increased (worsened), this may reflect a change in either mean airway pressure or FiO_2, in contrast to the PaO_2/FiO_2 ratio where mean airway pressure is ignored. Although the oxygenation index may be a superior 'integrated' index of the oxygenation efficiency of the lungs during mechanical ventilation, there are important gaps in our knowledge. We do not know the relative importance of incremental alterations of the three parameters, nor do we understand whether they have linear relationships. In this sense the formula is empiric, not derived. Finally, it is possible that certain conditions exist that render the oxygenation index unsuitable. For example, with excessive mean airway pressure leading to over inflation, the oxygenation index may become disproportionately higher. In such a situation, considering the oxygenation index only, without regard to its individual elements, could be interpreted as a worsening of the underlying physiology, suggesting that higher FiO_2 or mean airway pressure are required, as opposed to the correct option, i.e., lowering the mean airway pressure.

Measures Incorporating Global Perfusion

Global O_2 delivery (DO_2)

This parameter requires measurement of cardiac output and arterial oxygen content. This might be a logical target for oxygenation because it involves delivery apart from just oxygenation of blood, but it requires the presence of a pulmonary artery catheter, or other accurate measure of cardiac output. However, in many groups of critically ill patients (e.g., those with sepsis), cardiac output is extremely high. Thus, from the outset, provided SpO_2 is above say 90%, it is obvious that measures to increase global DO_2 do not have any bearing on normal physiology. Therefore, global DO_2 is often far greater than normal values before any titration is commenced. Furthermore, the clinician is interested in local conditions at the organ or cellular level, rather than global delivery.

Mixed venous O_2 saturation (SvO_2)

This reflects the difference between global DO_2 and global oxygen consumption (VO_2) and is a surrogate marker for oxygen extraction by the tissues. While theoretically attractive as a marker of true 'adequacy' of DO_2, the SvO_2 suffers from several difficulties. First, any faulty assumptions – see above – that apply to DO_2 apply also to SvO_2. Second, there are inherent flaws due to mathematical coupling that may invalidate SvO_2 as a measure of global VO_2. This flaw has been demonstrated by comparing calculated vs. measured VO_2 [4]. Finally, phenomena such as flow weighted averaging (e.g., minor contributions from vulnerable vascular beds are diluted in the global cardiac output), and non-contribution of specific tissue venous outflow, can render the global SvO_2 insensitive to local oxygen supply-demand imbalance.

Measures of Tissue Oxygenation

Gastric Tonometry

Of all the tonometric methods, gastric tonometry has been the best validated and several studies suggest that hemodynamic management driven by gastric tonometry is a logical approach in critically ill patients. The principles of tonometry are that gastric mucosal intracellular pH (pHi) is reflected in the gastric muscosal intracellular CO_2, which can be deduced using a variety of saline or aero-tonometric techniques. It has been suggested that correction for arterial CO_2 level, such that titration against ($PiCO_2$-$PaCO_2$) instead of titration against $PiCO_2$ alone, is optimal, in order to correct for fluctuations in arterial CO_2 tension. Gastric tonometry would ideally represent a composite marker of metabolic demands balanced against the local supply of tissues. In principle, this would be an excellent composite measure of oxygen content, delivery and consumption at the local level. However, the caveats include adequacy of sampling, regional variation, measurement and methodologic concerns, as well as the assumption that indeed the gastric mucosa truly reflects vulnerable tissue beds. The technique has been used in weaning from mechanical ventilation, but does not replace the established markers of weaning success (e.g., f/V_T ratio) [5]. Nonetheless, the differences in intramucosal oxygen supply-demand status associated with successful vs. failed weaning attempts underline the importance of integrated systemic markers of respiratory distress [5].

Near Infrared Spectroscopy (NIRS)

This is a technique that measures an aggregate index of tissue oxygenation and has been standardized for a variety of tissues including the brain10 [6]. NIRS reflects tissue oxygen status in a global manner but regional differences cannot be reliably deduced. In addition, it is not really understood what NIRS represents and the technology requires standardization on a regular basis. Although not reported in ARDS, it has been studied in neonatal respiratory failure to assess high frequency oscillatory ventilation (HFO) [7].

In summary, although all the above measures of oxygenation assessment are in use in critical care, there is really no good assessment as to what constitutes the optimal measure of tissue oxygenation. There does, however, appear to be a consensus that an oxygen saturation of > 90% is a reasonable target provided that it can be safely achieved. In the neonatal critical care literature, established criteria for extracorporeal membrane oxygenation (ECMO) are based on the oxygenation index, i.e., recognition of the concept that despite a toxic level of FiO_2 and damaging levels of mean airway pressure that the resultant PaO_2 (preductal) is inadequate for the neonatal brain. In adult critical care, such criteria are not as well established. Finally, although there are multiple modalities for monitoring and titration of tissue oxygenation on the horizon, the last consensus conference concluded that clinical assessment of oxygenation relied, for now, on bedside assessment [8].

Carbon Dioxide as a Target

Permissive Hypercapnia

Mechanical ventilation has traditionally been utilized to assist in the appearance of carbon dioxide as a respiratory waste gas. Limitation of V_T or inspiratory pressure to protect the lungs against excessive mechanical stretch was introduced, initially by Wung et al. [9] for neonatal hypoxic respiratory failure, and subsequently by Hickling et al. [10, 11]. In these situations, the $PaCO_2$ was allowed to become elevated, and the idea that mild to moderate hypercapnia was not necessarily a harmful entity but was worth tolerating in order to spare physical ventilator-induced lung injury (VILI) became popular. This was termed 'permissive hypercapnia' [10]. The limitations to hypercapnia have been reviewed in detail [12, 13] and the technique of permissive hypercapnia does appear to be associated with improved patient outcome, although this is not proven. The ranges of permissive hypercapnia that should be tolerated are difficult to assess. In Hickling's studies $PaCO_2$ values of over 13 kPa were noted in some patients (with concomitant pH values below 7.1) [10, 11]. In the ARDSNet study where low stretch ventilation was utilized, the mean CO_2 was higher in the low stretch group than in the high stretch group [14]. However, although statistically significant, the magnitude of the between-group difference was small, making the effect of $PaCO_2$ difficult to interpret.

Therapeutic Hypercapnia

A new concept has arisen in critical care investigation termed 'therapeutic hypercapnia'. This is defined as the deliberate induction of hypercapnia with the potential for therapeutic benefits over and above those that might be associated with a reduction of lung stretch [15, 16]. Multiple mechanisms have been suggested whereby elevated $PaCO_2$ *per se* might be associated with benefit in the critically ill.

Carbon Dioxide as a Ventilatory Target

Currently, laboratory – not clinical – evidence only exists suggesting that therapeutic hypercapnia might be beneficial. This however, must be seen in the light of potential detrimental effects. In terms of permissive hypercapnia, the primary target is V_T or airway pressure limitation, and the CO_2 is not seen as a target as much as a measure to be tolerated. Several clinical studies have shown beneficial effects of ventilatory strategies that involve the development of mild to moderate arterial hypercapnia [10, 11, 14, 17, 18]. Conversely, traditional studies of ARDS associated with limitation of V_T or inspiratory pressure have not shown a beneficial effect of hypercapnia, and one study suggested (although without direct evidence) that hypercapnic acidosis may increase the incidence of renal failure [19].

The experimental evidence relating to therapeutic hypercapnia can be divided into supportive and nonsupportive evidence. The supportive evidence is as follows:

- Pulmonary: a variety of lung models demonstrate that ambient hypercapnic acidosis protects against reperfusion injury [20], stretch induced injury *in vitro*, stretch induced injury *ex vivo* [21] and *in vivo* [22] as well as reperfusion injury *in vivo* [23].
- Central nervous system: In terms of brain protection, there is evidence that additional CO_2 protects against experimental neonatal cerebral ischemia [24].
- Cardiac: Nomura et al. have demonstrated that hypercapnic acidosis is associated with improved myocardial performance following ischemia-reperfusion [25].

In addition, the use of pH-stat CO_2 management during cardiopulmonary bypass (associated with increased administration of CO_2) results in improved cardiac and neurological parameters in children undergoing cardiopulmonary bypass for correction of congenital heart disease [26].

These potentially positive effects must be balanced by the emerging evidence of adverse effects. First, Holmes et al. have demonstrated that although hypercapnia increases retinal oxygenation, it may also increase neovascularization of the retina and thus predispose neonates to retinopathy of prematurity [27]. Although not the primary focus of their study, the more striking finding was the far higher mortality associated with the administration of CO_2. While this might not occur in adult subjects, or be relevant during mechanical ventilation, it is extremely disturbing and is thus far unexplained. Second, the issue of nitration is important. Nitration, resulting from the reaction of peroxynitrite with proteins (characteristically, on tyrosine residues), sometimes results in an alteration of protein function. Zhu et al. have demonstrated that in cultured epithelial cells, introduction of carbon dioxide increases nitration of surfactant protein-A and results in a worsening of the ability of that protein to aggregate lipids [28]. Important caveats include the fact that the solutions were all buffered to normal pH, and the study was not so much one of hypercapnia, as opposed to correction of hypocapnia. In addition, Lang et al. have demonstrated similar findings – increased nitration – in cultured epithelial cells stimulated by lipopolysaccharide (LPS) [29]. These last two studies may be particularly important because of the data demonstrating that nitrotyrosine formation in patients with ARDS is common, and is associated with adverse effects on complex plasma proteins involved in free radical scavenging and thrombosis [30]. Thus, while titrated hypercapnia may be tolerated by clinicians, it may not be universally tolerated by their patients; in the context of ARDS or critical illness these caveats must be borne in mind.

Hypercapnic Acidosis – Targets for Buffering

Hypercapnic acidosis is accompanied immediately by a degree of tissue buffering with chloride shift and elevation of extracellular bicarbonate. Following this, renal correction takes place and the pH is buffered toward 7.4. However, metabolic acidosis and/or renal failure are common in the critically ill and buffering mechanisms are frequently non-functional or inefficient. The situation can be worsened with dilutional acidosis from resuscitation with bicarbonate free fluids or infusion of total perenteral nutrition. Nonetheless, buffering has been recommended by many authors but its clinical value is unproven. In fact, there is evidence that it may be harmful. First, buffering of hypercapnic acidosis in *ex vivo* lung ischemia perfusion is associated with worsening of injury, i.e., ablation of the beneficial effects of hypercapnic acidosis in this model [31]. Second, although perhaps not applicable to hypercapnic acidosis, buffering of metabolic acidosis is associated with augmentation of introduction of endogenous acids [32] as has been demonstrated experimentally [33] and in diabetic ketoacidosis in humans. Finally, *in vitro* effects demonstrate that CO_2 augmented protein nitration may have been enhanced by buffering of the experimental medium [29,30].

In summary, there are advantages and disadvantages associated with experimental models of hypercapnia. Whereas moderate levels of hypercapnia have been associated with improved outcome, the hypercapnia is as a result of primary reductions of tidal pressure or volume. The potential for adverse outcome, and the lack of clinical study, suggests that whereas permissive hypercapnia may be an appropriate strategy, clinical application of deliberate (therapeutic) hypercapnia is not currently appropriate.

Hypocapnia During Mechanical Ventilation

Whereas hypercapnia may have direct or indirect beneficial effects as indicated above, hypocapnia has very few beneficial effects except in the setting of life threatening incipient brain stem herniation or (in neonates, particularly) critical pulmonary hypertension. Aside from these two definite beneficial applications [34], there are multiple adverse effects including tissue ischemia, impaired oxygenation and oxygen delivery, increased metabolic demand, bronchospasm, surfactant inactivation [34]. Thus, whereas hypercapnia may or may not be a worthwhile tradeoff against mechanical injury, hypocapnia in the absence of a specific indication is never an appropriate clinical target.

Positive End-Expiratory Pressure (PEEP)

Since its proposal by Alan K. Laws in Toronto in the late 1960s, and subsequent publication [35], there have been many descriptions of the titration of PEEP. For the bedside clinician, PEEP is utilized in an attempt to increase the FRC, and has the potential to achieve the following goals:
- Improved oxygenation (permitting lowered FiO_2)
- Improved compliance
- Improved hemodynamic status (reduced pulmonary vascular resistance, reduced left ventricular afterload)

- Reduced stretch-induced lung injury (and concomitant lung-to-systemic release of inflammatory factors)
- Elimination of auto-PEEP

While these goals are admirable, they need to be weighed in the context of the potential deleterious effects of excessive PEEP including:
- Barotrauma
- Reduced compliance (if over-inflated)
- Impaired hemodynamic status (reduced right – and maybe left – ventricular preload)

The effects of PEEP on oxygenation and hemodynamics occur rapidly with changes in PEEP, and, therefore, are well appreciated by any bed-side intensivist. An early attempt to titrate the beneficial effects of PEEP on oxygenation against the deleterious effects on hemodynamics represented one of the first attempts to integrate several key ICU parameters in ICU patients [36]. In terms of clinical trials of the application of PEEP in ARDS, three studies are especially important. Amato et al demonstrated that maintenance of PEEP at a level greater than the LIP in a PV curve, as well as utilizing small V_T, was associated with a significantly better survival compared with a strategy consisting of lower PEEP plus higher V_T [17]. Application of 'prophylactic' PEEP was not associated with improved outcome in ARDS [37], and preliminary data from a recently completely study suggest that use of PEEP to induce recruitment is not associated with improved outcome 10[38]. The full data from this study are not yet available, and it is not clear that the applied PEEP resulted in lung recruitment 10[38].

However, several issues have become prominent since then. First, patients with ARDS represent a heterogeneous population in terms of the etiology of their respiratory failure, as well as the 'morphology' of the lung injury. Although most acute forms of lung injury are similar at a microscopic (i.e., histologic) level, wider utilization of bedside respiratory mechanics and CT scanning [39] has increased our appreciation of different categories of ARDS [40]. Indeed Gattinoni et al. have suggested that the etiology of ARDS is related to the characterization of the subsequent lung mechanics, wherein 'pulmonary' etiology (e.g., aspiration, primary pneumonia) results in ARDS associated with consolidated, non-recruitable lung, whereas 'non-pulmonary' etiology (e.g., sepsis) results in recruitable lung [41]. Second, the protection against stretch-induced lung injury afforded by PEEP is largely accepted in the laboratory literature, spanning multiple experimental models of VILI [42, 43]. However, this is far from obvious in the clinical environment, given the mixed outcomes from clinical studies. In this context, timing may be extremely important. A recent clinical study [45], demonstrated that the ability to recruit lungs depends on the timing of the efforts: recruitment is easier in the setting of early lung injury, and is more difficult when injury is more established.

In a recent provocative article, Rouby et al. developed a paradigm for characterizing patients with ARDS [40]. In that paper, the authors outline the importance of early assessment of CT-based morphology and bedside compliance in patients with ARDS. Following this, they outline an approach to optimization of PEEP, based on the slope of the PV curve, as well as the values of the lower and upper inflection points [40]. The rationale for this approach is largely based on their division of ARDS into two basic populations. In cases with diffuse hyperdensities accompanied by a 'high' LIP (>5 cmH2O) and a 'non-compliant' PV curve (slope <<50 ml/cmH2O), higher levels of PEEP are likely to be necessary, and are unlikely to cause problematic hyperinflation. Conversely, where the hyperdensities are focal and accompanied by a 'low' LIP (<5 cmH2O) and a 'compliant' PV curve (slope >50 ml/cmH2O), lower levels of PEEP are likely to be optimal; however, higher levels are likely to cause hyperinflation with the potential for barotrauma.

Finally, the 'titration' of PEEP against either oxygenation (or recruitment) must take into account the experimental findings of Rimensberger et al. [46] who confirmed theoretical predictions based on the differences between the inspiratory *vs.* expiratory limbs of the PV curve. They reported that whereas high levels of airway pressure (PEEP or continuous positive airway pressure [CPAP]) may be required to 'open' collapsed lungs in an experimental model, far lower levels of PEEP are required to maintain this opened -'recruited'- state. Thus, the early need for high levels of PEEP may not be maintained. Thus, one should not set a high level of PEEP and leave the bedside. Rather, one should apply a high level of PEEP or CPAP (sometimes to very high levels as tolerated by the hemodynamic status), and when improved oxygenation is attained, convert to a lower (but still elevated) level of PEEP, and thereafter titrating downwards to a 'stable' level of PEEP. This process may need to be repeated to progressively higher levels of 'stable' PEEP if oxygenation deteriorates during downward titration of 'stable' PEEP. The clinician will only discover this for each patient by regular – and repeated – titration.

In summary, if oxygenation is the chosen surrogate for recruitment, regular titration of PEEP should be commenced early in the ICU course, and be guided by the morphology and mechanics.

Tidal Volume and Plateau Pressure

Recent clinical trials have provided contradictory results relating to the optimal V_T, plateau pressure, and associated PEEP [14, 17, 19, 47, 48]. Whereas three of these studies found no impact of ventilatory strategy on outcome, two studies did. The clearest evidence of effect has been provided by the studies of Amato et al. [17] and the ARDSnet group [14]. The study by Amato et al. reported that relatively low V_T combined with relatively high levels of PEEP resulted in significantly reduced mortality [17]. The ARDnet study reported that a 'low tidal volume' *vs.* a 'high tidal volume' strategy (as part of a comprehensive ventilatory management protocol that dictated FiO_2, plateau airway pressure, and PEEP) was associated with improved patient survival [14]. These two studies are the only randomized controlled trials that demonstrate that mechanical ventilation has an impact on mortality in ARDS, and as such, constitute critically important contributions to the critical care literature. Applying the 'best available' evidence, a clinician might be tempted to conclude that 'on aggregate', lower V_T is generally better than higher V_T. However, titration of V_T in ARDS based on such suppositions may be dangerous for three reasons. First, each of the studies had two experimental groups (only), so that the results are 'binary'. Therefore, we have no clinical basis for interpolation about 'intermediate' ventilatory targets, or for extrapolating towards extremes of V_T. Second, a recent meta-analysis [49] of these studies casts (disputed [50]) doubt on the reliability of the validity of the concerns about 'high' V_T (as opposed to high plateau pressure) and the benefits of 'low' V_T [49]. Finally, a large-scale Australian study of outcome in ARDS, reported (without presenting the data) that there was no correlation between V_T and mortality [51].

In summary, if the alternatives available to a clinician are either of the four treatment groups in the studies by Amato et al. [17] or the ARDSnet [14], then the clinician should definitely opt for one of the respective 'low stretch' group options. This is never the case, however, and the clinician should not at this stage decide that lower V_T is necessarily better for all ranges of V_T; therefore, V_T should not be continually titrated downwards in the absence of due regard to lung recruitment or adequacy of ventilation. Instead, avoidance of high V_T that result in elevated plateau pressures appears appropriate.

Cytokines

Since the late 1960s it has been recognized that lung stretch results in release of inflammatory mediators [52], and this was proposed as a mechanism of hemody-namic depression resulting from mechanical ventilation [53]. Recent work from multiple laboratories has suggested that adverse forms of mechanical ventilation are associated with pulmonary [54] or systemic [55] release of cytokines or bacterial products [56, 57]. From the clinical perspective, these findings have been confirmed, at least in principle. The ARDSnet study reported that systemic circulating interleukin (IL)-6 was higher in the 'high stretch' group [14], and an additional smaller study demonstrated that high PEEP combined with lower V_T resulted in lesser elevations in lung and circulating cytokine release [18]. Nonetheless, not all experimental evidence concurs with the hypothesis that adverse ventilatory strategy results in elevated cytokines [58].

Our group has recently reported that cytokine gene activation is associated with high stretch ventilation, but that such activation occurs well before the develop-ment of measurable physiologic lung impairment or before the appearance of pathologic changes in lung histology [59]. Taken together, these data suggest that in the future, plasma cytokine profile might provide an early-warning signal of impend-ing stretch-induced lung injury, thereby mandating a change in ventilatory strategy. In such a way circulating (or bronchoalveolar lavage) cytokines or bacterial products could function as a target for ventilatory titration.

Targeting the Long-term

Much of the foregone discussion has focussed on respiratory issues, or on the integrated physiology of O_2 delivery and CO_2 control. However, it is increasingly clear that patients do not die from hypoxia *per se* [60], or indeed from any particular impingement of pulmonary function, including overt barotrauma [61]. Furthermore, the overall ICU mortality from ARDS appears to be fairly consistent over the last decade, and pending a radical change in approach to mechanical ventilation or a new biologically driven therapy, it is difficult to envisage how mortality could improve significantly beyond the current range. Thus, clinicians should expand their focus from mortality statistics to the broader issues of morbidity and quality of life in those patients – the majority – who survive ARDS. Several groups have investigated these issues, and several pertinent findings have been described. The key causes of long-term morbidity disability relate to acquired neuromuscular impairment [62]. In addition, long-term depression and post-traumatic stress disorder may be associated with increased use of sedative or neuromuscular blocking drugs [63]. Finally, the use of low V_T –although associated with less mortality [14, 17] – does not appear to translate into less morbidity in survivors of ARDS [64]. Thus, it will be important for future investigators to explore the biologic basis for long-term disability, and investigate therapeutic and preventive approaches.

Conclusion: Trading Multiple Targets Against Each Other

Although we are rapidly accumulating knowledge about specific questions in critical care, we do not – and will never – have the answers to all possible clinical questions in ventilatory care, much less in critical care in general. Thus, randomized clinical trials will answer isolated questions, and the individual clinician will have to weigh the evidence as applied to specific scenarios. However, frameworks can be constructed to address clinical situations. In terms of targeting parameters in mechanical ventilation, the following approach might be useful:

1. Decide on the single most important immediate issue for the patient, and consider the following (illustrative) examples:
   - If the SpO_2 is less than 85%, then correction of hypoxemia would be the first priority.
   - On the other hand, if the $PaCO_2$ is 11 kPa in the setting of elevated intracranial pressure, then reduction of $PaCO_2$ would be a very high priority.
2. Prioritize among the following parameters or targets (oxygenation, $PaCO_2$, plateau pressure or V_T, hemodynamic depression, lung recruitment, patient-ventilator synchrony) and rank them in order of importance for the patient.
3. Decide on which parameters will be selected for clinical titration

In summary, the clinician needs to decide which parameter is of immediate – and subsequent – importance, and which scientific literature is applicable. In addition, he/she must decide on which 'trade-offs' are appropriate for the patient in question, and at what stage the benefits of targets such as oxygenation, perfusion, recruitment are worth the cost to the patient of attaining them.

References

1. Mao C, Wong DT, Slutsky AS, Kavanagh BP (1999) A quantitative assessment of how Canadian intensivists believe they utilize oxygen in the intensive care unit. Crit Care Med 27:2806–2811

2. Kavanagh BP (1998) Goals and concerns for oxygenation in acute respiratory distress syndrome. Curr Opin Crit Care 4:16–20
3. Bernard GR, Artigas A, Brigham KL, et al (1994) The American-European consensus conference on ARDS. Definitions, mechanisms, relevant outcomes, and clinical trial coordination. Am J Respir Crit Care Med 149:818–824
4. Phang PT, Cunningham KF, Ronco JJ, Wiggs BR, Russell JA (1994) Mathematical coupling explains dependence of oxygen consumption on oxygen delivery in ARDS. Am J Respir Crit Care Med 150:318–323
5. Maldonado A, Bauer TT, Ferrer M, et al (2000) Capnometric recirculation gas tonometry and weaning from mechanical ventilation. Am J Respir Crit Care Med 161:171–176
6. Obrig H, Villinger A (2003) Beyond the visible-imaging the human brain with light. J Cereb Blood Flow Metab 23:1–18
7. Schlosser RL, Voigt B, von Loewenich V (2000) [Cerebral perfusion in newborn infants treated with high-frequency oscillation ventilation]. Klin Padiatr 212:308–311
8. Conference C (1996) Tissue hypoxia. How to detect, how to correct, how to prevent. Am J Respir Crit Care Med 154:1573–1578
9. Wung JT, James LS, Kilchevsky E, James E (1985) Management of infants with severe respiratory failure and persistence of the fetal circulation, without hyperventilation. Pediatrics 76:488–494
10. Hickling KG, Henderson SJ, Jackson R (1990) Low mortality associated with low volume pressure limited ventilation with permissive hypercapnia in severe adult respiratory distress syndrome. Intensive Care Med 16:372–377
11. Hickling KG, Walsh J, Henderson S, Jackson R (1994) Low mortality rate in adult respiratory distress syndrome using low-volume, pressure-limited ventilation with permissive hypercapnia: a prospective study. Crit Care Med 22:1568–1578
12. Bidani A, Tzouanakis AE, Cardenas VJ, Jr., Zwischenberger JB (1994) Permissive hypercapnia in acute respiratory failure. JAMA 272:957–962
13. Feihl F, Perret C (1994) Permissive hypercapnia. How permissive should we be? Am J Respir Crit Care Med 150:1722–1737
14. The Acute Respiratory Distress Syndrome Network (2000) Ventilation with lower tidal volumes as compared with traditional tidal volumes for acute lung injury and the acute respiratory distress syndrome. N Engl J Med 342:1301–1308
15. Laffey JG, Kavanagh BP (1999) Carbon dioxide and the critically ill - too little of a good thing? Lancet 354:1283–1286
16. Laffey JG, Kavanagh BP (2000) Biological effects of hypercapnia. Intensive Care Med 26:133–138
17. Amato MB, Barbas CS, Medeiros DM, et al (1998) Effect of a protective-ventilation strategy on mortality in the acute respiratory distress syndrome. N Engl J Med 338:347–354
18. Ranieri VM, Suter PM, Tortorella C, et al (1999) Effect of mechanical ventilation on inflammatory mediators in patients with acute respiratory distress syndrome: a randomized controlled trial. JAMA 282:54–61
19. Stewart TE, Meade MO, Cook DJ, et al (1998) Evaluation of a ventilation strategy to prevent barotrauma in patients at high risk for acute respiratory distress syndrome. Pressure- and Volume-Limited ventilatory strategy. N Engl J Med 338:355–361
20. Shibata K, Cregg N, Engelberts D, Takeuchi A, Fedorko L, Kavanagh BP (1998) Hypercapnic acidosis may attenuate acute lung injury by inhibition of endogenous xanthine oxidase. Am J Respir Crit Care Med 158:1578–1584
21. Broccard AF, Hotchkiss JR, Vannay C, et al (2001) Protective effects of hypercapnic acidosis on ventilator-induced lung injury. Am J Respir Crit Care Med 164:802–806
22. Sinclair SE, Kregenow DA, Lamm WJ, Starr IR, Chi EY, Hlastala MP (2002) Hypercapnic acidosis is protective in an in vivo model of ventilator-induced lung injury. Am J Respir Crit Care Med 166:403–408

23. Laffey JG, Tanaka M, Engelberts D, et al (2000) Therapeutic hypercapnia reduces pulmonary and systemic injury following In vivo lung reperfusion. Am J Respir Crit Care Med 162:2287–2294
24. Vannucci RC, Towfighi J, Heitjan DF, Brucklacher RM (1995) Carbon dioxide protects the perinatal brain from hypoxic-ischemic damage: an experimental study in the immature rat. Pediatrics 95:868–874
25. Nomura F, Aoki M, Forbess JM, Mayer JE (1994) Effects of hypercarbic acidotic reperfusion on recovery of myocardial function after cardioplegic ischemia in neonatal lambs. Circulation 90:321–327
26. du Plessis AJ, Jonas RA, Wypij D, et al (1997) Perioperative effects of alpha-stat versus pH-stat strategies for deep hypothermic cardiopulmonary bypass in infants. J Thorac Cardiovasc Surg 114:991–1000
27. Holmes JM, Leske DA, Zhang S (1997) The effect of raised inspired carbon dioxide on normal retinal vascular development in the neonatal rat. Curr Eye Res 16:78–81
28. Zhu S, Basiouny KF, Crow JP, Matalon S (2000) Carbon dioxide enhances nitration of surfactant protein A by activated alveolar macrophages. Am J Physiol 278:L1025–L1031
29. Lang JD JR, Chumley P, Eiserich JP, et al (2000) Hypercapnia induces injury to alveolar epithelial cells via a nitric oxide-dependent pathway. Am J Physiol 279:L994–1002
30. Gole MD, Souza JM, Choi I, et al (2000) Plasma proteins modified by tyrosine nitration in acute respiratory distress syndrome. Am J Physiol 278:L961–967
31. Laffey JG, Engelberts D, Kavanagh BP (2000) Buffering hypercapnic acidosis worsens acute lung injury. Am J Respir Crit Care Med 161:141–146
32. Hood VL, Tannen RL (1998) Protection of acid-base balance by pH regulation of acid production. N Engl J Med 339:819–826
33. Abu Romeh S, Tannen RL (1986) Amelioration of hypoxia-induced lactic acidosis by super-imposed hypercapnea or hydrochloride acid infusion. Am J Physiol 250:F702–F709
34. Laffey JG, Kavanagh BP (2002) Hypocapnia. N Engl J Med 347:43–53
35. McIntyre RW, Laws AK, Ramachandran PR (1969) Positive expiratory pressure plateau: improved gas exchange during mechanical ventilation. Can Anaesth Soc J 16:477–486
36. Suter PM, Fairley B, Isenberg MD (1975) Optimum end-expiratory airway pressure in patients with acute pulmonary failure. N Engl J Med 292:284–289
37. Pepe PE, Hudson LD, Carrico CJ (1984) Early application of positive end-expiratory pressure in patients at risk for the adult respiratory-distress syndrome. N Engl J Med 311:281–286
38. NIH (2002) ALVEOLI study: at http://hedwig.mgh.harvard.edu/ardsnet/ards04.html.
39. Gattinoni L, Mascheroni D, Torresin A, et al (1986) Morphological response to positive end expiratory pressure in acute respiratory failure. Computerized tomography study. Intensive Care Med 12:137–142
40. Rouby JJ, Lu Q, Goldstein I (2002) Selecting the right level of positive end-expiratory pressure in patients with acute respiratory distress syndrome. Am J Respir Crit Care Med 165:1182–1186
41. Gattinoni L, Pelosi P, Suter PM, Pedoto A, Vercesi P, Lissoni A (1998) Acute respiratory distress syndrome caused by pulmonary and extrapulmonary disease. Different syndromes? Am J Respir Crit Care Med 158:3–11
42. Parker JC, Hernandez LA, Peevy KJ (1993) Mechanisms of ventilator-induced lung injury. Crit Care Med 21:131–143
43. Dreyfuss D, Saumon G (1998) Ventilator-induced lung injury: lessons from experimental studies. Am J Respir Crit Care Med 157:294–323
44. Grasso S, Mascia L, Del Turco M, et al (2002) Effects of recruiting maneuvers in patients with acute respiratory distress syndrome ventilated with protective ventilatory strategy. Anesthesiology 96:795–802
45. Suzuki H, Papazoglou K, Bryan AC (1992) Relationship between PaO2 and lung volume during high frequency oscillatory ventilation. Acta Paediatr Jpn 34:494–500

46. Rimensberger PC, Pristine G, Mullen BM, Cox PN, Slutsky AS (1999) Lung recruitment during small tidal volume ventilation allows minimal positive end-expiratory pressure without augmenting lung injury. Crit Care Med 27:1940–1945
47. Brower RG, Shanholtz CB, Fessler HE, et al (1999) Prospective, randomized, controlled clinical trial comparing traditional versus reduced tidal volume ventilation in acute respiratory distress syndrome patients. Crit Care Med 27:1492–1498
48. Brochard L, Roudot-Thoraval F, Roupie E, et al (1998) Tidal volume reduction for prevention of ventilator-induced lung injury in acute respiratory distress syndrome. The Multicenter Trail Group on Tidal Volume reduction in ARDS. Am J Respir Crit Care Med 158:1831–1838
49. Eichacker PQ, Gerstenberger EP, Banks SM, Cui X, Natanson C (2002) Meta-analysis of acute lung injury and acute respiratory distress syndrome trials testing low tidal volumes. Am J Respir Crit Care Med 166:1510–1514
50. Brower RG, Matthay M, Schoenfeld D (2002) Meta-analysis of acute lung injury and acute respiratory distress syndrome trials (letter). Am J Respir Crit Care Med 166:1515–1517
51. Bersten AD, Edibam C, Hunt T, Moran J (2002) Incidence and mortality of acute lung injury and the acute respiratory distress syndrome in three Australian States. Am J Respir Crit Care Med 165:443–448
52. Edmonds JF, Berry E, Wyllie JH (1969) Release of prostaglandins caused by distension of the lungs. Br J Surg 56:622–623
53. Berry EM, Edmonds JF, Wyllie H (1971) Release of prostaglandin E2 and unidentified factors from ventilated lungs. Br J Surg 58:189–192
54. Imai Y, Kawano T, Miyasaka K, Takata M, Imai T, Okuyama K (1994) Inflammatory chemical mediators during conventional ventilation and during high frequency oscillatory ventilation. Am J Respir Crit Care Med 150:1550–1554
55. Chiumello D, Pristine G, Slutsky AS (1999) Mechanical ventilation affects local and systemic cytokines in an animal model of acute respiratory distress syndrome. Am J Respir Crit Care Med 160:109–116
56. Murphy DB, Cregg N, Tremblay L, Engelberts D, Laffey JG, Slutsky AS, Romaschin A, Kavanagh BP (2000) Adverse ventilatory strategy causes pulmonary-to-systemic translocation of endotoxin. Am J Respir Crit Care Med 162:27–33
57. Nahum A, Hoyt J, Schmitz L, Moody J, Shapiro R, Marini JJ (1997) Effect of mechanical ventilation strategy on dissemination of intratracheally instilled Escherichia coli in dogs. Crit Care Med 25:1733–1743
58. Ricard JD, Dreyfuss D, Saumon G (2001) Production of inflammatory cytokines in ventilator-induced lung injury: a reappraisal. Am J Respir Crit Care Med 163:1176–1180
59. Copland I, Engelberts D, Kavanagh BP, Post M (2001) High stretch ventilation causes cytokine gene activation before injury. Am J Respir Crit Care Med 161:A164 (abst)
60. Montgomery AB, Stager MA, Carrico CJ, Hudson LD (1985) Causes of mortality in patients with the adult respiratory distress syndrome. Am Rev Respir Dis 132:485–489
61. Weg JG, Anzueto A, Balk RA, et al (1998) The relation of pneumothorax and other air leaks to mortality in the acute respiratory distress syndrome. N Engl J Med 338:341–346
62. Herridge MS, Cheung AM, Tansey CM, et al (2003) One-year outcomes in survivors of the acute respiratory distress syndrome. N Engl J Med 348:683–693
63. Nelson BJ, Weinert CR, Bury CL, Marinelli WA, Gross CR (2000) Intensive care unit drug use and subsequent quality of life in acute lung injury patients. Crit Care Med 28:3626–3630
64. Orme J Jr, Romney JS, Hopkins RO, et al (2003) Pulmonary function and health-related quality of life in survivors of acute respiratory distress syndrome. Am J Respir Crit Care Med 167:690–694

How to Detect VILI at the Bedside

P. P. Terragni, B. Chiaia, and V. M. Ranieri

Introduction

Mechanical ventilation is the main supportive therapy to re-establish sufficient oxygen supply to peripheral organs in patients with acute respiratory distress syndrome (ARDS). As with any therapy, mechanical ventilation may expose patients to side effects. Alveolar rupture and air leak, the so-called barotraumas, were recognized early as the main side effects of mechanical ventilation [1]. However, in 1974, Webb and Tierney showed that mechanical ventilation could also be responsible for ultra-structural injury, independent of air leaks [2]. The potential clinical implication of these data was not realized until a series of studies showed that, apart from the physical alveolar disruption, mechanical ventilation can induce further injury to the lung by increasing alveolar-capillary permeability through the overdistension of the lung (volutrauma) [3] and/or worsening lung injury through the tidal recruitment-derecruitment of the collapsed alveoli (atelectrauma) [4, 5], and lead to even more subtle injury manifested by the activation of the inflammatory process (biotrauma) [6-8]. All these experimental and clinical data led to the concept that all the patho-physiological mechanisms involved in ARDS (ventilation-perfusion mismatch and reduced compliance, lung edema, atelectasis, pulmonary inflammation) may be worsened by the mechanical stress caused by inappropriate ventilator settings. In the early nineties, an international consensus conference concluded that both tidal overdistension of normal alveoli and opening-closing of collapsed alveoli, contribute to a component of a progressive lung injury that arises not only from the disease process itself, but also from the impact of the ventilator patterns applied during the course of the disease [9]. Ventilator-induced lung injury (VILI) was therefore defined as acute lung injury (ALI) directly induced by mechanical ventilation [10, 11].

Although randomized clinical trials [8, 12, 13] have successfully demonstrated that a ventilatory strategy designed to minimize overdistension and opening-closing may reduce mortality in patients with ARDS, information regarding the biomechanical characteristics of stress applied to the ventilated lungs is still missing. VILI is, in fact, determined by the dynamic and continuous interaction between: a) the mechanical characteristics of the lung; and b) the ventilator settings. The relationship between these terms is conditioned by the dynamic variations in respiratory mechanics as determined by the status and evolution of the pathological process and by the consequences of ventilator parameters on the mechanical characteristics of the lung. Therefore, clinicians have to choose tidal volume (V_T), positive end-expiratory pressure (PEEP) and recruiting maneuvers assuming that the ventilator settings are not causing VILI but lacking a clinical tool able to identify whether the interaction between the currently used ventilator settings and the actual status of pulmonary mechanics results in mechanical stress or not.

The mechanical characteristics of animal models [4, 6, 14] and patients [15, 16] with ARDS have been investigated by the analysis of the static pressure-volume (PV) curve of the respiratory system. Bedside analysis of the PV curve provided most of the physiological rationale explaining the pulmonary injury due to VILI. The static PV curve is, in fact, characterized by a lower (LIP) and an upper (UIP) inflection point that are thought to represent the average critical opening pressure above which alveolar units start to re-open and the volume/pressure values above which stretching and overdistension start to occur, respectively [17]. Several studies have demonstrated that tidal inflation starting below the LIP on the PV curve leads to tidal recruitment/de-recruitment of previously collapsed alveoli while tidal ventilation occurring above the UIP results in pulmonary over-stretching both leading to a spectrum of pulmonary and systemic lesions such as air leaks [18], alterations in lung fluid balance [3], increases in endothelial and epithelial permeability [19, 20], severe tissue damage [4], and pulmonary [6] and systemic [11, 21] production of inflammatory mediators.

Because of this link between VILI and assessment of the PV curve, and in an effort to make the measurement of the PV curve available at the bedside, a growing interest in the development of new technologies and on the clinical interpretation of the PV curve has become evident in the last few years [22-30]. However, although a large number of experimental studies correlated PV curves to histological [4] and biological [6, 21] manifestations of VILI, only two randomized trials showed that a protective ventilatory strategy individually tailored to the PV curve minimized pulmonary and systemic inflammation [8] and decreased mortality in patients with ALI [12]. Furthermore, despite the fact that several studies have proposed new techniques to perform PV curves at the bedside [23, 24, 27], confirming that the LIP and UIP correspond to computed tomography (CT) scan evidence of atelectasis and overdistension [26, 28, 29] and demonstrating the ability of the PV curve to estimate alveolar recruitment with PEEP [15, 16], no large clinical studies have assessed whether such measurements can be performed in all ICUs as a monitoring tool to orient ventilator therapy.

This chapter will:
a) review the basic principles of mechanical stress;
b) discuss how to measure and interpret the *static* PV curve to minimize VILI;
c) revise the potential advantage of the use of *dynamic* PV curves to monitor, prevent and minimize VILI.

Mechanical Characteristics of VILI

Respiratory mechanics is classically partitioned into the relationships between pressure and volume (elastic mechanics) and the relationships between pressure and flow (resistive mechanics). Resistive and elastic mechanics is usually described at a `macro-level' using various geometrical bodies (e.g., octahedrons, dodecahedrons and combinations of spheroids, cones and ellipsoids) to describe the tri-dimensional structure of the alveolar region [31-33]. These models provide useful information on the gross mechanical behavior but cannot take into account the internal distribution of stresses within the alveolar wall. On the other hand, the mechanics of the alveolar tissue lies at the 'micro-level'. The alveolar septum is a tiny structural framework that insures a minimal barrier between air and blood, while a relatively enormous surface of contact is maintained for efficient gas exchange. It consists of a skeleton of fine collagen and elastin fibers that are interlaced with the capillary network [34]. This structural organization comprises a 'composite' made of extensible elastin fibers woven into non-extensible collagen networks, allowing the lung to inflate within the normal range also providing support and a high stiffness at limiting volumes. The study by Gefen et al. [35] aimed to overcome the limitations inherent to a 'macro' description, by describing the internal stresses in a two-dimensional slice of an alveolar sac. The authors found that significant stress concentrations arise in lungs with emphysema (up to 6 times the stresses of a normal lung) at a lung volume of 60% of the total capacity. This provides progressive damage to the elastin fibers during breathing cycles. The pioneering study by Mead et al. [36] developed a two-dimensional static model at the alveolar scale to investigate the mechanics of deformation of a non-homogeneous lung. However, this model does not take into in account that: a) alveolar deformation takes place at a three-dimensional level; b) the inter-dependence among the various scales of the anatomic and functional pulmonary structures (more than 20 scales are involved in the respiratory mechanics); c) the multi-physics of the process due to the coupling the air flow process with the mechanical deformations and the surface tension.

The Mechanics of Stress, Strain, and Elasticity in Solid Media

Basic principles of stress and deformation within solid bodies were originally described by Timoshenko [37]. Central to Timoshenko theory is the description of infinitesimal deformations within the solid body that can be described by continuum mechanics. This theory has been proved to be effective in many fields of engineering, including bio-engineering, e.g., for the design of hip prostheses, dental implants and tubular stents. In the presence of soft tissues, however, the theory must be enriched by removing the hypothesis of small deformations and considering explicitly large strains and finite displacements of the body points. This provides cumbersome analytical models, of less immediate physical explanation than the infinitesimal theory. In the following, the elementary concepts of the infinitesimal theory will be outlined, in order to get the physical insight into continuum mechanics and create the basis for a correct nomenclature of the mechanical quantities.

The basic concepts of the so-called continuum mechanics are the concepts of *strain* and *stress*. In order to measure the deformation field within a solid body, the so-called strain tensor (ε) needs to be introduced. Such a quantity is defined at any

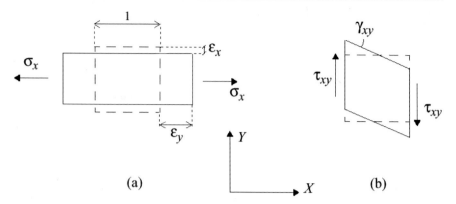

Fig. 1. Normal stresses and normal strains (a); shear stresses and distortions (b) in the XY plane.

point of the medium and, in a cartesian space, is a function of the three axes X, Y, Z and of the normal (n) to a generic plane which the deformation is referred to. It is formally a symmetric 3x3 matrix, with three normal strain ε corresponding to elongation in the X, Y, Z directions (which provide volume changes in the body) and three tangential strains γ corresponding to shape distortions of the infinitesimal volume around the considered point (Fig. 1). The strains are non-dimensional quantities, i.e., normal strains represent the deformation of the oriented fibers divided by the initial length of the fiber, whereas tangential strains represent angular variations with respect to $\pi/2$. Without going into the details, it can be shown that, at any point of the body, there exist three orthogonal principal directions that do not alter their orientation during deformation and are subjected only to the (normal) principal strains. In order to calculate the (elastic) energy that is stored in the body in correspondence to a certain strain field, the static counterpart of strain is introduced and is named the stress tensor [σ]. The stress field is tensorial because the stress vector, defined at any point P of the medium, depends also on the plane considered to which the components are referred (Fig. 2). In perfect correspondence to the strain tensor, [σ] is a symmetric matrix made of three *normal stresses* σ acting in the X, Y, Z directions (e.g., acting orthogonal to the planes defined by the normal vectors parallel to X, Y, Z) and of three tangential or *shear stresses* τ. These quantities have the physical dimension of pressures, i.e., forces per unit area. When the stress vector is orthogonal to the plane, we speak of a principal plane, and the stress coincides with its normal component. In the general case, there will also be the tangential components in the plane. As can be deduced from Figure 1, normal stresses σ (which can be positive, or tensile, and negative or compressive) work for the corresponding normal strains ε (respectively, fiber elongation or contraction), whereas shear stresses τ are coupled to the angular distortions γ. It should be noted that the stress is an abstract entity, i.e., it is a quantity that cannot be measured directly. On the contrary, strains are measurable, and therefore experimental measures of stresses rely on the direct evaluation of the strains. Accurate measurements of strains on soft (biologic) tissues, like the lung tissue, are currently a major challenge from the technological point of

Fig. 2. Definition of the stress vector t_n and of its normal and tangential components referred to the sectional plane.

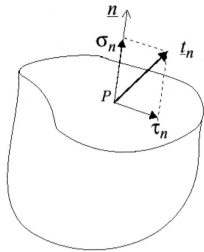

view, both due to relatively large deformation of tissues and to their irregular shapes.

The relation between stresses and strains is called the *constitutive law* of the material. All solid materials possess to a certain extent the property of elasticity, i.e., if external forces producing deformation of a structure do not exceed a certain limit, the deformation disappears with the removal of the forces. This implies that the strain energy is totally recovered, i.e., the material does not dissipate energy in any form. Elastic materials are modeled by means of a constitutive relation between stress and strain, i.e., by a functional form $[\sigma]=[\sigma(\varepsilon)]$.

Lung Tissue as a Cellular Material

The determination of the stress and strain fields within the lung represents an awkward task in mechanics. This is due to the large deformations (compared to traditional structural materials) and to the hierarchical structure of the lung, with more than 20 levels of scales characterized by specific meso- and micro-structures, each with well-defined geometrical characteristics [34]. The first 16 levels, starting from the trachea down to the terminal bronchioles, constitute the conductive zone, where flow occurs to and from the lungs. From level 17 to level 24 (corresponding to the almost 300,000,000 alveoli with capillaries lying in their septae), the so-called respiratory zone, gas exchange occurs and the effects of air velocity are negligible. At the scale of alveoli, the surface tension of the surfactant is comparable to the mechanical actions, thereby complicating even further the scenario. The mechanical interdependence of airways and alveoli within the lung has probably been designed with the aim to support uniform expansion of air spaces. In non-uniformly expanded lungs, the effective pressure differs from trans-pulmonary pressure, giving rise to shear stresses and consequent synergetic enhancement of the pathologies.

It is well known that solid materials suffer mostly due to shear stresses rather than to normal stresses. Shear stresses or the elastic energy due to distortions are responsible for material crisis according to the widely used criteria of material's strength (e.g., Tresca or von Mises criteria, [37]). Stresses in the pulmonary tissue, however, cannot be described by a continuous field, as is commonly done in continuous homogeneous media and has been briefly described in the previous section. A more precise description of lung mechanics, from the point of view of the alveolar tissue, must be pursued by means of more complicated theories such as the theory of cellular materials, which can account for the multiscale character of the stress/strain fields [38]. As is schematically shown in Figure 3, the mechanics of cellular materials explicitly considers the constituent geometry of the structures,

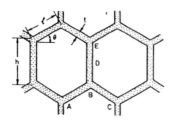

Fig. 3. Elementary deformation pattern of a cellular sub-structure subjected to mechanical loading.

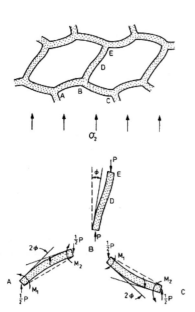

at a certain level of observation. From a mathematical point of view, such a discretization can be considered as an approximation of the continuum theory although, in reality, there are profound differences. Shear stresses, for instance, arise in the alveolar walls not only under the action of shear forces (Fig. 3), but also in the presence of normal forces, due to the microstructural characteristics. From the pictures, it appears evident how, in the absence of adequate surface tension and consequent homogeneous distension of the alveoli, the forces exerted by the surrounding sacs tend to induce distortion of the septae of the sick alveoli, enhancing their tendency to collapse.

The Use of the Static PV Curve to Minimize VILI

Patients with ARDS are characterized by a reduction in the range of volume excursion, because of the reduction in the ventilating units, and a smaller change in volume for unit of change in pressure. The initial part of the PV curve, at very low lung volume, is therefore considerably flatter than the rest of the curve, showing the amount of pressure required to open collapsed peripheral alveoli. This 'lower inflection point' separates a tract of the curve with bad elastic properties from the tract characterized by optimal elastic properties. After this initial tract, the curve presents a linear section in which the open alveoli are ventilated. Then the PV curve flattens again at values of V_T lower than those observed in normal subjects. This 'upper inflection point' indicates that stretching and overdistension of at least some alveolar structures is occurring.

Lower Inflection Point

Inflation of an excised lung requires a critical opening pressure to be applied in order to re-expand the collapsed alveoli [39]. This critical pressure appears on the PV curve as the pressure corresponding to the sudden change in slope of the curve after the initial inflation. In normal subjects, this critical opening pressure amounts to ~20 cmH$_2$O. Similarly, in patients with ARDS, the inspiratory PV curve shows a LIP, that is the sudden change in slope occurring at the onset of tidal inflation, when the applied pressure varies between 10-20 cmH$_2$O. This shows that in ARDS the vast majority of the lung is collapsed at the beginning of inspiration. The pressure corresponding to the LIP should therefore represent the minimal level of PEEP that should be applied in order to have tidal inflation within an open lung. Considering that ARDS and ALI are conditions of in-homogeneous lung parenchyma, CT densities are more concentrated in dependent lung regions, where there is a more positive pleural pressure if compared with nondependent regions (0 cmH$_2$O and –3, –5 cmH$_2$O, respectively). The influence of this vertical gradient in pleural pressure in the supine position, may be enhanced by the gravitational distribution of edema.

Upper Inflection Point

The decrease of the PV curve slope indicates the end of alveolar recruitment, the beginning of alveolar overdistension and so the maximal alveolar pressure that should be applied to obtain the maximal amount of alveolar recruitment. In normal subjects, the UIP is reached at a lung volume that is 85-90% of TLC (total lung capacity); in patients with ARDS, UIP occurs at a much lower volume. An increase in pressure above the UIP only gives overdistension without any other increase in volume, with a maximal stretch of lung aerated areas.

Techniques to Assess Static PV Curve

Super-syringe technique

This is the first technique used to assess the status of elastic properties of the respiratory system in mechanically ventilated ALI/ARDS patients in supine position sedated and paralyzed, to permit the slow inflation of the lung with a predetermined gas volume of oxygen. The inflated volume is 100-200 ml. The syringe stops for 2-3 sec, then the respiratory system is inflated with intermittent pause until a volume of 25 ml/kg or an airway pressure of 40 cmH$_2$O is reached. With this technique it is easy to detect the lower and upper inflection points but, on the other hand, paralysis, sedation and disconnection of the patient from the ventilator are required.

Rapid airway occlusion technique

This technique is based on a single-breath occlusion at different inflations during mechanical ventilation. With inspiratory flow constant, different volumes are achieved. Each occlusion is maintained until a plateau in the open airways pressure is obtained thus representing the static pressure of the total respiratory system. Using different volumes the static PV curve can be constructed. Advantages of this technique include no need for patient disconnection and the ability to identify the elastic properties of the respiratory system as determined by the actual volume. In addition, the measurement does not require special devices. However, patients must be paralyzed and sedated and curves are not immediately available since single data points need to be first collected and recorded and than plotted; identification of LIP and UIP is not easy.

Constant flow technique

This method is based on the assumption that when inspiratory flow is constant during passive inflation the rate of change in the airway opening pressure is related to the elastance of the respiratory system and the resistive components are nil. There is no need to disconnect the patient from the ventilator, special devices are not required and results are available at the bedside; lower and upper inflection points are usually easily identified. Yet, this method requires paralysis, sedation and only few ventilators are equipped with such a monitoring tool.

In patients with ARDS, the rapid airway occlusion technique (static PV curve) provides the same information as the constant flow technique (with a flow of 3 l/min) regarding the elastic properties of the respiratory system, whereas the PV curve obtained by the 9 l/min constant flow is slightly shifted to the right [27]. The slopes of the PV curves and the LIP are not different between all methods, indicating that the resistive component induced by administering a constant flow equal to or less than 9 l/min is not of clinical relevance. However, all methods have an intrinsic risk of adverse effects, including hypoxemia at low lung volumes and de-recruitment at low levels of PEEP [26-28]. Other problems include hemodynamic changes (decrease of venous return) or complications related to sedation or paralysis required to obtain the characteristics of passive mechanic of respiratory system. For all these reasons, PV curves are not usually obtained in the routine clinical assessment [39].

A non-linear model of respiratory mechanics in ARDS has recently been used to verify the physiological interpretation of the LIP and UIP and to examine their potential use in the clinical setting to set mechanical ventilation [30, 40]. This analysis showed that: i) the initial increase in slope of the PV curve indicates the minimal pressure at which alveolar recruitment starts to occur rather than the maximum level of PEEP able to provide maximum recruitment. Under these circumstances, a PEEP level equal to the LIP underestimates the optimal level of PEEP able to minimize end-expiratory alveolar collapse; ii) the decrease in the slope of the PV curve does not indicate the beginning of alveolar overdistension but the end of alveolar recruitment. According to this mathematical model, the UIP is therefore unrelated to alveolar overdistension being caused by the decrease in the rate of alveolar recruitment during lung inflation. Under these circumstances, the LIP will indicate the maximal alveolar pressure that should be applied to obtain the maximal amount of alveolar recruitment. Animal and clinical experiments are consistent with these data and have shown that recruitment occurs throughout the entire lung inflation from end-expiratory lung volume to TLC rather than being an 'all or none' phenomenon [41, 42].

Analysis of the Dynamic Pressure-time Curve during Constant Flow: A 'Stress Index' to Minimize VILI

We recently proposed that the use of the static PV curve could be replaced by the analysis of the dynamic airway opening pressure-time profile during constant-flow inflation [43]. In 19 patients with ALI we previously found that a downward concavity on the pressure-time profile during constant flow inflation corresponded to a static PV curve with a distinct LIP and a continuous increase in compliance (i.e., progressive recruitment with inflating volume) [15]. On the other hand, an upward concavity on the pressure-time profile during constant flow inflation corresponded to a static PV curve with a distinct UIP and a continuous reduction in compliance (i.e., progressive overdistension with inflating volume) [15]. Based on these results we raised the hypothesis that analysis of the shape of the pressure-time curve during constant flow inflation could identify the presence of tidal recruitment and/or tidal overinflation and, therefore, allow a non-invasive and continuous assessment of mechanical stress due to non appropriate ventilator settings.

During constant flow conditions and if resistances are constant, airway opening pressure (Pao) changes linearly with time when compliance does not change with increasing lung volume. When compliance decreases, Pao is concave upward and when compliance increases Pao is concave downward with respect to the time axis [15, 44-46]. Such an analysis of the pressure-time relationship is based on the assumption that during volume controlled ventilation with a constant flow inflation, the rate of change pressure is related to the changes in pulmonary compliance [15, 44-46]. Under these circumstances, the Pao profile as function of inspiratory time (t) can be described by a power equation (Fig. 4):

$$Pao = a \cdot t^b + c.$$

The coefficient a is a scaling factor, c is the pressure value at $t = 0$. The coefficient b is a dimensionless number that describes the shape of the pressure-time curve and that can, therefore, identify and quantify mechanical stress (stress index): a stress index = 1 means that the pressure time curve is linear and compliance remains constant throughout out tidal inflation; a stress index < 1 indicates that the pressure time curve has a downward concavity due to the tidal increase in compliance therefore identifying stress due to tidal recruitment; a stress index > 1

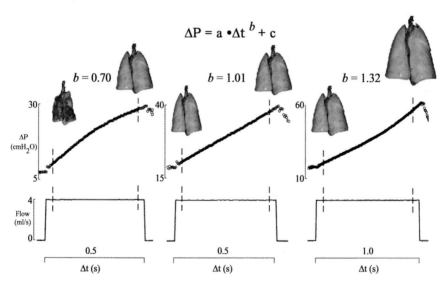

Fig. 4. The conceptual illustration of the dynamic pressuretime (P-t) curve. Based on the power equation $P_L = a \cdot t^b + c$; $b = 0,5$ produces a convex P-t curve, indicating continuing recruitment; $b = 1$ produces a straight P-t line, indicating no alveolar continuing recruitment or overdistension; and $b = 1,5$ produces a concave P-t curve, indicating alveolar overdistension. The power equation was applied to the transpulmonary pressure (PL) signal during a constant inspiratory flow (vertical bars) (modified from [43] with permission).

indicates that the pressure time curve has an upward concavity due to the tidal reduction in compliance, therefore, identifying stress due to tidal overinflation. This analysis requires several assumptions:

- a stiff chest wall may influence estimation of the upward/downward concavity on the dynamic pressure-time curve [44].
- in more complex conditions, the pressure-time curve may be characterized by a sigmoidal shape with an initial downward concavity due to alveolar opening, followed by a linear portion and a final downward concavity due to alveolar overdistension. Under these circumstances, it would be best to fit the power equation first to the initial portion of the curve (to set PEEP) and then to the second portion of the curve (to set V_T).
- on a theoretical basis, the time course of applied pressure during constant flow inflation should be characterized by an immediate step change due to the resistive components, abruptly followed by the progressive increase in pressure reflecting the changes in pulmonary compliance [45]. However, on- and off flow transients may be due to pendelluft (i.e., the time required to achieve a steady-state flow to each alveolar unit with different time constants) [47], viscoelasticity [30, 48] and the time required by the ventilator to initiate and to stop delivery of constant flow [15]. The first part of the pressure events must therefore be discarded, and only the portion on the pressure-time relationship corresponding to constant flow remains valid.
- a high sampling frequency of the recorded signals is required to achieve an adequate dynamic recording of airway pressure with no phase lag at high frequency.
- resistive and viscoelastic contributions to airway pressure are assumed constant over the range of changes in lung volume. Some of these factors may explain the relative low specificity (i.e., a relevant number of false positive) of the dynamic pressure-time profile to detect VILI.

The 'stress index' approach was initially tested in an isolated rat lung model of ARDS [43]. A significant ($p < 0.0001$) U-shaped relationship between individual values of stress index and pulmonary histologic damage and pulmonary concentration of pro-inflammatory cytokines was found; the lowest values of histologic injury score and cytokine concentration were systematically associated with a stress index around 1 (Fig. 5). The threshold value for the stress index that discriminated best between lungs with and without histologic and inflammatory evidence of VILI ranged between 0.90–1.10. For such threshold values, the sensitivity of the stress index to identify non-injurious ventilatory strategy was 1.00. In a second study [49] we examined the impact of different ventilatory strategies on the development of ischemia-reperfusion injury following lung transplantation and evaluated whether a ventilatory strategy aimed at maintaining a stress index of 1 would minimize pathophysiological indices of ARDS in the setting of lung transplantation. In a rat lung transplant model, animals were randomized into two groups defined by the ventilatory strategy during the early reperfusion period: 1) Conventional mechanical ventilation in which the transplanted lung was ventilated with a V_T equal to 50% of the inspiratory capacity of the left lung and a low PEEP; 2) Minimal mechanical stress ventilation in which the transplanted lung was

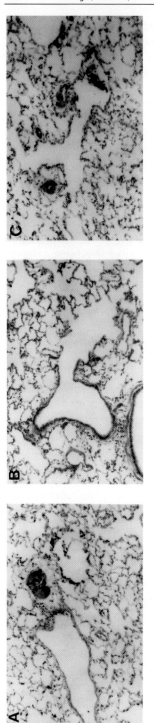

Fig. 5. Histological images of lung parenchyma in animal ARDS models; ventilation corresponding to (A) Stress Index < 1 (B) Stress Index = 1 (C) Stress Index > 1. Normal histology was found only in animals ventilated with a Stress Index = 1 (B), while in animals ventilated with Stress Index < and > 1 (A, C) hyaline membranes, epithelial damage and inflammatory cell infiltration were evident.

ventilated with a V_t equal to 20% of the inspiratory capacity of the left lung and PEEP adjusted according to the shape of the pressure-time curve to obtain a stress index of 1. After 3 hours of reperfusion, oxygenation from the transplanted lung was significantly higher in animals ventilated with a stress index of 1 than in animals ventilated with conventional ventilation. In addition, elastance, cytokine levels, and morphologic signs of injury were significantly lower in the group ventilated with a stress index of 1. This study demonstrates that the mode of mechanical ventilation used in the early phase of reperfusion of the transplanted lung can influence ischemia-reperfusion injury, and a protective ventilatory strategy based on a stress index of 1 can lead to improved lung function after lung transplantation. In a rabbit ARDS model, Nakane et al. [50] compared the efficacy in minimizing VILI of a ventilatory strategy aimed to maintain a stress index of 1 to the National Institute of Health (NIH) protective ventilatory strategy [13]. Animals were randomly ventilated for 3 hours using one of the following ventilatory strategies: SI group: V_T 6ml/kg, PEEP adjusted so that b = 1; NIH group: V_T 6ml/kg,, PEEP set according to the table created by NIH ARDSNet; Injurious group: V_T 10–12 ml/kg, PEEP 1–2, FiO_2 was adjusted so that PaO_2 was 55–80 in all groups. Respiratory mechanics worsened with time only in animals ventilated with the NIH and the injurious ventilatory strategies while they were maintained at baseline levels only in animals ventilated with a stress index of 1. After 3 hours of mechanical ventilation, lung homogenate concentration of interleukin (IL)-8 in the dependent region was significantly lower in animals protected by VILI using the SI strategy than in animals protected using the NIH strategy; histological examination showed a significantly lower incidence of VILI in the SI compared to the other groups.

In eight pigs, lung injury was induced with lung lavage [51]. Each animal was ventilated in random order with three ventilator settings aimed to obtain a stress index =1, a stress index > 1, and a stress index < 1. At the end of each experimental condition we measured respiratory mechanics, gas exchange and quantified tidal recruitment and tidal overinflation with spiral CT scan and multiple inert gas elimination technique (MIGET). CT evidence of intratidal alveolar collapse and/or overdistension were mirrored by the stress index. Preliminary data in patients with ARDS [52, 53] show that the use of the stress index is feasible also in the clinical scenario and that, compared to the gold standard protective ventilatory strategy (NIH protocol), patients ventilated with a stress index of 1 have lower elastance and higher recruitment of collapsed alveoli.

Other groups have independently confirmed and expanded these findings. In 20 paralyzed children with ARDS, Neve and coworkers showed that the analysis of the profile dynamic pressure time curve during constant flow ventilation permits detection of hyperinflation and has a good agreement with the results of the static PV curve [54]. Gama de Abreu and coworkers in a rabbit model of unilateral ARDS confirmed that the analysis of the pressure time curve during constant flow ventilation allows detection of the optimal protective strategy also during one-lung ventilation [55]. These data, therefore, suggest that the shape of the dynamic inspiratory pressure-time profile during constant flow inflation (stress index) allows prediction of a ventilatory strategy that minimizes the occurrence of VILI. Modern ventilators are able to deliver excellent square-wave inspiratory flow profiles, and are also equipped with monitoring tools that are able to provide on-line, dynamic pressure-time curves; however, further clinical studies will be required to confirm the utility of this approach to set protective ventilatory strategies and minimize VILI.

Conclusion

The main supportive therapy in ARDS patients is mechanical ventilation. As with any therapy, mechanical ventilation has side effects, and may induce lung injury (VILI). The mechanical factors responsible for VILI are though to be related to tidal recruitment/de-recruitment of previously collapsed alveoli and/or pulmonary over-distention. The PV curve of the respiratory system in patients as well as in animal models of ALI has a characteristic sigmoid shape, with a LIP corresponding to the pressure/end-expiratory volume required to initiate recruitment of collapsed alveoli, and an UIP corresponding to the pressure/end-inspiratory volume at which alveolar overdistension occurs. 'Protective' ventilatory approaches have therefore set out to minimize mechanical injury by using the PV curve to individualize PEEP (PEEP above the LIP) and V_T (by setting end-inspiratory volume/pressure below the UIP) since a large number of experimental studies have correlated PV curves to histological and biological manifestations of VILI and two randomized trials showed that a protective ventilatory strategy individually tailored to the PV curve minimized pulmonary and systemic inflammation and decreased mortality in patients with ALI. However, despite the fact that several studies have: a) proposed new techniques to perform PV curves at the bedside; b) confirmed that the LIP and UIP correspond to CT scan evidence of atelectasis and overdistension; and c) demonstrated the ability of the PV curve to estimate alveolar recruitment with PEEP, no large studies have assessed whether such measurement can be performed in all ICUs as a monitoring tool to orient ventilator therapy. Preliminary experimental and clinical studies show that the shape of the dynamic inspiratory pressure-time profile during constant flow inflation (stress index), allows prediction of a ventilatory strategy that minimizes the occurrence of VILI.

References

1. Macklin MT, Macklin CC (1944) Malignant interstitial emphysema of the lungs and mediastinum as an important occult complication in many respiratory disease and other conditions: an interpretation of the clinical literature in the light of laboratory experiment. Medicine 23:281–352
2. Webb HH, Tierney DF (1974) Experimental pulmonary edema due to intermittent positive pressure ventilation with high inflation pressures. Protection by positive end-expiratory pressure. Am Rev Respir Dis 110:556–565
3. Dreyfuss D, Soler P, Basset G, Saumon G (1988) High inflation pressure pulmonary edema. Respective effects of high airway pressure, high tidal volume, and positive end-expiratory pressure. Am Rev Respir Dis 137:1159–1164
4. Muscedere JG, Mullen JB, Gan K, Slutsky AS (1994) Tidal ventilation at low airway pressures can augment lung injury. Am J Respir Crit Care Med 149:1327–1334
5. Slutsky AS (1999) Lung injury caused by mechanical ventilation. Chest 116:9S–15S

6. Tremblay L, Valenza F, Ribeiro SP, Li J, Slutsky AS (1997) Injurious ventilatory strategies increase cytokines and c-fos m-RNA expression in an isolated rat lung model. J Clin Invest 99:944–952

7. Tremblay LN, Slutsky AS (1998) Ventilator-induced injury: from barotrauma to biotrauma. Proc Ass Am Physicians 110:482–488

8. Ranieri VM, Suter PM, Tortorella C, et al (1999) Effect of mechanical ventilation on inflammatory mediators in patients with acute respiratory distress syndrome: a randomized controlled trial. JAMA 282:54–61

9. American Thoracic Society International Consensus Conference (1999) Ventilator-associated lung injury in ARDS. Am J Respir Crit Care Med 160:2118–2124

10. Slutsky AS (1993) Mechanical ventilation. Chest 10:1833–1859

11. Slutsky AS, Tremblay LN (1998) Multiple system organ failure. Is mechanical ventilation a contributing factor? Am J Respir Crit Care Med 157:1721–1725

12. Amato MB, Barbas CS, Medeiros DM, et al (1998) Effect of a protective-ventilation strategy on mortality in the acute respiratory distress syndrome. N Engl J Med 338:347–354

13. Acute Respiratory Distress Syndrome Network (2000) Ventilation with lower tidal volumes as compared with traditional tidal volumes for acute lung injury and the acute respiratory distress syndrome. N Engl J Med 342:1301–1308

14. Martin-Lefreve L, Roupie E, Dreyfuss D, Saumon G (1998) Can respiratory system pressure-volume (PV) curve analysis predict the occurrence of volutrauma? Am J Respir Crit Care Med 157:A693 (abst)

15. Ranieri VM, Giuliani R, Fiore T, Dambrosio M, Milic-Emili J (1994) Volume-pressure curve of the respiratory system predicts effects of PEEP in ARDS: "occlusion" versus "constant flow" technique. Am J Respir Crit Care Med 149:19–27

16. Ranieri VM, Eissa NT, Corbeil C, et al (1991) Positive end-expiratory pressure on alveolar recruitment and gas exchange in patients with the adult respiratory distress syndrome. Am Rev Respir Dis 144:544–551

17. Brochard L (1997) Respiratory pressure-volume curves. In: Tobin MJ (ed) Principles and Practice of Intensive Care Monitoring. McGraw-Hill, New York, pp:597–616

18. Tobin MJ (2001) Advances in mechanical ventilation. N Engl J Med 344:1986–1996

19. Dreyfuss D, Basset G, Soler P, Saumon G (1985) Intermittent positive-pressure hyperventilation with high inflation pressures produces pulmonary microvascular injury in rats. Am Rev Respir Dis 132:880–884

20. Broccard AF, Hotchkiss JR, Kuwayama N, et al (1998) Consequences of vascular flow on lung injury induced by mechanical ventilation. Am J Respir Crit Care Med 157:1935–1942

21. Chiumello D, Goesev P, Slutsky AS (1999) Mechanical ventilation affects local and systemic cytokines in an animal model of acute respiratory distress syndrome. Am J Respir Crit Care Med 160:109–116

22. Liu JM, De Robertis E, Blomquist S, Dahm PL, Svantensson C, Jonson B (1999) Elastic pressure-volume curves of the respiratory system reveal a high tendency to lung collapse in young pigs. Intensive Care Med 25:1140–1146

23. Jonson B, Richard JC, Straus C, Mancebo J, Lemaire F, Brochard L (1999) Pressure-volume curves and compliance in acute lung injury: evidence of recruitment above the lower inflection point. Am J Respir Crit Care Med 159:1172–1178

24. Servillo G, Svantesson C, Beydon L, et al (1997) Pressure-volume curves in acute respiratory failure: automated low flow inflation versus occlusion. Am J Respir Crit Care Med 155:1629–1636

25. Jonson B, Svantesson C (1999) Elastic pressure-volume curves: what information do they convey? Thorax 54:82–87

26. Vieira SR, Puybasset L, Lu Q, et al (1999) A scanographic assessment of pulmonary morphology in acute lung injury. Significance of the lower inflection point detected on the lung pressure-volume curve. Am J Respir Crit Care Med 159:1612–1623

27. Lu Q, Vieira SR, Richecoeur J, et al (1999) A simple automated method for measuring pressure-volume curves during mechanical ventilation. Am J Respir Crit Care Med 159:275–282

28. Vieira SR, Puybasset L, Richecoeur J, et al (1998) A lung computed tomographic assessment of positive end-expiratory pressure-induced lung overdistension. Am J Respir Crit Care Med 158:1571–1577

29. Puybasset L, Cluzel P, Chao N, Slutsky AS, Coriat P, Rouby JJ (1998) A computed tomography scan assessment of regional lung volume in acute lung injury. The CT Scan ARDS Study Group. Am J Respir Crit Care Med 158:1644–1655

30. Hickling KG (1998) The pressure-volume curve is greatly modified by recruitment. A mathematical model of ARDS lungs. Am J Respir Crit Care Med 158:194–202

31. Fung YC (1988) A model of lung structure and its validation. J Appl Physiol 64:2132–2142

32. Kimmel E, Budiansky B (1990) Surface tension and the dodecahedron model for lung elasticity. J Biomech Eng 112:160–167

33. Denny E, Schroter RC (1995) The mechanical behavior of a mammalian lung alveolar duct model. J Biomech Eng 117:254–261

34. Weibel ER (1963) Morphometry of the Human Lung. Springer-Verlag, Berlin

35. Gefen A, Elad D, Shiner RJ (1999) Analysis of stress distribuition in the alveolar septa of normal and simulated emphysematic lungs. J Biomech 32:891–897

36. Mead J, Takishima T, Leith D (1970) Stress distribuition in lungs: a model of pulmonary elasticity. J Appl Physiol 28:596–608

37. Timoshenko S (1934) Theory of Elasticity. McGraw-Hill, New York

38. Gibson LJ, Ashby MF (1997) Cellular Solids: Structure and Properties. 2nd ed. Cambridge University Press, Cambridge

39. Ranieri VM, Slutsky AS (1999) Respiratory physiology and acute lung injury: the miracle of Lazarus. Intensive Care Med 25:1040–1043

40. Hickling KG (2001) Best compliance during a decremental, but not incremental, positive end-expiratory pressure trial is related to open-lung positive end-expiratory pressure: a mathematical model of acute respiratory distress syndrome lungs Am J Respir Crit Care Med 163:69–78

41. Crotti S, Mascheroni D, Caironi P, et al (2001) Recruitment and derecruitment during acute respiratory failure: a clinical study. Am J Respir Crit Care Med 164:131–140

42. Pelosi P, Goldner M, McKibben A, et al (2001) Recruitment and derecruitment during acute respiratory failure: an experimental study. Am J Respir Crit Care Med 164:122–130

43. Ranieri, VM, Zhang H, Mascia L, et al (2000) Pressuretime curve predicts minimally injurious ventilatory strategy in an isolated rat lung model. Anesthesiology 93:1320–1328

44. Ranieri VM, Brienza N, Santostasi S, et al (1997) Impairment of lung and chest wall mechanics in patients with acute respiratory distress syndrome: role of abdominal distension. Am J Respir Crit Care Med 156:10821091

45. Bates JHT, Rossi A, Milic-Emili J (1985) Analysis of the behavior of the respiratory system with constant inspiratory flow. J Appl Physiol 58:18401848

46. D'Angelo E, Robatto FM, Calderini E, et al (1991) Pulmonary and chest wall mechanics in anesthetized paralyzed humans. J Appl Physiol 70:26022610

47. Eissa NT, Ranieri VM, Chasse M, Robatto FM, Braidy J, Milic-Emili J (1991) Analysis of the behaviour of the respiratory system in ARDS patients: Effects of flow, volume and time. J Appl Physiol 70:27192729

48. Jonson B, Beydon L, Brauer K, Mansson C, Valind S, Grytzell H (1993) Mechanics of respiratory system in healthy anesthetized humans with emphasis on viscoelastic properties. J Appl Physiol 75:132140

49. De Perrot M, Imai Y, Volgyesi GA, et al (2002) Effect of ventilator-induced lung injury on the development of reperfusion injury in a rat lung transplant model. J Thorac Cardiovasc Surg 124:1137–1144

50. Nakane M, Imai Y, Kajikawa O, et al (2002) Stress index strategy: Analysis of dynamic airway opening pressure-time curve may be a useful tool to protect rabbits from VILI. Am J Respir Crit Care Med 165:A680 (abst)

51. Grasso S, Terragni P, Mascia L, et al (2002) Dynamic airway pressure/time curve (stress index) in experimental ARDS. Intensive Care Med 28:A727 (abst)

52. Grasso S, Mascia L, Trotta T, et al (2000) Dynamic airway pressure/time curve analysis to realize lung protective ventilatory strategy in ARDS patients. Intensive Care Med 26:A449 (abst)

53. Grasso S, Mascia L, Capobianco S, et al (2000) Protective ventilatory strategy: "NIH" vs "Static P-V curves" vs "Stress Index" protocol. Intensive Care Med 26:A619 (abst)

54. Neve V, de la Roque ED, Leclerc F, et al (2000) Ventilator-induced overdistension in children: dynamic versus low-flow inflation volume-pressure curves. Am J Respir Crit Care Med 162:139–147

55. Gama de Abreu M, Heintz M, Heller A, Szechenyi R, Albrecht DM, Koch T (2003) One-lung ventilation with high tidal volumes and zero positive end-expiratory pressure is injurious in the isolated rabbit lung model. Anesth Analg 96:220–228

Lung Morphology in ARDS:
How it Impacts Therapy

J. J. Rouby and C. R. de A Girardi

Introduction

In patients with acute respiratory distress syndrome (ARDS), ventilatory support is aimed at re-establishing lung aeration in order to provide adequate arterial oxyenation and CO_2 elimination. Tidal inflation provides inspiratory lung recruitment and renewal of alveolar gas whereas positive end-expiratory pressure (PEEP) prevents expiratory derecruitment. Hypotheses and concepts proposed to explain the loss of aeration characterizing the injured lung directly impact the optimization of the ventilatory strategy aimed at re-establishing adequate gas exchange and avoiding ventilator-induced lung injury (VILI). One of the major advances in the understanding of the mechanisms of aeration loss has been the possibility of directly measuring lung volumes of gas and tissue and the distribution of lung aeration using lung computed tomography (CT) [1]. The current and well-accepted view of the ARDS lung relies on the 'sponge theory' where alveolar collapse plays a pivotal role: the injured lung collapses under his own weight according to gravity [2] and 'opening' pressures of the lung increase from the sternum to the diaphragm in the supine position [3]. The respiratory effects of mechanical ventilation are thought to act according to the 'opening and collapse hypothesis': tidal volume (V_T) participates in 'lung reopening' if insufficient PEEP does not prevent end-expiratory lung collapse by counteracting entirely the 'superimposed pressure' resulting from the increased lung weight. Lung barotrauma appears as the direct result of repetitive opening and collapse of lung units as demonstrated experimentally; the high local pressure stress applied to collapsed lung units induces bronchiolar lesions [4] and the systemic release of inflammatory cytokines that participates in multiorgan failure and death [5, 6]. As a consequence, the logical ventilatory strategy is to 'keep the lung fully open' by increasing PEEP [7] and reducing V_T to avoid 'lung volutrauma', another form of VILI [8].

This theory that views the ARDS lung mainly as a 'collapsed' lung, is largely invalidated by recent experimental data [9, 10], is far from supported by CT data obtained in the whole lung, and is difficult to reconcile with the pathophysiology of ARDS [11] and the theoretical concepts governing alveolar inflation and collapse [12]. In addition, it does not fit experimental and clinical studies showing that VILI is made for a good part of bronchiolar and alveolar distension [13, 14]. Last but not least, the reappraisal of mechanisms of aeration loss and VILI directly impacts the ventilatory strategy and questions the concept of keeping the lung fully open at end-expiration.

The aim of the present chapter is to review how the mechanisms and the distribution of aeration loss in ARDS (lung morphology) impact ventilatory strategy and the prevention of VILI.

The Computed Tomographic Assessment of Lung Aeration

CT of the whole lung allows the accurate assessment of lung volumes (gas and tissue) and lung aeration. With the last generation of CT scanners, contiguous CT sections can be obtained from the apex to the diaphragm in less than 10 seconds with a spatial resolution of CT images as high as 0.2 mm^3. Overall lung volume (gas + tissue) is computed as the number of voxels present in a given lung region. Because the lung parenchyma is composed of gas and tissue with physical density close to water density, it is possible to compute for any pulmonary region, the volume of gas, the volume of tissue and the volumic distribution of lung aeration [15, 16]. Classically, lung aeration is quantified in 4 categories:

1. normal aeration, defined by CT attenuations ranging between 900 and 500 HU (aeration ranging between 90 and 50%)
2. overinflation, defined by CT attenuations < –900 HU (aeration > 90%)
3. insufficient aeration, defined by CT attenuations ranging between –100 HU and –500 HU (aeration ranging between 10% and 50%),
4. non-aeration, defined by CT attenuations greater than –100 HU (aeration < 10%).

The initial mandatory step of the quantitative analysis is the manual delineation of the lung parenchyma. Then, lung volumes and pulmonary aeration can be measured using softwares like Osiris from the University of Geneva and Lungview from our Institution [17]. Of particular interest is the color encoding system present in the Lungview software that attributes a specific color to overinflated, normally, poorly and non-aerated lung areas according to their CT attenuations [18]. At end-expiration, the normal lung aeration ranges between 50 and 90% [16, 19]. Lung tissue volume is approximately 1 liter, representing 30% of the end-expiratory lung volume and is equally distributed between right and left upper and lower lobes [16]. Functional residual capacity (FRC) is around 2 liters, representing 70% of the overall lung volume and is smaller in the left lung than in the right lung due to the presence of the heart in the left hemithorax. In addition, end-expiratory gas volume is slightly smaller in lower lobes than in upper lobes.

Protein-rich pulmonary edema, increased extravascular lung water, lung infection and lung inflammation increase lung tissue in ARDS. A massive loss of aeration is also a prominent feature of the acutely injured lung. When the loss of aeration is isolated, without excess lung tissue, it reflects atelectasis resulting from the mechanical compression or obstruction of distal bronchioles [20]. When the loss of aeration is associated with an increase in lung tissue, it likely reflects 'alveolar flooding' resulting from the replacement of alveolar gas by edema and/or inflammation. Excess lung tissue can be detected in a given patient by comparison to the amount of lung tissue normally present in the corresponding lung region of healthy humans [21].

Alveolar recruitment resulting from PEEP, sigh, or recruitment maneuvers can be measured as the re-aeration of non-aerated lung regions according to the opening and collapse hypothesis [22–24] – it does not take into consideration re-aeration of poorly ventilated lung regions – or as the re-aeration of poorly and non-aerated lung regions if the hypothesis of alveolar flooding is taken into consideration [18]. Of peculiar importance is the requirement for assessing alveolar recruitment on the whole lung. As reported in supine patients with ARDS, alveolar recruitment resulting from PEEP predominates in non-dependent and cephalic lung regions, is rather limited in the diaphragmatic region and can even be negative (alveolar derecruitment) caudally to the diaphragmatic cupola [20, 25]. As a consequence, assessing alveolar recruitment on a single juxta-diaphragmatic CT section often underestimates recruitment of the whole lung. In contrast, because apical and juxta-hilar CT sections are more representative of upper lobes than of lower lobes, assessing alveolar recruitment on three CT sections often overestimates recruitment of the whole lung [26].

A lung aeration > 90% – corresponding to CT attenuations ≤ -900 HU is considered as the threshold separating inflation from overinflation defined as an excess of alveolar gas as compared to lung tissue [19]. Lung emphysema complicating chronic obstructive pulmonary disease (COPD) and characterized by lung overinflation and vascular destruction is also characterized by CT attenuations < -900 HU [27, 28]. Pulmonary overinflation resulting from mechanical ventilation predominates in caudal and nondependent lung regions [20]. As a consequence, assessing lung overinflation in patients with ARDS requires the analysis of the whole lung including CT sections caudal to the diaphragmatic cupola.

The Different Lung Morphology Patterns in Acute Respiratory Distress Syndrome

The Distribution of Aeration Loss and Excess Tissue in Patients with ARDS

The diffuse injury of the alveolar-capillary membrane that characterizes the ARDS lung, produces a high-permeability type pulmonary edema. The resulting increase in lung tissue detected on CT [16] is distributed from the apex to the diaphragmatic cupola, predominant in the upper lobes and frequently associated with a massive loss of aeration [20]. In caudal parts of the lung, although the regional loss of aeration is always massive, the excess lung tissue is absent or minimum in one-third of lower lobes [16]. Inversely, although the excess lung tissue is constantly observed in the cephalic parts of the lung, the aeration remains either partially preserved or entirely normal in two-third of upper lobes.

In the supine position at zero end-expiratory pressure (ZEEP), the degree of aeration of the upper lobes determines the lung morphology and the radiological pattern. In a minority of patients with ARDS, the loss of aeration is massive and equally distributed within the lung parenchyma (Fig. 1). In such patients with diffuse and bilateral CT attenuations, arterial hypoxemia is severe and the mortality

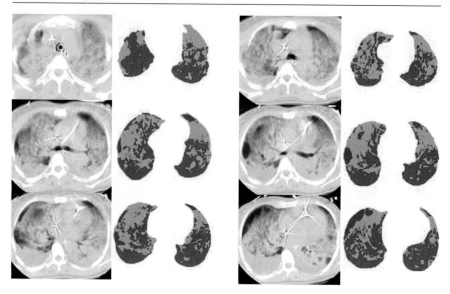

Fig. 1. Six CT sections obtained at zero end-expiratory pressure (ZEEP) in a 40-year old patient with ARDS secondary to posttraumatic peritonitis and characterized by a diffuse loss of aeration. On the right side of each CT section, the corresponding lung aeration is represented using a color code included in the software Lungview. Nonaerated lung regions characterized by CT attenuations ranging between 0 and –100 Hounsfield units (HU) are colored in black. Poorly aerated lung regions characterized by CT attenuations ranging between –100 and –500 HU are colored in light gray. Normally aerated lung regions characterized by CT attenuations ranging between –500 and –900 HU are colored in dark gray. At ZEEP, less than 10% of the lung is normally aerated. The loss of aeration is homogeneously distributed between upper and lower lobes and there is a moderate increase in lung tissue: gas volume in upper lobes = 135 ml (normal values = 1636 319 ml), gas volume in lower lobes = 190 ml (normal values = 1391 367 ml), tissue volume in upper lobes = 616 ml (normal values = 461 68 ml), tissue volume in lower lobes = 530 ml (normal values = 482 89 ml).

rate is above 70%. A primary insult to the lung is the most frequent cause of ARDS. The typical radiological presentation is of bilateral and diffuse hyperdensities resulting in 'white lungs' [16, 21]. In the majority of patients with ARDS, the aeration of upper lobes is either entirely or partially preserved despite a regional excess of lung tissue and the loss of aeration involves predominantly lower lobes. When aeration loss in the lower lobes is caused by alveolar flooding, a marked increase in lung tissue is observed, the overall lobar volume is preserved (Fig. 2) and bilateral radiological densities of the lower quadrants are present erasing the diaphragmatic cupola. When the regional loss of aeration is caused by compression atelectasis, a moderate, or no, increase in lung tissue is observed, the overall lower lobe volume is markedly reduced (Fig. 3), and bilateral radiological densities of the lower quadrants are discrete leaving apparent the diaphragmatic cupola. In such patients with 'focal' CT attenuations, arterial oxygenation impairment is severe contrasting with the lack of extensive radiological abnormalities and the mortality rate is around 40% [21].

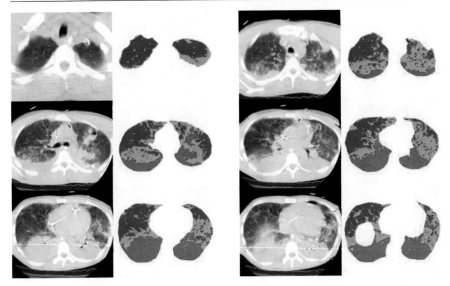

Fig. 2. Six CT sections obtained at zero end-expiratory pressure (ZEEP) in a 23-year old patient with ARDS secondary to pulmonary contusion and characterized by an unevenly distributed loss of lung aeration (some regions of the upper lobes remain normally aerated). On the right side of each CT section, the corresponding lung aeration is represented using a color code included in the software Lungview. Nonaerated lung regions characterized by CT attenuations ranging between 0 and –100 Hounsfield units (HU) are colored in black. Poorly aerated lung regions characterized by CT attenuations ranging between –100 and –500 HU are colored in light gray. Normally aerated lung regions characterized by CT attenuations ranging between –500 and –900 HU are colored in dark gray. At ZEEP, 30% of the lung is normally aerated. The loss of aeration predominates in lower lobes and there is a marked increase in lung tissue homogeneously distributed between upper and lower lobes: gas volume in upper lobes = 995 ml (Normal values = 1636 319 ml), gas volume in lower lobes = 212 ml (Normal values = 1391 367 ml), tissue volume in upper lobes = 1182 ml (Normal values = 461 68 ml), tissue volume in lower lobes = 1166 ml (Normal values = 482 89 ml).

Interestingly, in lung regions located caudally to the diaphragmatic cupola, compression atelectasis becomes predominant [20]. In deeply sedated patients lying supine, the diaphragm behaves as a passive structure that moves upward in the rib cage [25] and transmits to lower lobes the increased abdominal pressure resulting from abdominal surgery and/or abdominal trauma. It has to be outlined that the lung injury itself can increase abdominal pressure. It is well known, since the mid 1940s, that abdominal pain and distension can be the revealing signs of an acute lung injury [29]. In fact, caudal and dependent parts of the lungs are not only compressed by the abdominal content [25] but also by the heart [30] and the possible pleural effusion. In lung regions located beneath the heart, the loss of aeration is massive and significantly greater than in lung regions located outside the ventricles' limits [30]. Despite the lack of left ventricular failure, the heart is enlarged and heavier in ARDS patients compared to healthy volunteers [30]. Myocardial edema, hyperdynamic profile and pulmonary hypertension-induced

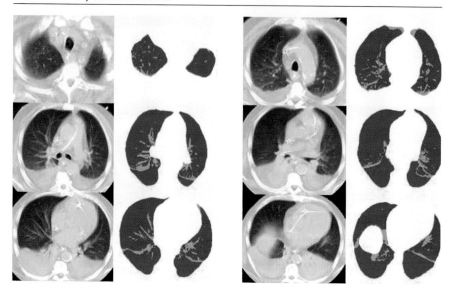

Fig. 3. Six CT sections obtained at zero end-expiratory pressure (ZEEP) in a 73-year old patient with ARDS caused by a massive bronchopneumonia and characterized by an unevenly distributed loss of lung aeration. On the right side of each CT section, the corresponding lung aeration is represented using a color code included in the software Lungview. Nonaerated lung regions characterized by CT attenuations ranging between 0 and –100 Hounsfield units (HU) are colored in black. Poorly aerated lung regions characterized by CT attenuations ranging between –100 and –500 HU are colored in light gray. Normally aerated lung regions characterized by CT attenuations ranging between –500 and –900 HU are colored in dark gray. At ZEEP, the loss of aeration concerns exclusively the lower lobes where the increase in lung tissue is moderate: gas volume in lower lobes = 14 ml (Normal values = 1391 367 ml) and tissue volume in lower lobes = 634 ml (Normal values = 482 89 ml). In contrast, upper lobes remain normally aerated despite a marked increase in lung tissue: gas volume in upper lobes = 1629 ml (Normal values = 1636 319 ml) and tissue volume in upper lobes = 1053 ml (Normal values = 461 68 ml). The regional distribution of lung volumes clearly shows that the visual impression of 'normal' upper lobes is misleading. The lack of apparent sternovertebral gradient of aeration in upper lobes despite a 128% increase in regional lung tissue does not fit the 'sponge' theory.

right ventricular dilation are potential mechanisms that may contribute to the increased cardiac mass and dimensions in ARDS patients. Finally, in the supine position, there is a nondependent to dependent decrease in regional aeration that is maximum in the juxta-diaphragmatic parts of the rib cage [20, 25]. Lung tissue structures including pulmonary vessels are squeezed by the different forces acting on caudal parts of the ribcage, a compression that likely limits the plasma leakage through the injured alveolar-capillary barrier and explains why compression atelectasis becomes predominant beyond the diaphragmatic cupola.

It was initially believed that the overall volume of the ARDS lung was preserved because the loss of gas was exactly compensated by the excess lung tissue [1]. This hypothesis, based on CT data obtained from single CT sections, has not been verified in the whole lung: multiple CT sections clearly demonstrate that the cephalocaudal dimensions of the ARDS lung are markedly reduced essentially at the expense of the lower lobes [25]. In fact, the ARDS lung is made of a combination of alveolar flooding, interstitial inflammation and atelectasis. In cephalic parts of the lung where external compressive forces are absent, alveolar flooding, when present, induces a massive loss of aeration with a conservation of the overall lung volume [16]. In contrast, in caudal parts of the lungs where external compressive forces abdominal content, cardiac mass, and pleural fluid effusion - are maximum in the supine position, a reduction of the overall lung volume of the lower lobes is frequently observed depending on the relative importance of alveolar flooding and compression atelectasis. This view of the ARDS lung has therapeutic consequences: re-establishment of lung aeration providing adequate gas exchange can be achieved not only by increasing intrathoracic pressure but also by relieving the external forces compressing lower lobes by adequate body positioning. At a given PEEP level, prone and semi-recumbent positions allow the recruitment of caudal lung regions by partially relieving heart and abdominal compressions [31, 32].

Consequences of Lung Morphology on Respiratory Pressure-Volumes (PV) Curves

When the lung is characterized by a diffuse loss of aeration at ZEEP, the PV curve is essentially a lung recruitment curve and does not reflect lung mechanics of the 'baby' lung gas as previously believed [3, 33]. During the inflation procedure, each ml of gas penetrating within the respiratory system contributes to alveolar recruitment either by improving the aeration of poorly aerated lung regions and/or by reinflating nonaerated areas: the lung recruitment is equal to PEEP-induced increase in FRC. The lower inflection point (LIP), which is usually prominent and well defined, corresponds to the pressure above which alveolar recruitment increases linearly with airway pressure. The initial part of the PV curve the starting compliance is generally flat, indicating that a minimum pressure is required to reaerate the injured lung. The first ml of gas delivered to the respiratory system penetrates primarily into poorly aerated lung regions. Very likely, these lung regions are characterized by a gas-liquid interfaces within the alveolar space which alter regional lung mechanics and explain the low starting compliance. Then, with the progressive reaeration of nonaerated lung regions, lung recruitment starts to be substantial and the chord compliance (the slope of the PV curve in its linear portion) becomes higher than the starting compliance. Experimentally, a LIP can be caused either by the reopening of collapsed lung areas or by the reinflation of an edematous lung in which all units are open [34–36]. By itself, the presence of a prominent LIP is not an indication of the mechanisms of lung aeration loss and alveolar recruitment. The upper inflection point (UIP) indicates the end of alveolar recruitment and the pressure above which alveolar overinflation commences. The slope of the PV curve determines the potential for recruitment. At the early stage of ARDS, the potential for recruitment is important in patients with diffuse loss of aeration [20]. As expected, the slope of the PV curve decreases with PEEP, attesting that the lung is progressively recruited [37, 38]. Interestingly, 90% of ARDS characterized by a diffuse loss of aeration is caused by a direct insult to the lung and the hypothesis raised of a marginal recruitment in primary ARDS [39] has not been substantiated by further studies [18, 20, 37, 40].

When the loss of aeration is focally distributed at end-expiration, the interpretation of the PV curve is much more complex. Lung recruitment of nonaerated lung regions as well as the mechanical properties of the parts of the remaining normally aerated at ZEEP both contribute to the PV curve. The lower and upper inflection points are either absent or little prominent. The starting compliance is usually steep, indicating that lung volume immediately increases at low pressures; normally aerated parts of the lung are inflated and distended long before the recruitment of nonaerated lung regions commences. In the linear part of the PV curve, distension and recruitment occur simultaneously in different parts of the lung. At high pressure, overinflation of the aerated lung may appears whereas lung recruitment of nonaerated lung regions continues. These two opposite effects explain why the UIP is either absent or very progressive in many of these patients. Similar reasoning can be applied to the LIP that is most often absent or progressive [16]. During the initial insufflation, normally aerated lung regions are the first to be inflated at low pressures long before the nonaerated parts of lung are recruited. As a consequence, in ARDS patients with focal loss of aeration, keeping the plateau inspiratory pressure lower than the UIP does not protect against lung overinflation. Similarly, the slope of the PV curve reflects not only the potential for recruitment but also the elastance of the aerated lung.

In Patients with ARDS, the Lung Morphology determines the Radiological Presentation and the Response to PEEP

Except in patients with a 'diffuse' lung morphology whose radiographic and CT aspects are often concordant showing bilateral 'white lungs', the bedside frontal chest radiograph is misleading in the majority of patients with ARDS. In a series of 70 patients, bedside frontal chest radiography correctly identified lung morphology in 41% of the patients only, the highest rate of error being observed in patients with 'focal' ARDS [21]. Surprisingly, in some severely hypoxemic patients, the frontal bedside chest radiograph may remain grossly normal: only a few basal hyperdensities can be identified and indirect signs suggesting a major reduction in the volume of lower lobes such as the visualization of the small fissura immediately above the right diaphragmatic cupola are present. This radiological presentation, which often confuses the clinician, generally corresponds to nonaerated and partially atelectatic lower lobes which stand on the posterior face of the diaphragm and caudally to the diaphragmatic cupola. In contrasting with the apparent preservation of lung aeration on the frontal chest radiograph, lung CT always shows a major lung volume loss predominating in lower lobes and explaining the severe impairment of arterial oxygenation [21]. In fact, the aeration present on frontal chest radiography concerns essentially upper lobes, which, paradoxically, are also characterized by a substantial increase in lung tissue.

Because a substantial proportion of the lung parenchyma remains normally aerated at ZEEP in the majority of ARDS patients [16], regional lung compliances are unevenly distributed [20]. Very often, upper lobes are more compliant than lower lobes and the initial increase in intrathoracic pressure distends cephalic lung regions before recruiting nonaerated pulmonary areas [20, 41]. Increasing the intrathoracic pressure by increasing PEEP often overinflates the aerated lung regions while, concurrently, nonaerated areas begin to be recruited [19, 20, 41, 42]. These results have been experimentally observed in dogs with oleic acid-injured lungs where regional lung volumes were measured using the parenchymal marker techniques [9, 10]. In the minority of patients whose ARDS is characterized by a diffuse and bilateral loss of aeration, the risk of overinflation appears more limited [18, 20, 41]. The lack of normally aerated lung regions at ZEEP explains why PEEP greater than 10 cmH2O does not induce any detectable lung overinflation [41]. The most severe forms of lung infection, pulmonary contusion, aspiration pneumonia fat embolism, amniotic embolism, and near drowing are characterized by a 'diffuse' loss of lung aeration whereas less severe forms of primary ARDS show a more 'focal' distribution of the aeration loss [20, 21]. Most of secondary ARDS cases are characterized by a 'focal' loss of aeration [21]. As shown in a series of 69 patients with ARDS [20], primary and secondary ARDS patients do not differ as far as basal cardiorespiratory parameters, cardiorespiratory effects of PEEP, and survival are concerned. The response to PEEP is not influenced by the nature of lung injury primary or secondary as previously suggested [39] but rather by the lung morphology which depends on the severity of lung injury.

The rationale for selecting the 'right' PEEP level is based on the experimental and clinical finding that lung overinflation and alveolar recruitment occur simultaneously in many patients or animals with ARDS [43]. The optimal PEEP for a given patient can be defined as the PEEP allowing optimization of arterial oxygenation without introducing a risk of oxygen toxicity and VILI [43]. In the majority of ARDS patients in whom significant parts of the lungs remain normally aerated at ZEEP, the PEEP trial should range between 5 and 12 cmH2O in order to avoid overinflation of aerated lung regions that would inevitably result from the application of higher PEEP required to keep the lung fully aerated at end-expiration. In other words, most injured lungs cannot be entirely reaerated without introducing a risk of VILI. In the minority of patients without a single lung region normally aerated at ZEEP, high PEEP can be safely applied without overinflating other parts of the lung [19, 20, 41] and the concept of keeping the lung fully aerated may be accepted [7]. In both situations, the use of periodic sighs could be useful [38, 44, 45]. CT studies have provided evidence that at a given PEEP level, end-expiratory aeration is markedly dependent on the preceding inspiratory plateau pressure: the higher the inspiratory plateau pressure, the more the PEEP prevents end-expiratory lung derecruitment [3].

Mechanisms of Aeration Loss and their Influence on VILI

The loss of aeration characterizing the ARDS lung is classically explained according to the 'sponge' model developed from CT scan studies performed on a single juxta-diaphragmatic CT section: the increased tissue mass causes the lung to collapse under its own weight [46] creating a sternovertebral gradient of aeration. The validity of this hypothesis implies that the pulmonary edema remains purely interstitial because the presence of fluid within the alveolar space prevents alveolar collapse. It also implies a decrease in the overall lung volume because, for anatomical reasons, the increase in the interstitial volume cannot compensate entirely the decrease in the alveolar volume resulting from alveolar collapse. Recently, in accordance with pathophysiological concepts and human histological data [11], Hubmayr outlined the fact that very likely the ARDS lung is derecruited because it is filled with fluid, not collapsed [12]. In a canine oleic acid-induced ARDS model, Martynowicz et al. found no evidence of collapse of dependent lung units and were unable to demonstrate any opening and collapse of lung units with mechanical ventilation using the parenchymal marker technique [9, 10]. The authors logically concluded that the presence of liquid and foam in alveoli and conducting airways was the mechanism causing the loss of lung aeration [36]. Surprisingly, the distribution of 'threshold opening pressures' of the injured lung was recently described in a similar model of canine oleic acid-induced lung [3] where lung collapse is not present because alveoli are flooded with hemorrhagic edema.

In patients with ARDS, CT data obtained from the whole lung are also difficult to reconcile with the opening and collapse theory. If aeration loss is explained by the 'sponge' model, the loss of overall lung volume should be predominantly observed in upper lobes in patients lying supine since the excess lung tissue predominates in cephalic parts of the injured lung [16]. In fact, a marked reduction of the end-expiratory volume of lower lobes is often observed in patients with ARDS whereas the volume of upper lobes is not reduced [16, 25]. In some patients, the end-expiratory volume of upper lobes is even increased when compared to healthy controls [16] as experimentally observed in oleic acid-injured lungs. In patients with 'white lungs' (diffuse CT attenuations), there is a massive loss of aeration in the upper lobes that is largely compensated by a marked increase in lung tissue, resulting in a slight increase in the overall lobar lung volume [16]. These data clearly suggest that alveolar flooding rather than lung collapse is the primary mechanism for lung derecruitment in upper lobes. In contrast, partial lung collapse is always present in the lower lobes and likely results from an external compression by the abdominal compartment and the heart [30]. It seems hazardous to incriminate the excessive lung weight as a causative factor for the loss of aeration in the lower lobes since substantial increases in lung tissue are not associated with lung collapse in the upper lobes. In fact, the sternovertebral gradient of aeration likely results from the anatomical superposition of upper and lower lobes in the supine position, the cephalocaudal gradient of aeration being the most important determinant causing the partial collapse of lower lobes.

As outlined recently [12], VILI is predominantly composed of overinflation of aerated lung regions if lung recruitment results from the displacement of the air-fluid interface from distal airways to the alveolar space. If the reopening and collapse of terminal bronchioles is the mechanism of lung recruitment, then VILI should predominantly involve the distal bronchioles in dependent lung areas. Human data on VILI injury have reported both overinflation of aerated lung areas and bronchial distension in nonaerated lung regions [13]. Recently, these lesions were reproduced in ventilated piglets with *Escherichia coli* pneumonia, a model of 'focal' ARDS where alveoli are fluid filled and not collapsed [14]. Such results suggest that both mechanisms – partial reversal of alveolar flooding in the upper and lower lobes and partial reopening of collapsed lung areas in the lower – lobes are likely involved in mechanical ventilation-induced lung recruitment. However, very likely, lung collapse of caudal parts of the lung in the supine position does not result from the increased lung weight but from the external compression of lower lobes by the heart and the abdomen. This external compression explains why pressures much greater than 15 cmH2O the average anteroposterior lung dimension are required to fully reaerate the ARDS patient's lower lobes.

Conclusion

CT data obtained in patients with ARDS lying supine show that a majority of them have substantial parts of their upper lobes that remain normally aerated at ZEEP. In contrast, aeration loss is always massive in caudal parts of the lungs and, because an external compression is exerted on lower lobes by the heart, the abdomen and the presence of pleural effusion, juxta-diaphragmatic lung regions are often entirely atelectatic. One of the most intriguing results from CT studies of the whole lung is that marked increases in lung tissue are not automatically associated with a massive loss of aeration. The hypothesis that the injured lung collapses under its own weight is not supported by recent experimental and human data. Very likely, the aeration loss in ARDS is mainly resulting from alveolar flooding by edema fluid and/or inflammatory infection. As a consequence, human VILI is basically characterized by alveolar overinflation of aerated lung areas. The uneven distribution of the aeration loss in a majority of patients with ARDS, creates a risk of overinflating normally aerated lung areas when high PEEP is implemented for recruiting nonaerated lung regions. In other words, the injured lung of the majority of ARDS patients cannot be kept fully aerated at end-expiration without overinflating some parts of the lungs. These data form the rationale for selecting the right PEEP level, which should be a compromise between the benefits of lung recruitment and the risks of lung overdistension. Adequate body positioning by reversing the external compression on lower lobes appears an attractive complement to PEEP for re-establishing lung aeration in ARDS.

Acknowledgments. We would like to give special thanks to Priscyla Girardi who actively contributed to the present manuscript. Cassio Girardi was the recipient of a scholarship provided by the Ministère Français des Affaires Etrangères (ref 359530G/P330281D).

References

1. Gattinoni L, Pelosi P, Pesenti A, et al (1991) CT scan in ARDS; clinical and physiopathological insights. Acta Anaesthesiol Scand 35 (Suppl 95):87–96
2. Gattinoni L, Caironi P, Pelosi P, Goodman LR (2001) What has computed tomography taught us about the acute respiratory distress syndrome? Am J Respir Crit Care Med 164:1701–1711

3. Pelosi P, Goldner M, McKibben A, et al (2001) Recruitment and derecruitment during acute respiratory failure: an experimental study. Am J Respir Crit Care Med 164:122–130
4. Muscedere JG, Mullen JB, Gan K, Slutsky AS (1994) Tidal ventilation at low airway pressures can augment lung injury. Am J Respir Crit Care Med 149:1327–1334
5. Tremblay L, Valenza F, Ribeiro SP, Li J, Slutsky AS (1997) Injurious ventilatory strategies increase cytokines and c-fos m-RNA expression in an isolated rat lung model. J Clin Invest 99:944–952
6. Slutsky AS (2001) Basic science in ventilator-induced lung injury: implications for the bedside. Am J Respir Crit Care Med 163:599–600
7. Lachmann B (1992) Open up the lung and keep the lung open. Intensive Care Med 18:319–321
8. Dreyfuss D, Saumon G (1998) Ventilator-induced lung injury: lessons from experimental studies. Am J Respir Crit Care Med 157:294–323
9. Martynowicz MA, Walters BJ, Hubmayr RD (2001) Mechanisms of recruitment in oleic acid-injured lungs. J Appl Physiol 90:1744–1753
10. Martynowicz MA, Minor TA, Walters BJ, Hubmayr RD (1999) Regional expansion of oleic acid-injured lungs. Am J Respir Crit Care Med 160:250–258
11. Ware LB, Matthay MA (2000) The acute respiratory distress syndrome. N Engl J Med 342:1334–1349
12. Hubmayr RD (2002) Perspective on lung injury and recruitment: a skeptical look at the opening and collapse story. Am J Respir Crit Care Med 165:1647–1653
13. Rouby JJ, Lherm T, Martin de Lassale E, et al (1993) Histologic aspects of pulmonary barotrauma in critically ill patients with acute respiratory failure. Intensive Care Med 19:383–389
14. Goldstein I, Bughalo MT, Marquette CH, Lenaour G, Lu Q, Rouby JJ (2001) Mechanical ventilation-induced air-space enlargement during experimental pneumonia in piglets. Am J Respir Crit Care Med 163:958–964
15. Gattinoni L, Pesenti A, Torresin A, et al (1986) Adult respiratoy distress syndrome profiles by computed tomography. J Thorac Imag 1:25–30
16. Puybasset L, Cluzel P, Gusman P, Grenier P, Preteux F, Rouby JJ (2000) Regional distribution of gas and tissue in acute respiratory distress syndrome. I. Consequences for lung morphology. CT Scan ARDS Study Group. Intensive Care Med 26:857–869
17. Malbouisson LM, Preteux F, Puybasset L, Grenier P, Coriat P, Rouby JJ (2001) Validation of a software designed for computed tomographic (CT) measurement of lung water. Intensive Care Med 27:602–608
18. Malbouisson LM, Muller JC, Constantin JM, Lu Q, Puybasset L, Rouby JJ (2001) Computed tomography assessment of positive end-expiratory pressure-induced alveolar recruitment in patients with acute respiratory distress syndrome. Am J Respir Crit Care Med 163:1444–1450
19. Vieira S, Puybasset L, Richecoeur J, et al (1998) A lung computed tomographic assessment of positive end-expiratory pressure-induced lung overdistension. Am J Respir Crit Care Med 158:1571–1577
20. Puybasset L, Gusman P, Muller J-C, et al (2000) Regional distribution of gas and tissue in acute respiratory distress syndrome - part 3: Consequences for the effects of positive end expiratory pressure. Intensive Care Med 26:1215–1227
21. Rouby JJ, Puybasset L, Cluzel P, Richecoeur J, Lu Q, Grenier P (2000) Regional distribution of gas and tissue in acute respiratory distress syndrome. II. Physiological correlations and definition of an ARDS Severity Score. CT Scan ARDS Study Group. Intensive Care Med 26:1046–1056
22. Gattinoni L, Pesenti A, Avalli L, Rossi F, Bombino M (1987) Pressure-volume curve of total respiratory system in acute respiratory failure. Computed tomographic scan study. Am Rev Respir Dis 136:730–736
23. Gattinoni L, D'Andrea L, Pelosi P, Vitale G, Pesenti A, Fumagalli R (1993) Regional effects and mechanism of positive end-expiratory pressure in early adult respiratory distress syndrome. JAMA 269:2122–2127

24. Gattinoni L, Pesenti A, Bombino M, et al (1988) Relationships between lung computed tomographic density, gas exchange, and PEEP in acute respiratory failure. Anesthesiology 69:824–832

25. Puybasset L, Cluzel P, Chao N, et al (1998) A computed tomography assessment of regional lung volume in acute lung injury. Am J Respir Crit Care Med 158:1644–1655

26. Lu Q, Malbouisson LM, Mourgeon E, Goldstein I, Coriat P, Rouby JJ (2001) Assessment of PEEP-induced reopening of collapsed lung regions in acute lung injury: are one or three CT sections representative of the entire lung? Intensive Care Med 27:1504–1510

27. Gevenois PA, Vuyst P, Maertelaer V, et al (1996) Comparison of computed density and microscopic morphometry in pulmonary emphysema. Am J Respir Crit Care Med 154:187–192

28. Gould GA, Macnee W, Mclean A, et al (1988) CT measurements of lung density in life can quantitate distal airspace enlargement – An essential defining feature of human emphysema. Am Rev Respir Dis 137:380–392

29. Mondor H (1940) Diagnostics urgents Abdomen. Masson Editeur, Paris

30. Malbouisson LM, Busch CJ, Puybasset L, Lu Q, Cluzel P, Rouby JJ (2000) Role of the heart in the loss of aeration characterizing lower lobes in acute respiratory distress syndrome. CT Scan ARDS Study Group. Am J Respir Crit Care Med 161:2005–2012

31. Gattinoni L, Pelosi P, Vitale G, Pesenti A, D'andrea L, Mascheroni D (1991) Body position changes redistribute lung computed tomographic density in patients with acute respiratory failure. Anesthesiology 74:15–23

32. Richard JC, Maggiore SM, Michard F, et al (1999) Upright positioning (UP) in patients with Acute Lung Injury (ALI). Am J Respir Crit Care Med 159:A 695 (abst)

33. Hickling KG (1998) The pressure-volume curve is greatly modified by recruitment. A mathematical model of ARDS lungs. Am J Respir Crit Care Med 158:194–202

34. Suki B, Andrade JS, Jr., Coughlin MF, et al (1998) Mathematical modeling of the first inflation of degassed lungs. Ann Biomed Eng 26:608–617

35. Martin-Lefevre L, Ricard JD, Roupie E, Dreyfuss D, Saumon G (2001) Significance of the changes in the respiratory system pressure-volume curve during acute lung injury in rats. Am J Respir Crit Care Med 164:627–632

36. Wilson TA, Anafi RC, Hubmayr RD (2001) Mechanics of edematous lungs. J Appl Physiol 90:2088–2093

37. Jonson B, Richard JC, Straus C, Mancebo J, Lemaire F, Brochard L (1999) Pressure-volume curves and compliance in acute lung injury: evidence of recruitment above the lower inflection point. Am J Respir Crit Care Med 159:1172–1178

38. Richard JC, Maggiore SM, Jonson B, Mancebo J, Lemaire F, Brochard L (2001) Influence of tidal volume on alveolar recruitment. Respective role of PEEP and a recruitment maneuver. Am J Respir Crit Care Med 163:1609–1613

39. Gattinoni L, Pelosi P, Suter PM, Pedoto A, Vercesi P, Lissoni A (1998) Acute respiratory distress syndrome caused by pulmonary and extrapulmonary disease. Different syndromes? Am J Respir Crit Care Med 158:3–11

40. Rialp G, Betbese AJ, Perez-Marquez M, Mancebo J (2001) Short-term effects of inhaled nitric oxide and prone position in pulmonary and extrapulmonary acute respiratory distress syndrome. Am J Respir Crit Care Med 164:243–249

41. Vieira SR, Puybasset L, Lu Q, et al (1999) A scanographic assessment of pulmonary morphology in acute lung injury. Significance of the lower inflection point detected on the lung pressure-volume curve. Am J Respir Crit Care Med 159:1612–1623

42. Dambrosio M, Roupie E, Mollet JJ, et al (1997) Effects of positive end-expiratory pressure and different tidal volumes on alveolar recruitment and hyperinflation. Anesthesiology 87:495–503

43. Rouby JJ, Lu Q, Goldstein I (2002) Selecting the right level of positive end-expiratory pressure in patients with acute respiratory distress syndrome. Am J Respir Crit Care Med 165:1182–1186

44. Pelosi P, Cadringher P, Bottino N, et al (1999) Sigh in acute respiratory distress syndrome. Am J Respir Crit Care Med 159:872–880

45. Van Der Kloot TE, Blanch L, Youngblood AM, et al (2000) Recruitment maneuvers in three experimentals models of acute lung injury. Effects on lung volume and gas exchange. Am J Respir Crit Care Med 161:1485–1494
46. Pelosi P, D'andrea L, Pesenti A, Gattinoni L (1994) Vertical gradient of regional lung inflation in adult respiratory distress syndrome. Am J Respir Crit Care Med 149:8–13

ARDS/VILI: Therapy

Recruitment Maneuvers in ARDS

V. N. Okamoto, J. B. Borges, and M. B. P. Amato

Introduction

After a decade of evolving concepts about mechanical ventilation in patients with acute lung injury (ALI) and acute respiratory distress syndrome (ARDS), it is now indisputable that reducing lung stretch by limiting the end-inspiratory lung volume powerfully impacts on the outcome of such patients [1, 2]. However, uncertainty remains concerning the relative role of the maintenance of the end-expiratory volume in the context of ALI/ARDS. The avoidance of lung collapse and cyclic reopening may probably determine further benefit on patient outcome but it is a much more complex hypothesis to be tested in randomized clinical trials than the simple reduction of lung stretch [3].

In this chapter, we review the evidence that air space collapse is a major feature of ALI/ARDS and that the presence of lung collapse, either persistent or cyclic, is detrimental. We also comment on the difficulties involved in the testing of a comprehensive protective strategy in the clinical arena.

Evidence of Air Space Collapse in ALI/ARDS

The presence of inhomogeneous aeration in mechanically ventilated patients was first described in tomographic studies of normal subjects during anesthesia [4, 5]. Animal studies proved that these consolidated areas were constituted by atelectatic tissue, with collapsed or folded lung units causing pulmonary shunt and impaired gas exchange [6, 7]. Soon after, the same phenomenon was also observed in a larger extent in computerized tomography (CT) studies of ARDS patients [8].

The finding of non-aerated tissue on gravity dependent lung regions gave rise to theoretical concepts that were later tested in clinical trials. The first was the 'baby lung' concept, which credited the low compliance of the respiratory system observed in ARDS patients to the reduced volume of normally aerated tissue but not to a homogeneously stiff lung parenchyma [9].

Additional insights came from tomographic studies in different ventilator settings. Gattinoni and colleagues observed that increasing levels of positive end-expiratory pressure (PEEP) caused decrements in non aerated tissue, suggesting that these non aerated areas were not liquid or debris-filled alveoli, but collapsed air spaces [9]. They postulated that the collapse occurred due to the increased weight of the edematous lung over its lowermost regions and therefore could be recruited when the resultant of collapsing forces was opposed by positive airway pressure [10]. This 'superimposed pressure theory' implies that the lung skeleton is loose and flexible enough to behave as a liquid body, i.e., the parenchymal stresses are much more determined by the lung weight than by shape of the chest wall [11].

In physical terms, a liquid and a solid body differ in their static response to shearing stress: unlike a solid, a liquid body does not sustain shearing stress. In practical terms, a liquid-like behavior means that the weight of the lung is supported from its base, with the lowermost regions of the lung supporting the weight of the whole column of tissue on top of it. Such transmission of pressures imply that, at a given vertical plane, the pressure at the outer surface of alveolar walls equals density multiplied by the height of the column of tissue above. Microgravity and acceleration experiments performed in fast-jet aircrew support this concept. When submitted to increased acceleration, with an increased inertial force from sternum to spine, the aircrew men experienced airway collapse with trapped gases at the lung bases. By breathing 100% oxygen under those conditions, they developed visible atelectasis in the X-ray of lung bases. This airspace collapse was produced during 3G (3 x gravity) forces, which means that the lung weight increased by 3 times. This increment approximates the weight gain generated by the interstitial lung edema commonly found in ARDS [12, 13].

In a study of ALI/ARDS patients, Tsubo et al. demonstrated the presence of densities in the left lung regions in more than half of his patients using transesophageal echocardiography (TEE). End-expiratory pressures of 5, 10 and 15 cmH2O were applied in some patients, resulting in reduction in the densities associated with the improvement in the PaO2/FiO2 [14].

In a series of CT studies in ARDS patients, Gattinoni and colleagues documented the occurrence of cyclic collapse and reopening during tidal breaths. Increasing PEEP from 0 to 20 cmH2O minimized these occurrences even in patients with heavy and edematous lungs [15]. Clinical studies using serial compliance assessments or pressure volume (PV) loops initiated at different PEEP levels also suggested that tidal recruitment and derecruitment were quite common in patients under mechanical ventilation [16-18]. Once more, very high PEEP levels were necessary to avoid them.

In summary, evidence from various sources has pointed to the presence of dependent collapse caused by the increased lung weight and compression. If one accepts the theory that collapse promotes lung injury, those findings should attract the attention of intensivists.

The 'Fluid and Foam' Hypothesis

Recently, the concept that the liquid-like behavior of the lung is responsible for the vertical gradient of tomographic densities has been challenged on the basis of the so-called limitations of CT [19]. Briefly, the quantitative analysis of CT sections is based on the density number assigned to voxels (the CT unit of volume) inside a region of interest. Each voxel usually embraces hundreds of alveolar units. As the CT density number represents the composite of the density distribution within the voxel, it cannot distinguish between alveolar collapse and alveolar flooding [13]. For instance, when explaining how PEEP could decrease the amount of consolidated areas in the CT images, some authors have argued that the addition of PEEP could expand further those lung units already open, decreasing the mean density of the given region of interest without any recruitment of the flooded areas. Furthermore, the addition of PEEP could displace fluid-filled alveoli along the craniocaudal axis, putting them out of the initial plane of interest, with additional decrease of the mean density.

The studies supporting this challenging hypothesis are based on the parenchymal marker technique, which is claimed to measure regional lung volumes directly by means of transthoracic implants of metal beads in the caudal lobes. By measuring the distance among the beads (i.e., the volume outlined by groups of 4 of them), Martynovicz and colleagues did not observe any reduction in the functional residual capacity (FRC) of dependent lung regions measured soon after the development of oleic-acid injury in dogs [20]. These authors concluded that this phenomenon was not compatible with the presence of alveolar collapse consequent to the superimposed pressure and that alveolar flooding would be the responsible mechanism for the phenomenon. The absence of significant phase lag between dependent and non-dependent lung regions during inspiration was also interpreted as a strong argument against the superimposed pressure gradient. If the opening pressures were determined by the superimposed pressures, one should expect a vertical wave of recruitment across the parenchyma, with the dependent regions popping open much later during inspiration, only after the achievement of very high inspiratory pressures.

Finally, the authors challenge the concept that high energy dissipation (with stress concentration on the terminal bronchioles) is involved in the recruitment process. They considered that liquid bridges interspersed with trapped air might occlude the branching network of open airways. Under this condition, opening pressures would be dissipated on a series of curved menisci spread over the bronchial tree, and local stresses on the lining epithelial cells would be negligible [19, 20]. In that case, ventilator-induced lung injury (VILI) could only be caused by overdistension of already aerated alveoli, rather than by shear stresses in airways as they open. In simpler words: if the 'liquid and foam' argument were correct, recruitment maneuvers would be pointless.

More than Foam

It is important to stress here that, according to extensive experimental evidence, collapse and flooding are not mutually exclusive. In fact, it is very likely that the collapse of lung units favors plasma transudation from the capillaries of collapsed septa. We believe that much of the 'liquid and foam' controversy quoted above could be avoided by adopting a straightforward definition of recruitment: the aeration of a previously collapsed, flooded or folded unit, enough to promote some gas exchange. A flooded unit can also be recruited, as commonly occurs during partial liquid ventilation, with bubbles of air filling the alveolar space, surrounded by a thick liquid layer. The recruitment achieved at end inspiration may vanish at end expiration, especially when the surfactant properties are impaired or the unit is flooded. Still, this transient aeration may be enough to increase arterial oxygenation or CO_2 elimination.

By accepting this simple definition, two important consequences follow concerning the mechanics of recruitment (now broadly considering a flooded or truly collapsed unit). First, according to the interdependence models of the lung skeleton, the flooding of a central alveolus may attenuate the alveolar wall stress caused by the expansion of surrounding units, but it does not eliminate it. According to the original conception of interdependence, the stresses are created by non uniform expansion and not exclusively by complete atelectasis [21]. Second, the progression of a bubble of air inside a liquid filled airway can still cause a lot of stress, especially at the level of the lining epithelial cells of bronchioles, as demonstrated by studies from Bilek and co-workers [22].

Having arisen from a single group of experiments in dogs, submitted to the peculiar preparation of oleic acid lung injury, the conclusions of the experiments supporting the foam hypothesis contrast with overwhelming evidence coming from studies using sophisticated imaging techniques. Not sharing the so-called limitations of conventional CT, these studies strongly suggest the ubiquitous occurrence of dependent collapse, associated with loss of regional lung volume, in patients with ALI.

For instance, recent investigations using electrical impedance tomography (EIT), a bedside imaging technique representing a much thicker slice of lung tissue (10-15 cm), have corroborated the findings of the CT studies in animal models of lung injury. Briefly, EIT is based on the detection of variations in electrical tissue impedance. As changes in thoracic impedance are linearly related to changes in air volume [23], this tool is very appealing as a monitoring device for mechanical ventilation, where imbalances in ventilation are well known [24]. In a lung lavage model of ALI, pressure-volume and pressure-impedance curves were compared during lung inflation with the constant flow technique [25]. The pressure-volume and the pressure-impedance curves were significantly correlated (r^2=0.76; p<.005). There was an identifiable lower inflection point (LIP) in both curves for the nine pigs studied. The LIP of the pressure-impedance curve was within 2 cmH_2O of the LIP of the pressure-volume curve. By defining gravity-oriented regions of interest on the EIT images, it was possible to identify regional lower inflection points of each region of interest. Not surprisingly, the dependent regions showed a higher regional inflection point in the pressure-impedance curve. These findings were compatible with the presence of collapse in the dependent lung region and with an opening pressure gradient of 9 cmH_2O across the vertical axis, exactly as predicted by the superimposed pressure theory.

Direct proof of the existence of tidal recruitment and collapse comes also from *in vivo* microscopy of subpleural alveoli. In normal lungs, this technique has demonstrated that there is little change in the alveolar volume during tidal ventilation [26] despite the large change in overall lung volume. The authors suggested that the recruitment of new units instead of alveolar inflation was the predominant phenomenon taking place during lung expansion. On the contrary, in a surfactant deactivation model of lung injury, a dramatic increase in alveolar size was observed at end inspiration, with partial or total expiratory collapse [27]. This observation is in agreement with the classic propositions of Mead that in non uniformly expanded lungs the effective distending pressure can be much higher than the global transpulmonary pressure, leading to inspiratory overinflation of air spaces neighboring collapsed or flooded alveoli [21].

Corroborating those findings, studies with fluorescent-quenching PO_2 probes clearly demonstrated enormous oscillations in PaO_2 associated with tidal inflation/deflations in a lung lavage model producing alveolar instability. The temporary occurrence of massive shunt at end-expiration strongly suggested the existence of tidal recruitment/derecruitment. Interestingly, these oscillations in PaO_2 decreased with the addition of PEEP [28].

We believe that the skepticism against CT as a tool to diagnose lung collapse and recruitment tends to dissipate as advances in the technique permit scanning of the whole lung at acceptable radiation levels and increased spatial resolution. Recent volumetric scanning of the whole lung, apex-to-diaphragm, have cast light on the concerns expressed above (i.e., that non aerated regions might be displaced on the craniocaudal axis by increments of PEEP, causing a misleading reduction in densities). For instance, Lu and coworkers confirmed a reduction of non aerated tissue after PEEP increments in a quantitative analysis embracing the whole lung [29]. Our own experience with this technique reinforced the latter findings. In a spiral tomographic study of 11 ALI/ARDS patients [30, 31], we observed a dramatic reduction of non aerated tissue in the apex-to-diaphragm CT scans after a stepwise and intensive recruitment maneuver. This reduction was very well correlated with an increase in PaO_2, compatible with a reduction in the shunt fraction to less than 10%.

Rouby and coworkers have also demonstrated that the total lung volume of patients with ARDS, assessed by spiral/volumetric CT scan, is severely reduced when compared to normal subjects. This remained so even after PEEP application (10 cmH_2O) with substantial reduction in the amount of high-density zones. By considering that the total lung volume assessed by CT encompasses tissue, liquid and air, and that the tissue plus liquid components are usually increased, a profound reduction of FRC must have occurred. These results were in evident opposition to the 'flooding hypothesis' and the experiments with the parenchymal marker technique in oleic-acid induced lung injury, in which the authors reported maintenance of regional FRC.

As an additional finding to these complete volumetric CT studies, two recent investigations have suggested that a craniocaudal gradient is negligible in patients or animal models of ARDS and, therefore, the displacement of fluid densities towards the caudal regions cannot be evoked as an explanation for the density changes caused by PEEP - as observed in single CT slices [32, 33].

Finally, in contrast to the results in dogs, we have recently demonstrated the unequivocal presence of phase-lag between dependent versus non-dependent zones in patients with ARDS or ALI (Fig. 1). As indicated above, the existence of phase-lag along the gravity axis is very suggestive of a true vertical gradient of opening/collapsing pressures, confirming the predictions of the superimposed pressure theory.

In summary, the majority of evidence points to the existence of true air space collapse on the dependent lung regions in ALI/ARDS patients, with a marked loss

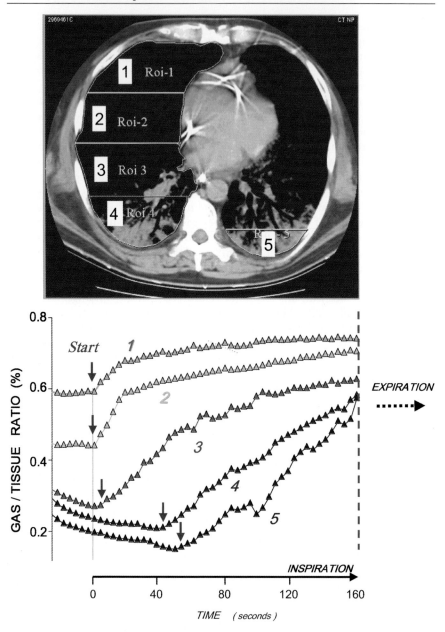

Fig. 1. A sequence of dynamic CT scanning obtained in a patient with ARDS. During a slow inflation maneuver at constant flow rate (1 l/min), sequential CT scans (every 2 seconds) in the same thoracic plane were obtained. After splitting the lung area into five regions of interest (ROI), as indicated in the top part of the figure, the average gas/tissue ratio for each ROI was plotted against time. As shown, after suffering a small deflation (suggestive of complete airway blockage), dependent zones start to inflate only after a delay of more than 40 seconds. The delay was proportional to the superimposed pressure gradient.

of regional lung volume, as predicted by the superimposed pressure theory. Obviously, some alveolar flooding may also occur, but not as the predominant phenomenon in the clinical setting. In opposition to the 'liquid and foam' hypothesis, we also believe that the eventual presence of some flooding does not simplify the matter and should not attenuate our concerns about VILI. The expected shear stress applied on the terminal airway or among adjacent alveoli with different opening pressures seems to be very high, regardless of whether the alveoli are flooded or truly collapsed.

Evidence of Detrimental Effects of Air Space Collapse

Putting aside the practical problems related to the clinical implementation of lung recruitment, there is experimental evidence of a beneficial effect associated to the maintenance of end-expiratory volume at every level of observation.

On the cellular level, the consequences of controlled deformation on the alveolar epithelial viability were assessed in an *in vitro* model [34]. In this model, repetitive stretching of alveolar epithelial cells was more damaging than tonically held deformations. For the same maximum deformation, any reduction of the amplitude of cell deformation (obtained by increasing the tonic or sustained deformation during the relaxation phase) significantly reduced damage as compared with full range or large-amplitude deformations. These data suggest that prevention of cyclic air space deflation to low volumes followed by re-expansion by means of enough end-expiratory pressure might reduce injury.

The reopening of a collapsed airway was modeled experimentally and computationally by means of the progression of a bubble in a narrow fluid-occluded channel with a lining of viable pulmonary epithelial cells, as mentioned above [22]. This model was valid both for collapsible or rigid-fluid-filled airways and demonstrated that the mechanical stresses during airway reopening causes injury to epithelial cells, ultimately resulting in cell death and epithelial detachment. High surface tension forces at the lining layer seemed to amplify those phenomena. However, even when considering healthy airways and normal lungs, recent studies have suggested that, during airway reopening, there is enough stress to cause problems along periods as short as 6 hours of mechanical ventilation [35]. The airway collapse in this study was simply promoted by muscle paralysis, increasing the pleural pressures preferentially at the dependent zones.

In vivo microscopy demonstrated that PEEP stabilized alveoli in the model of surfactant deactivation with tween [36]. After enough PEEP, tidal ventilation resembled an almost normal pattern of alveolar inflation. A study to determine if this nearly normal appearance is also related to less release of inflammatory cytokines is currently under way (Gary Nieman, personal communication).

At a broader level of observation of the lung function, which includes pulmonary mechanics, oxygenation, pressure-volume curves, histology and production of inflammatory cytokines, a protective effect of PEEP was demonstrated in all the studies that kept a similar end-inspiratory pressure in the comparison group. Webb and Tierney first demonstrated that 10 cmH$_2$O PEEP was protective when applied during ventilation with 45 cmH$_2$O peak pressure. They showed better oxygenation, compliance and absence of alveolar edema in comparison with the huge alterations observed in the group ventilated with 45 cmH2O peak pressure and zero PEEP [37]. This finding was consistent with the subsequent work of Dreyfuss et al., who also demonstrated that the ultra structure of the alveolar epithelium was preserved in a group of rats ventilated with 45 cmH2O peak pressure and 10 cmH2O PEEP [38]

However, in all these *in vivo* experiments it was difficult to isolate the effect of PEEP in preventing injury because of the impossibility of maintaining similar blood flow and oxygenation between the comparison groups. To overcome this problem, Muscedere and colleagues developed an *ex vivo* non-perfused model of lung injury induced by lung lavage [39]. They demonstrated that low volume ventilation could worsen previous lung injury and that PEEP above the LIP of the pressure volume curve did prevent damage. In a subsequent study with a similar *ex vivo* model, Tremblay showed that a group of rats ventilated with tidal volume (V_T) of 15 ml/kg and PEEP of 10 cmH2O (peak pressure around 56 cmH2O) suffered less injury than both a group ventilated with V_T 40 ml/kg and zero PEEP (peak pressure around 46 cmH2O) and a group with V_T 15 ml/kg and zero PEEP (peak pressure around 30 cmH2O). The static compliance curves of the moderate volume/ high PEEP group were not shifted to the right after two hours of ventilation, which markedly occurred in both zero PEEP groups. The final concentrations of tumor necrosis factor (TNF)-α, interleukin (IL)-1β, IL-6, macrophage inflammatory protein (MIP)-2, interferon (IFN)-γ and IL-10 in the lung lavage were also lower in the PEEP group [40]. This finding, although criticized [41], was consistent with subsequent investigation in a sheep model of lung injury induced by repeated lavage [42]. Takeuchi et al. [42] demonstrated higher levels of messenger RNA for IL-1β and IL-8 in lung lavage sheep ventilated with PEEP titrated according to oxygenation (around 16 cmH2O) when compared to two other PEEP-titration strategies based on the pressure-volume curve, in which PEEP was around 22 and 26 cmH2O. The plateau pressure was slightly higher in the two latter groups, implying that the prevention of lung collapse played a pivotal role in lung protection, even at the cost of a somewhat higher plateau pressure.

Nonetheless, in our opinion, comparisons between high frequency oscillation ventilation (HFOV) and conventional ventilation provide the most compelling histological evidence of lung protection through a strategy aiming at the maintenance of a high expiratory lung volume. In an *in vivo* rabbit model of lung lavage, Hamilton demonstrated that HFOV after a sustained inflation of 25–30 cmH2O was associated with a PaO2 around 400 mmHg during 5 and 20 hours. The conventional ventilation group also received the same sustained inflation, but was later submitted to lower mean airway pressures and progressed with deterioration on oxygenation and death within 20 hours. On histological examination, the lungs ventilated with HFOV showed less prominent epithelial sloughing and necrosis and much less hyaline membrane formation [43]. In a complementary study, the same group compared two strategies of HFOV. The HFOV strategy aiming at a high lung volume applied whatever airway pressure necessary to achieve a PaO2 > 350 mmHg. This strategy was associated with less epithelial damage than both HFOV employing lower mean airway pressures and conventional ventilation [44].

Extending further these results, Rimensberger ventilated surfactant-depleted rabbits, demonstrating that a volume recruitment strategy during small V_T ventilation (using conventional frequencies) plus lung volumes above a critical closing pressure is as protective as HFOV at similar lung volumes [45]. These findings strongly suggest that the mainstay of a comprehensive protective ventilation is the maintenance of the alveolar volume.

Obviously, when the maintenance of end-expiratory lung volumes results in unavoidable increment of end-inspiratory pressures because of the constraints of CO_2 removal the net result of such a strategy will depend on the range of pressures applied, and the peculiarities of the animal model studied. However, two consistent findings in the literature should be noted:

a) When considering studies comparing animals submitted to equivalent end-inspiratory pressures, there is almost no exception for the protective effects of PEEP,

b) Even in studies where PEEP caused some increment in end-inspiratory pressures (compared to the control group), a beneficial net effect was still demonstrated by several of them, depending on the range of pressures applied and on the animal preparation.

Evidence and Limitations of Recent Clinical Trials

The recent randomized clinical studies [1, 2, 46–48] on lung protective ventilation gave rise to much debate. Some important aspects require further comment in this chapter. Although the five studies addressed the consequences of the 'baby lung theory' by limiting the end-inspiratory pressure, only the Brazilian study applied a first-intention strategy to prevent cyclic collapse and reopening [1]. The chosen PEEP-titration method at the time was the inspiratory pressure volume curve. PEEP was set at 2 cmH2O above the LIP (Pflex) of a pressure volume curve obtained before randomization. This PEEP strategy was applied on the protective ventilation arm after a recruitment maneuver with continous positive airways pressure (CPAP) of 35 to 40 cmH2O for 40 seconds. On that occasion, we believed that nearly maximal recruitment and aeration could be achieved with this strategy. Later investigation suggested, however, that the term 'open lung approach' needed some review.

The theoretical limitations of the inspiratory pressure volume curve as a PEEP titration method to prevent airspace collapse have been extensively discussed [49] (Fig. 2). Much less appreciated, however, was the inefficacy of a '40x40' CPAP maneuver to achieve total lung recruitment (defined as shunt fraction< 10%) in ALI/ARDS patients.

The most direct evidence of the incompleteness of the above recruitment strategy is our own subsequent work [30, 31]. We compared oxygenation and the presence of non-aerated tissue on CT scans of ALI/ARDS patients under two conditions: a) PEEP = Pflex + 2 cmH2O after a recruitment maneuver with CPAP of 40 cmH2O, and b) PEEP at a higher level (titrated though a decremental PEEP protocol) after a stepwise and intensive recruitment maneuver achieving plateau inspiratory pressures beyond 40 cmH2O (Fig. 3). What became clear after those experiments is that the opening/collapsing pressures found in the adult lung with ARDS are much higher than the predictions of the superimposed pressure theory alone, suggesting the existence of superposed collapsing forces like active surface

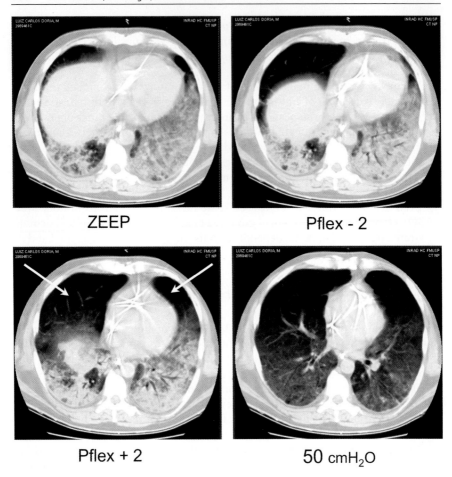

Fig. 2. A sequence of dynamic CT scanning obtained in a patient with ARDS, in a similar protocol to figure 1. Representative slices at airway pressures slightly below or slightly above an easily identifiable Pflex are shown. As can be observed, the crossing of Pflex coincides with the aeration of a large area in the non-dependent lung regions, but still accompanied by a large amount of collapse at the dependent lung regions.

tension forces, increased abdominal pressures, or maybe some other unknown factors [50]. Second, although there was some reasonable correlation between Pflex (usually corresponding to the opening pressures of the non-dependent lung regions – Fig. 2) and the expiratory closing pressures, a full recruitment strategy would require a more advanced approach.

As recruitment is also a time-dependent phenomenon, a final point to be considered here is that although clearly insufficient along the first hours of ventilation, our recruiting maneuvers and the subsequent PEEP levels in the Brazilian ARDS trial may have been enough to achieve a much higher lung recruitment over

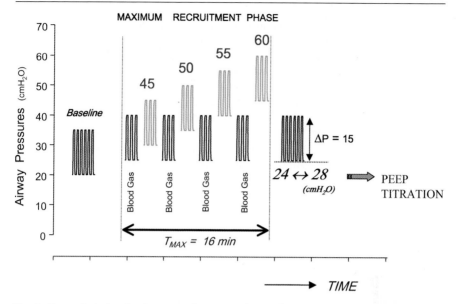

Fig. 3. Protocol design for lung recruitment. Each step lasts approximately 2 minutes and represents pressure controlled mechanical ventilation (I:E = 1:1, RR = 10 cycles/min). Note that later steps are optional, depending on the results of blood-gases during the controlled mechanical ventilation period at PEEP = 25 cmH2O. The detection of PaO2 values above 350 mmHg during this period was considered as indicator of near-maximum recruitment (less than 10% collapse) and the subsequent steps were aborted. Subsequently the patient initiated the PEEP titration phase, trying to detect the minimum PEEP capable of keeping PaO2 levels within 95% of the maximum value obtained.

the days. This cannot be proved retrospectively since we did not make serial measurements of the shunt fraction of our patients.

While the importance of preventing lung overinflation is now indisputable, the impact of preventing cyclic air space collapse and reopening is much more difficult to test. Our own study, as discussed above, is an example of the intrinsic difficulty in determining if the lung is recruited or not. Large randomized clinical trials of other ventilatory strategies aiming at alveolar recruitment and stabilization might have suffered from this same drawback. In a multicenter randomized trial of prone positioning in ARDS/ALI patients [51], an improvement in PaO2/FiO2 was observed in the prone position, which could not be sustained when the patient was positioned back to the supine position. It is tempting to speculate that insufficient PEEP was applied when back to the supine position, not enough to maintain the recruitment achieved during the prone position period. It is also worth considering whether or not full lung recruitment was achieved with the prone strategy. Another example of how ventilator handling may be influential on study results can be drawn from the comparison of two recent large randomized clinical studies of HFOV in infants. One of them demonstrated a beneficial effect of HFOV on mortality or development of bronchodysplasia [52], while the other did not [53]. As well observed in the editorial accompanying both studies [54], Johnson et al.

[53] found a higher rate of death and bronchodysplasia associated with the same type of oscillator that Courtney et al. [52] used successfully. A likely explanation for those opposite results would be the fact that the authors used the same ventilator quite differently, applying a different sequence of maneuvers and making different uses of the lung volume history.

Although the theoretical concept "open up the lung and keep it open" is most appealing [55], we believe still that it could not be tested broadly in the clinical setting of the adult patient with ALI/ARDS for several reasons summarized below:

1. Few instruments are capable of estimating the amount of collapsed lung tissue at the bedside. Many authors have stressed the limitations of respiratory mechanics measurements for this purpose [9, 27, 28, 49, 56]. In this context, we are enthusiastic about the potentials of EIT to detect imbalances in regional ventilation [24] (Fig. 4), the very phenomenon we want to avoid in a comprehensive protective strategy. The use of intrarterial blood gas analysis for titration of recruitment maneuvers and PEEP may prove to be a reasonable alternative for the bedside, especially when the amount of hypoxic vasoconstriction is negligible (a frequent scenario in the acute phase of ARDS, but not afterwards). It must be emphasized that we do not regard oxygenation as a clinical parameter to be met, but as a marker of a low shunt fraction, and thus, total lung recruitment. This approach is very different to that adopted in the unpublished ALVEOLI study, where different PEEP-FiO2 arrangements were proposed in order to reach a target oxygenation for both arms of the study.

2. The recruitment maneuver using CPAP= 40 cmH2O is not effective in obtaining total lung recruitment. We developed a stepwise and intensive recruitment maneuver using tidal ventilation with a fixed driving pressure and increasing PEEP levels, titrated according to the intrarterial blood gases to achieve total lung recruitment (Fig. 3). The objective of this maneuver is to reach a shunt fraction below 10% (defined as $PaO_2 > 350$ mmHg at $FiO_2 = 1.0$). This permits PEEP titration on the outer envelope of the deflation limb of the PV curve [49] at a reasonably low risk of barotrauma (Fig. 5).

3. The use of high PEEP levels poses the risk of transient overinflation of nondependent lung regions and barotrauma, as well as hemodynamic instability due to transmission of the applied pressures to the heart and great vessels [57]. However, our clinical impression is that the above mentioned stepwise maneuver is surprisingly well tolerated. As others, we have observed that the more collapsed the lung tissue, the lower the transmission of the applied airway pressure to the heart and great vessels. Therefore, the first recruitment steps are usually well tolerated in this stepwise approach, with some few problems only in the later steps (the highest steps are necessary only for very few patients, since the majority get full recruitment in the first 2 or 3 steps). Another theoretical argument in favor of this stepwise approach – as opposed to the 'single pulse' approach [58] is the reasoning that high pressures will only be employed when the parenchyma is already more homogeneous, avoiding transient peaks in transpulmonary pressure and decreasing the risks for barotrauma (Fig. 5). A clinical study is under way to clarify this issue. Preliminary data point to the occurrence of transient hypotension, in a similar degree to that observed in a safety study of a less aggressive, yet far less effective recruitment maneuver [59].

PEEP = 0 cmH₂O

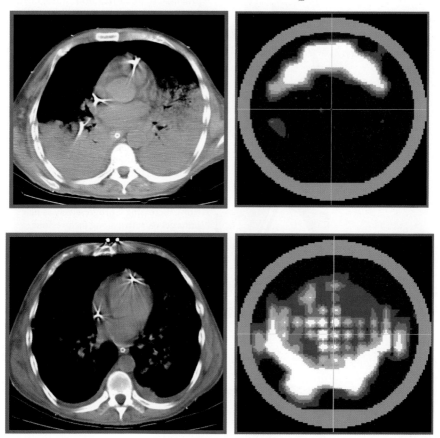

PEEP = 30 cmH₂O

Fig. 4. Tomographic images obtained at zero end-expiratory pressure (ZEEP, top) and after the application of 30 cmH₂O PEEP (bottom). Electric impedance tomography (EIT) images are presented on the right, whereas the corresponding CT images (obtained at the same PEEP level) are represented in the left side of the figure. The EIT images represent the ventilation map during tidal breaths. Brighter areas indicate pixels with larger impedance variations (larger alveolar ventilation) during tidal breaths. Excessive, as well as insufficient PEEP levels, caused uneven ventilation. Excessive PEEP caused preferential ventilation in the dependent lung zones (because of the relative overdistension of non-dependent lung zones). Insufficient PEEP caused dependent collapse with preferential ventilation towards the patent airspaces at the non-dependent 'baby-lung'.

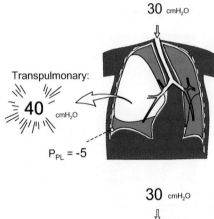

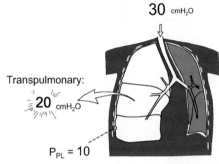

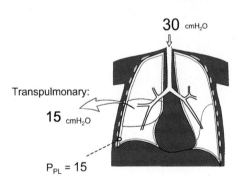

Fig. 5. Illustration of the rationale for the proposed stepwise recruitment maneuver (see figure 3). Observe that the same airway pressure (30 cmH$_2$O) can result in quite different transpulmonary pressures, depending on the total amount of collapsed tissue (see the 3 different lung conditions from top to bottom). When collapse is prevalent (top), the overall pleural pressure results very low and the local transpulmonary pressures (measured across the few opened areas) increase significantly. The risk of overdistension is very high at this condition, especially if one considers a single step - high pressure recruiting maneuver. Contrarily, we propose the application of lower pressures at this moment (top), increasing it progressively as new units get recruited along the previous steps. For instance, the patient represented at the bottom of the figure could stand a much higher plateau pressure than the patient at the top.

The risks of a recruitment maneuver should be comparable to the risks of a pulse-therapy, where the benefits in the long run are expected to outweigh the short-term risks. This is why the recruitment maneuver should be self-limited and as short as possible, taking advantage of the benefits collected during the resting period. That is also the reason why we do not believe that sighs should be proposed as recruiting maneuvers [60, 61]. Sighs provide a transient benefit in oxygenation by tidal recruitment, but they play no role in stabilizing the alveoli. They also lack any perspective of long-term benefit, since the patient is repetitively exposed to an injurious pattern of ventilation.

Conclusion

The avoidance of air space collapse and reopening, along with the avoidance of overdistension should be viewed as the primary goal of the ventilatory approach of the ALI/ARDS patient. The short-term use of high airway pressures as a boost to achieve an open lung status may prove to be important in the clinical setting of ALI/ARDS patients. Experimental evidence demonstrates the protective effect of the maintenance of the end-expiratory volume, as discussed in this chapter. Nonetheless, the testing of this broader concept is hampered by difficulties in detecting lung collapse and recruitment at the bedside. For this reason, we are awaiting the development of bedside technologies capable of detecting imbalances in regional ventilation. Furthermore, we are also evaluating the safety and efficacy of a stepwise recruitment maneuver based on the above-mentioned concepts regarding the pressure volume relationships. The rationale for this strategy carries an analogy with the concept of pulse-therapy, in the sense of being a balance between a short-term risk (i.e., the recruiting phase), which is expected to be minimal, and the consequent effect of maintaining the end-expiratory volume, which is expected to be a step forward in the management of ALI/ARDS patients.

References

1. Amato MB, Barbas CS, Medeiros DM, et al (1998) Effect of a protective-ventilation strategy on mortality in the acute respiratory distress syndrome. N Engl J Med 338:347–354
2. ARDSNet (2000) Ventilation with lower tidal volumes as compared with traditional tidal volumes for acute lung injury and the acute respiratory distress syndrome. N Engl J Med 342:1301–1308
3. Dries DJ, Marini JJ (2002) Optimized positive end-expiratory pressure - an elusive target. Crit Care Med 30:1159–1160
4. Damgaard-Pedersen K, Qvist T (1980) Pediatric pulmonary CT-scanning. Anaesthesia-induced changes. Pediatr Radiol 9:145–148
5. Brismar B, Hedenstierna G, Lundquist H, Strandberg A, Svensson L, Tokics L (1985) Pulmonary densities during anesthesia with muscular relaxation—a proposal of atelectasis. Anesthesiology 62:422–428
6. Hedenstierna G, Lundquist H, Lundh B, et al (1989) Pulmonary densities during anaesthesia. An experimental study on lung morphology and gas exchange. Eur Respir J 2:528–535
7. Nyman G, Funkquist B, Kvart C, et al (1990) Atelectasis causes gas exchange impairment in the anaesthetised horse. Equine Vet J 22:317–324
8. Gattinoni L, Mascheroni D, Torresin A, et al (1986) Morphological response to positive end expiratory pressure in acute respiratory failure. Computerized tomography study. Intensive Care Med 12:137–142
9. Gattinoni L, Pesenti A, Avalli L, Rossi F, Bombino M (1987) Pressure-volume curve of total respiratory system in acute respiratory failure. Computed tomographic scan study. Am Rev Respir Dis 136:730–736
10. Gattinoni L, D'Andrea L, Pelosi P, Vitale G, Pesenti A, Fumagalli R (1993) Regional effects and mechanism of positive end-expiratory pressure in early adult respiratory distress syndrome. JAMA 269:2122–2127
11. Pelosi P, D'Andrea L, Vitale G, Pesenti A, Gattinoni L (1994) Vertical gradient of regional lung inflation in adult respiratory distress syndrome. Am J Respir Crit Care Med 149:8–13

12. Glaister DH (2001) Effects of aceleration on the lung. In: Prisk GK, West JB (eds) Gravity and the Lung: Lessons from Microgravity, 1st edn. Marcel Dekker Inc., New York, pp 39–74
13. Gattinoni L, Caironi P, Pelosi P, Goodman LR (2001) What has computed tomography taught us about the acute respiratory distress syndrome? Am J Respir Crit Care Med 164:1701–1711
14. Tsubo T, Sakai I, Suzuki A, Okawa H, Ishihara H, Matsuki A (2001) Density detection in dependent left lung region using transesophageal echocardiography. Anesthesiology 94:793–798
15. Gattinoni L, Pelosi P, Crotti S, Valenza F (1995) Effects of positive end-expiratory pressure on regional distribution of tidal volume and recruitment in adult respiratory distress syndrome. Am J Respir Crit Care Med 151:1807–1814
16. Katz JA, Ozanne GM, Zinn SE, Fairley HB (1981) Time course and mechanisms of lung-volume increase with PEEP in acute pulmonary failure. Anesthesiology 54:9–16
17. Dambrosio M, Roupie E, Mollet JJ, et al (1997) Effects of positive end-expiratory pressure and different tidal volumes on alveolar recruitment and hyperinflation. Anesthesiology 87:495–503
18. Jonson B, Richard JC, Straus C, Mancebo J, Lemaire F, Brochard L (1999) Pressure-volume curves and compliance in acute lung injury: evidence of recruitment above the lower inflection point. Am J Respir Crit Care Med 159:1172–1178
19. Hubmayr RD (2002) Perspective on lung injury and recruitment: a skeptical look at the opening and collapse story. Am J Respir Crit Care Med 165:1647–1653
20. Martynowicz MA, Minor TA, Wilson TA, Walters BJ, Hubmayr RD (1999) Effect of positive end-expiratory pressure on regional lung expansion of oleic acid-injured dogs. Chest 116:28S–29S
21. Mead J, Takishima T, Leith D (1970) Stress distribution in lungs: a model of pulmonary elasticity. J Appl Physiol 28:596–608
22. Bilek AM, Dee KC, Gaver DP 3rd (2003) Mechanisms of surface-tension-induced epithelial cell damage in a model of pulmonary airway reopening. J Appl Physiol 94:770–783
23. Adler A, Amyot R, Guardo R, Bates JH, Berthiaume Y (1997) Monitoring changes in lung air and liquid volumes with electrical impedance tomography. J Appl Physiol 83:1762–1767
24. Frerichs I (2000) Electrical impedance tomography (EIT) in applications related to lung and ventilation: a review of experimental and clinical activities. Physiol Meas 21:R1–21
25. Kunst PW, Bohm SH, Vazquez de Anda G, et al (2000) Regional pressure volume curves by electrical impedance tomography in a model of acute lung injury. Crit Care Med 28:178–183
26. Carney DE, Bredenberg CE, Schiller HJ, et al (1999) The mechanism of lung volume change during mechanical ventilation. Am J Respir Crit Care Med 160:1697–1702
27. Schiller HJ, McCann UG 2nd, Carney DE, Gatto LA, Steinberg JM, Nieman GF (2001) Altered alveolar mechanics in the acutely injured lung. Crit Care Med 29:1049–1055
28. Baumgardner JE, Markstaller K, Pfeiffer B, Doebrich M, Otto CM (2002) Effects of respiratory rate, plateau pressure, and positive end- expiratory pressure on PaO2 oscillations after saline lavage. Am J Respir Crit Care Med 166:1556–1562
29. Lu Q, Malbouisson LM, Mourgeon E, Goldstein I, Coriat P, Rouby JJ (2001) Assessment of PEEP-induced reopening of collapsed lung regions in acute lung injury: are one or three CT sections representative of the entire lung? Intensive Care Med 27:1504–1510
30. Borges JB, Caramez MPR, Gaudêncio AMAS, et al (2000) Looking for the best PEEP: spiral CT analysis, mechanical and physiological parameters (abstract). Am J Respir Crit Care Med 161:A48 (abst)
31. Borges JB, Caramez MPR, Gaudêncio AMAS, et al (2000) Lung recruitment at airway pressures beyond 40 cmH2O: physiology, mechanics and spiral CT analysis (abstract). Am J Respir Crit Care Med 161:A48 (abst)
32. Borges JB, Janot GF, Okamoto VN, et al (2003) Is there a true cephalocaudal lung gradient in ARDS? Am J Respir Crit Care Med 167 (abst)
33. Neumann P, Berglund JE, Mondejar EF, Magnusson A, Hedenstierna G (1998) Effect of different pressure levels on the dynamics of lung collapse and recruitment in oleic-acid-induced lung injury. Am J Respir Crit Care Med 158:1636–1643.

34. Tschumperlin DJ, Oswari J, Margulies AS (2000) Deformation-induced injury of alveolar epithelial cells. Effect of frequency, duration, and amplitude. Am J Respir Crit Care Med 162:357–362

35. D'Angelo E, Pecchiari M, Baraggia P, Saetta M, Balestro E, Milic-Emili J (2002) Low-volume ventilation causes peripheral airway injury and increased airway resistance in normal rabbits. J Appl Physiol 92:949–956

36. McCann UG 2nd, Schiller HJ, Carney DE, Gatto LA, Steinberg JM, Nieman GF (2001) Visual validation of the mechanical stabilizing effects of positive end- expiratory pressure at the alveolar level. J Surg Res 99:335–342

37. Webb HH, Tierney DF (1974) Experimental pulmonary edema due to intermittent positive pressure ventilation with high inflation pressures: protection by positive end-expiratory pressure. Am Rev Respir Dis 110:556–565

38. Dreyfuss D, Soler P, Basset G, Saumon G (1988) High inflation pressure pulmonary edema. Respective effects of high airway pressure, high tidal volume and positive end-expiratory pressure. Am Rev Respir Dis 137:1159–1164

39. Muscedere JG, Mullen JBM, Slutsky AS (1994) Tidal ventilation at low airway pressures can augment lung injury. Am J Respir Crit Care Med 149:1327–1334

40. Tremblay L, Valenza F, Ribeiro SP, Li J, Slutsky AS (1997) Injurious ventilatory strategies increase cytokines and c-fos m-RNA expression in an isolated rat lung model. J Clin Invest 99:944–952

41. Ricard JD, Dreyfuss D, Saumon G (2001) Production of inflammatory cytokines in ventilator-induced lung injury: a reappraisal. Am J Respir Crit Care Med 163:1176–1180

42. Takeuchi M, Goddon S, Dolhnikoff M, et al (2002) Set positive end-expiratory pressure during protective ventilation affects lung injury. Anesthesiology 97:682–692

43. Hamilton PP, Onayemi A, Smyth JA, et al (1983) Comparison of conventional and high-frequency ventilation: oxygenation and lung pathology. J Appl Physiol 55:131–138

44. McCulloch PR, Forkert PG, Froese AB (1988) Lung volume maintenance prevents lung injury during high frequency oscillatory ventilation in surfactant-deficient rabbits. Am Rev Respir Dis 137:1185–1192

45. Rimensberger PC, Pache JC, McKerlie C, Frndova H, Cox PN (2000) Lung recruitment and lung volume maintenance: a strategy for improving oxygenation and preventing lung injury during both conventional mechanical ventilation and high-frequency oscillation. Intensive Care Med 26:745–755

46. Stewart TE, Meade MO, Cook DJ, et al (1998) Evaluation of a ventilation strategy to prevent barotrauma in patients at high risk for acute respiratory distress syndrome. Pressure- and Volume-Limited Ventilation Strategy Group. N Engl J Med 338:355–361

47. Brochard L, Roudot-Thoraval F, Roupie E, et al (1998) Tidal volume reduction for prevention of ventilator-induced lung injury in acute respiratory distress syndrome. The Multicenter Trial Group on Tidal Volume reduction in ARDS. Am J Respir Crit Care Med 158:1831–1838

48. Brower RG, Shanholtz CB, Fessler HE, et al (1999) Prospective, randomized, controlled clinical trial comparing traditional versus reduced tidal volume ventilation in acute respiratory distress syndrome patients. Crit Care Med 27:1492–1498

49. Hickling KG (2002) Reinterpreting the pressure-volume curve in patients with acute respiratory distress syndrome. Curr Opin Crit Care 8:32–38

50. Marini JJ ,Amato MB (2000) Lung recruitment during ARDS. Minerva Anestesiol 66:314–319

51. Gattinoni L, Tognoni G, Pesenti A, et al (2001) Effect of prone positioning on the survival of patients with acute respiratory failure. N Engl J Med 345:568–573

52. Courtney SE, Durand DJ, Asselin JM, Hudak ML, Aschner JL, Shoemaker CT (2002) High-frequency oscillatory ventilation versus conventional mechanical ventilation for very-low-birth-weight infants. N Engl J Med 347:643–652

53. Johnson AH, Peacock JL, Greenough A, et al (2002) High-frequency oscillatory ventilation for the prevention of chronic lung disease of prematurity. N Engl J Med 347:633–642

54. Stark AR (2002) High-frequency oscillatory ventilation to prevent bronchopulmonary dysplasia—are we there yet? N Engl J Med 347:682–684
55. Lachmann B (1992) Open up the lung and keep the lung open. Intensive Care Med 18:319–321
56. Hickling KG (2001) Best compliance during a decremental, but not incremental, positive end-expiratory pressure trial is related to open-lung positive end-expiratory pressure: a mathematical model of acute respiratory distress syndrome lungs. Am J Respir Crit Care Med 163:69–78
57. Grasso S, Mascia L, Del Turco M, et al (2002) Effects of recruiting maneuvers in patients with acute respiratory distress syndrome ventilated with protective ventilatory strategy. Anesthesiology 96:795–802
58. Villagra A, Ochagavia A, Vatua S, et al (2002) Recruitment maneuvers during lung protective ventilation in acute respiratory distress syndrome. Am J Respir Crit Care Med 165:165–170
59. Lapinsky SE, Aubin M, Mehta S, Boiteau P, Slutsky AS (1999) Safety and efficacy of a sustained inflation for alveolar recruitment in adults with respiratory failure. Intensive Care Med 25:1297–301
60. Pelosi P, Cadringher P, Bottino N, et al (1999) Sigh in acute respiratory distress syndrome. Am J Respir Crit Care Med 159:872–880
61. Patroniti N, Foti G, Cortinovis B, et al (2002) Sigh improves gas exchange and lung volume in patients with acute respiratory distress syndrome undergoing pressure support ventilation. Anesthesiology 96:788–794

Spontaneous Breathing During Ventilatory Support in Patients with ARDS

C. Putensen, R. Hering, and H. Wrigge

Introduction

Traditionally, controlled mechanical ventilation via an artificial airway has been provided to completely unload the patient from the work of breathing and to assure adequate gas exchange during the acute phase of respiratory insufficiency until the underlying respiratory dysfunction has resolved [1]. Discontinuation of mechanical ventilation is determined mainly by clinical and often subjective judgment or standardized weaning protocols and is accomplished with partial ventilatory support supplementing spontaneous breathing or T-tube trials. Not surprisingly, gradual discontinuation with partial ventilatory support has been shown to be only beneficial in patients with difficulties in tolerating unassisted spontaneous breathing. Although introduced as weaning techniques, partial ventilatory support modes have become standard techniques for primary mechanical ventilatory support in more and more intensive care units (ICUs).

Interaction Between Spontaneous Breathing and Mechanical Ventilation

The evolution of pathophysiologic knowledge and technology has resulted in a variety of new ventilatory modalities and techniques designed to augment alveolar ventilation, decrease the work of breathing, and improve gas exchange. However, new ventilatory support modalities are only likely to result in a significant clinical improvement if the method differs from previous techniques [2–4]. In the absence of large-scale comparative studies, the clinician is often left to decide for himself whether, when, and how to employ these ventilatory modalities to support a patient's inadequate attempts at spontaneous breathing.

Modulation of Tidal Volume (V_T) through Mechanical Support of each Breath-assisted Ventilation

Every inspiratory effort should be mechanically supported by the ventilator. Independent of different ventilatory modes, an increase in the patient's respiratory rate will result in more mechanical support. Stable spontaneous breathing and a sensitive synchronization mechanism are essential preconditions in these modes to ensure adequate alveolar ventilation and reduced work of breathing. This principle is applied during assist controlled ventilation (ACV) [5], pressure support ventilation (PSV) [6, 7], proportional assist ventilation (PAV) [8] and automatic tube compensation (ATC) [9].

Modulation of Minute Ventilation (V_E) with Intermittent Application of Mechanical Breaths in Addition to Non-assisted Spontaneous Breathing

In these modes, mechanical ventilator support is constant and independent of the patient's inspiratory efforts. Increased ventilatory demand does not result in any change in the level of mechanical support. However, by regulating the mechanical ventilatory rate, variable support of spontaneous breathing is possible. In the event of apnea, at least set V_E will be applied. However, since the patient can only breathe spontaneously between the mechanical breaths, the opportunity for free spontaneous breathing decreases as the rate of mechanical ventilation increases. This principle is applied during intermittent mandatory ventilation (IMV) [2].

Modulation of V_E by Switching Between Two CPAP-Levels

Time cycled switching between two levels of continuous positive airway pressure (CPAP) allows unrestricted spontaneous breathing in any phase of the mechanical ventilatory cycle. Changes in ventilatory demand do not result in any change in the level of mechanical support. Adjusting ventilatory rate and ventilation pressures allows infinitely variable support of spontaneous breathing. This principle is applied during airway pressure release ventilation (APRV) [10, 11] and bilevel positive airway pressure (BiPAP) [12].

Ventilatory Support Modalities Combining Several of the Techniques Described Above

Commercially available ventilators offer combinations of ventilatory support modalities such as IMV+PSV, IMV+ATC, BiPAP+PSV, BiPAP+ATC, and PAV+ATC. Very few of these combinations of ventilatory modalities have been shown to be advantageous in the treatment of patients [13]. In contrast, it remains doubtful whether simply combining different modalities of ventilation results in the addition of their positive effects [14]. It cannot be ruled out that proven physiological effects of one mode of ventilation might be minimized or even abolished by combining it with another method.

Benefits of Maintained Spontaneous Breathing

Pulmonary Gas Exchange

Radiological studies have demonstrated that spontaneous ventilation is preferably directed to the dependent well perfused lung regions [15]. During spontaneous breathing, the posterior muscular sections of the diaphragm move more than the anterior tendon plate [15]. Consequently, in patients in the supine position, the dependent lung regions tend to be better ventilated during spontaneous breathing. If the diaphragm is relaxed, it will be moved by the weight of the abdominal cavity and the intraabdominal pressure (IAP) towards the cranium and the mechanical V_T will be distributed more to the non-dependent, less perfused lung regions [16] (Fig. 1). Recent results demonstrate that the posterior muscular sections of the diaphragm move more than the anterior tendon plate when large breaths or sighs are present during spontaneous breathing [17].

Computed tomography (CT) of patients with acute respiratory distress syndrome (ARDS) has demonstrated radiographic densities corresponding to alveolar collapse localized primarily in the dependent lung regions, while the non-dependent lung regions are well aerated [18, 19]. Intrapulmonary shunting has been found to correlate with the amount of non-aerated lung tissue [20] and to account entirely for the arterial hypoxemia observed during ARDS [21]. These radiographic densities have been attributed to alveolar collapse caused by the superimposed pressure on the lung and a cephalad shift of the diaphragm most evident in dependent lung areas during mechanical ventilation [22]. The cephalad shift of the diaphragm may be even more pronounced in patients with extrapulmonary induced ARDS, in whom an increase in IAP is invariably observed. Persisting with spontaneous breathing has been considered to improve distribution of ventilation to dependent lung areas and, thereby, ventilation-perfusion (V/Q) matching, presumably by diaphragmatic contraction opposing alveolar compression [23, 24]. This theory is supported by CT radiographic observations in anesthetized patients demonstrating that contractions of the diaphragm favor distribution of ventilation to dependent, well perfused lung areas and decrease atelectasis formation during phrenic nerve stimulation [25].

Spontaneous breathing   Mechanical ventilation

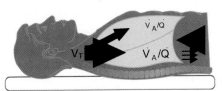 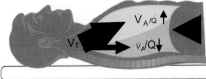

Fig. 1. Tidal ventilation distributed in the lungs during spontaneous and mechanical ventilation. V_T: tidal volume

APRV/BiPAP with spontaneous breathing   APRV/BiPAP without spontaneous breathing

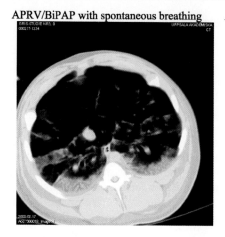 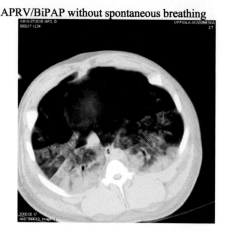

Fig. 2. Computed tomography of a lung region above the diaphragm in a pig with oleic acid induced lung injury during APRV/BiPAP with and without spontaneous breathing while maintaining airway pressure limits equal. (These investigations were done in collaboration with Göran Hedenstierna's laboratory at the University of Uppsala, Sweden).

Spontaneous breathing with APRV/BiPAP in pigs with oleic acid-induced lung injury was associated with less atelectasis formation in end-expiratory spiral CT of the whole lungs and in scans above the diaphragm (Fig. 2) [26]. Although other inspiratory muscles may also contribute to improvement in aeration during spontaneous breathing, the cranio-caudal gradient in aeration, aeration differences, and the marked differences in aeration in regions close to the diaphragm between APRV/BiPAP with and without spontaneous breathing suggest a predominant role of diaphragmatic contractions on the observed aeration differences [26]. These experimental findings are supported by observations using electro impedance tomography to estimate regional ventilation in patients with ARDS during APRV/BiPAP with and without spontaneous breathing. Spontaneous breathing with APRV/BiPAP is associated with better ventilation in the dependent well perfused lung regions and the anterior lung areas. When spontaneous breathing during APRV/BiPAP is abolished, mechanical ventilation is directed entirely to the less perfused non-dependent lung areas (Fig. 3).

In patients with ARDS, spontaneous breathing of 10 to 30% of the total V_E during APRV/BiPAP with equal airway pressure limits or V_E accounted for an improvement in V/Q matching and arterial oxygenation (Fig. 4) [24]. These results confirm earlier investigations in animals with induced lung injury [27–29] demonstrating improvement in intrapulmonary shunt and arterial oxygenation during spontaneous breathing with APRV/BIPAP. Increase in arterial oxygenation in conjunction with greater pulmonary compliance may be explained by recruitment of previously non-ventilated lung areas. Clinical studies in patients with ARDS show that spontaneous breathing during APRV/BiPAP does not necessarily lead to instant improvement in gas exchange but to a continuous improvement in oxygenation within 24 hours after the start of spontaneous breathing [30].

CPAP   APRV   PCV
                 with spontaneous breating

ventral   ventral   ventral

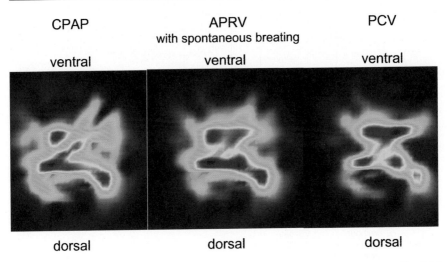

dorsal   dorsal   dorsal

Fig. 3. Electroimpedance tomography used to estimate regional ventilation in patients with ARDS during CPAP and APRV/BiPAP with and without spontaneous breathing. Spontaneous breathing with CPAP is associated with better ventilation in the dependent well perfused lung regions. Spontaneous breathing with APRV/BiPAP is associated with better ventilation in the dependent well perfused lung regions and the anterior lung areas. When spontaneous breathing during APRV/BiPAP is abolished mechanical ventilation is directed entirely to the less perfused non-dependent anterior lung areas.

Although PSV also has been used in certain patients with ARDS [31] it did not produce significant improvement in intrapulmonary shunt, V/Q matching or gas exchange when compared to controlled mechanical ventilation in a previous study [24]. This is in agreement with the results of Cereda and coworkers demonstrating comparable gas exchange in patients with acute lung injury (ALI) during controlled mechanical ventilation and PSV [31]. Apparently, spontaneous contribution on a mechanically assisted breath was not sufficient to counteract V/Q maldistribution of positive pressure lung insufflations. One possible explanation might be that inspiration is terminated by the decrease in gas flow at the end of inspiration during PSV [6]. This may reduce ventilation in areas of the lung with a slow time constant [32].

In patients with multiple trauma at risk of developing ARDS, spontaneous breathing maintained with APRV/BiPAP resulted in lower venous admixture and better arterial blood oxygenation over an observation period of more than 10 days as compared to controlled mechanical ventilation with subsequent weaning [33] These results show clearly that, even in patients requiring ventilatory support, maintained spontaneous breathing can counteract the progressive deterioration in pulmonary gas exchange.

In the clinical routine, APRV/BiPAP is frequently combined with PSV or ATC to compensate at least partially the resistance of the endotracheal tube although improvement in gas exchange in patients with ARDS was only demonstrated during

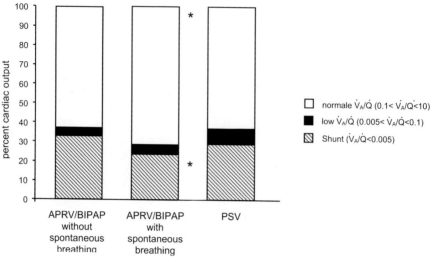

Fig. 4. Spontaneous breathing during APRV/BiPAP accounted for a decrease in blood flow to shunt units (V/Q<0.005) and an increase in perfusion of normal V/Q units (0.1< V/Q <10), without creating low V/Q areas (0.05< V/Q <0.1). PSV had no effect on the pulmonary blood flow distribution when compared to controlled mechanical ventilation (APRV/BiPAP without spontaneous breathing). *p < 0.05 compared with APRV/BiPAP without spontaneous breathing

APRV/BiPAP with unassisted spontaneous breathing. In patients with ARDS, ATC during APRV unloaded considerably the inspiratory muscle load and increased alveolar ventilation without deteriorating cardiorespiratory function. Apparently, transient lowering of airway pressures (Paw) during expiration with ATC did not promote alveolar collapse or worsen gas exchange in patients with ALI when superimposed on APRV/BiPAP. Unfortunately, data demonstrating the advantageous of APRV/BiPAP combined with PSV are lacking.

Cardiovascular Effects

When cardiac function is normal, the filling of the right and left ventricle during diastole is the predominant determinant of the stroke volume and cardiac output. Positive pressure ventilation increases intrathoracic pressure, which in turn reduces the venous return to the heart [34]. In normo- and hypovolemic patients, this produces reduction in right- and left-ventricular filling and results in decreased stroke volume, cardiac output and oxygen delivery (DO_2). To normalize systemic blood flow during mechanical ventilation, intravascular volume often needs to be increased and/or the cardiovascular system needs pharmacological support. Reducing mechanical ventilation to a level which provides adequate support for existing spontaneous breathing should help to reduce the cardiovascular side effects of ventilatory support [35].

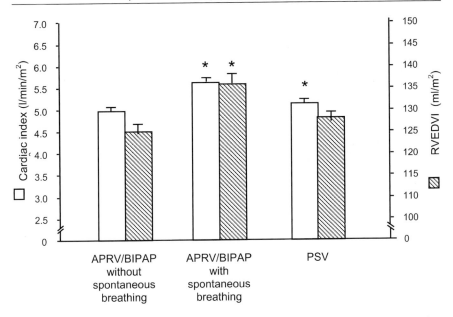

Fig. 5. Spontaneous breathing during APRV/BiPAP was associated with an increase in cardiac index. Simultaneous rise in right ventricular end-diastolic volume index (RVEDVI) during spontaneous breathing with APRV/BiPAP indicates improved venous return to the heart. *p< 0.05 compared to APRV/BiPAP without spontaneous breathing

Periodic reduction of intrathoracic pressure resulting from maintained spontaneous breathing during mechanical ventilatory support promotes the venous return to the heart and right- and left-ventricular filling, thereby increasing cardiac output and DO_2 [36]. Experimental [27, 29, 37, 38] and clinical [24, 30, 36] studies show that during APRV/BiPAP with spontaneous breathing of 10 to 40 % of total V_E at unchanged V_E or airway pressure limits results in an increase in cardiac index (Fig. 5). Simultaneous rise in right ventricular end-diastolic volume during spontaneous breathing with APRV/BiPAP indicates improved venous return to the heart [24]. In addition, the outflow from the right ventricle which depends mainly on the lung volume which is the major determinant of pulmonary vascular resistance may benefit from a decrease in intrathoracic pressure during APRV/BiPAP [24]. In contrast, ventilatory support of each individual inspiration with PSV and identical airway pressures produces no increase or small increase in cardiac index [24]. The increase in cardiac index observed during PSV when compared to controlled mechanical ventilation was a function of the pressure support level. This indicates that during assisted inspiration with PSV, spontaneous respiratory activity may not decrease intrathoracic pressures sufficiently to counteract the cardiovascular depression of positive airway pressure. Räsänen et al. [39] documented that a changeover from CPAP to spontaneous breathing with APRV/BiPAP did not affect cardiac output and tissue DO_2. In contrast, a similar ventilatory support with controlled mechanical ventilation reduced the stroke volume and DO_2.

Patients with left-ventricular dysfunction may not benefit from augmentation of the venous return to the heart and increased left-ventricular afterload as a result of reduced intrathoracic pressure. Therefore, switching abruptly from controlled mechanical ventilation to PSV with simultaneous reduction in airway pressure can lead to decompensation of existing cardiac insufficiency [40]. Räsänen et al. [41, 42] demonstrated the need of adequate ventilatory support and CPAP levels in patients with respiratory and cardiogenic failure. However, providing that spontaneous breathing receives adequate support and sufficient CPAP is applied, the maintenance of spontaneous breathing should not prove disadvantageous and, therefore, is not contraindicated even in patients with acute myocardial infarction or cardiac failure [41–44].

Oxygen Supply and Demand Balance

The concomitant increase in cardiac index and PaO$_2$ during APRV/BiPAP improved the relationship between tissue oxygen supply and demand because oxygen consumption remained unchanged despite the work of spontaneous breathing (Fig. 6). In accordance with previous experimental [28] and clinical findings [24], total oxygen consumption is not measurably altered by adequately supported spontaneous breathing in patients with low lung compliance. An increased DO$_2$ with unchanged oxygen consumption resulted in an improved relationship between tissue oxygen supply and demand as reflected by a significant decrease in

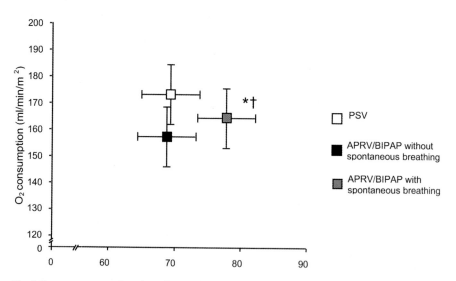

Fig. 6. Oxygen consumption plotted versus oxygen delivery during APRV/BiPAP with and without spontaneous breathing and during inspiratory assistance with PSV. Oxygen consumption was determined by indirect calorimetry. *p< 0.05 compared to APRV/BiPAP without spontaneous breathing; †< 0.05 compared to PSV

oxygen extraction rate and higher mixed venous PO_2, which also may have contributed to the higher PaO_2.

Organ Perfusion

By reducing cardiac index and the venous return to the heart, mechanical ventilation can have a negative effect on the perfusion and functioning of extrathoracic organ systems.

In the kidney, reduction in cardiac index and venous return causes, via a sympatho-adrenergic reaction, vasoconstriction of the afferent renal arterioles with reduction and redistribution of the renal blood flow from the cortical to the juxtaglomerular nephrons. This reduces the glomerular filtration rate and sodium excretion. Increase in venous return and cardiac output, due to the periodic fall in intrathoracic pressure during spontaneous inspiration, should significantly improve kidney perfusion and function during partial ventilatory support. In patients with ARDS, spontaneous breathing with IMV leads to an increase in glomerular filtration rate and sodium excretion [45, 46]. Compatible with these results, in patients with ARDS, kidney perfusion and glomerular filtration rate increase during spontaneous breathing with APRV/BiPAP as compared to pressure-limited ventilation with equal [47] airway pressure limits or V_E. Although cardiac index has been highest during mechanical ventilation with low V_T resulting in hypercapnia, kidney perfusion and glomerular filtration rate were lower than during spontaneous breathing with APRV/BiPAP (Fig. 7). This indicates that maintained spontaneous breathing is favorable for the perfusion and function of the kidney in patients requiring ventilatory support due to severe pulmonary dysfunction.

Reduction of cardiac output and venous return causes, via a sympatho-adrenergic reaction, vasoconstriction and lower blood flow in the portal vein and thereby in the liver and the splanchnic area. Preliminary data in patients requiring ventilatory support for ALI suggest that maintained spontaneous breathing may be beneficial for the liver function [48]. In addition, using colored microspheres in pigs with oleic acid-induced lung injury spontaneous breathing during APRV/BiPAP may be advantageous for the perfusion of the splanchnic area [48].

Suppression of Spontaneous Breathing

Suppressing spontaneous breathing activity during controlled mechanical ventilation can be achieved by hyperventilation, deep sedation or muscle relaxation. Hyperventilation in conjunction with respiratory alkalosis may result in a drop in cardiac output, cerebral vasoconstriction, increased oxygen consumption, bronchoconstriction and V/Q mismatch [49–51]. Analgosedation sufficient to suppress respiratory efforts is known to cause significant cardio-vascular depression. In addition, it may take longer for the patient to wake up following the long-term use of sedatives and analgesics [52]. Using muscle relaxants to facilitate adaptation to controlled mechanical ventilation is also open to question. An increasing number of reports claim that the long-term application of muscle relaxants during control-

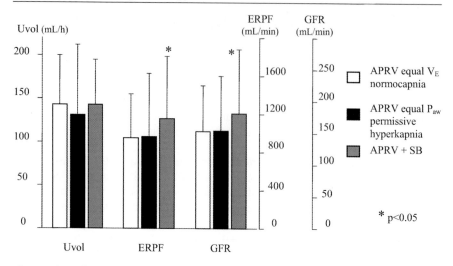

Fig. 7. Urine volume (Uvol), effective renal plasma flow (ERPF), and glomerular filtration rate (GFR) during airway pressure release ventilation with and without spontaneous breathing. During APRV without spontaneous breathing adjusted to produce equal minute ventilation (V_E) (normocapnia) while when APRV without spontaneous breathing was administered with equal airway pressure limits (Paw) (permissive hypercapnia).

led mechanical ventilation in the ICU can lead to muscular atrophy, damage to the neuromuscular end-plate and other muscle function disorders and can, therefore, delay or even prevent weaning from mechanical ventilation [53–55].

Analgosedation

As well as ensuring sufficient pain relief and anxiolysis, analgosedation is used to adapt the patient to mechanical ventilation [52, 56]. The level of analgosedation required during controlled mechanical ventilation is equivalent to a Ramsay score between 4 and 5, that is a deeply sedated patient unable to respond when spoken to and having no sensation of pain. During partial ventilatory support a Ramsay score between 2 and 3 can be targeted, i.e., an awake, responsive and cooperative patient [56]. In a retrospective study in about 600 heart surgery patients, and in a prospective investigation in patients with multiple trauma, maintaining spontaneous breathing with APRV/BiPAP lead to significantly lower consumption of analgesics and sedatives compared to initial use of controlled mechanical ventilation followed by weaning with partial ventilatory support [33, 57]. Obviously a large part of analgosedation is used exclusively to adapt patients to controlled mechanical ventilation. The higher doses of analgesics and sedatives used to adapt patients to controlled mechanical ventilation require higher doses of vasopressors and positive inotrops to maintain cardiovascular function stable [33]. Both from a medical and from an economic point of view it would therefore appear sensible to provide mechanical support with spontaneous breathing.

Setting Ventilation Pressures and Tidal Volumes

Mechanical ventilation with PEEP titrated above the lower inflection pressure of a static pressure-volume (V/P) curve and low V_T has been suggested to prevent tidal alveolar collapse at end-expiration and overdistension of lung units at end-inspiration during ARDS [58]. This lung-protective ventilatory strategy has been found to improve lung compliance, venous admixture, and PaO_2 without causing cardiovascular impairment in ARDS [58]. Recently, a lung protective mechanical ventilation using V_T of not more than 6 ml/kg ideal body weight has been shown in large-scale clinical trials to improve outcome in patients with ARDS [58, 59]. Based on these results the CPAP levels during APRV/BiPAP should be titrated to prevent end-expiratory alveolar collapse and tidal alveolar overdistension [58, 59]. In our investigations, CPAP levels were always adjusted. When CPAP levels during APRV/BiPAP were adjusted according to a lung-protective ventilatory strategy occurrence of spontaneous breathing improved cardiorespiratory function without affecting total oxygen consumption due to the work of breathing in patients with ARDS [24]. These data clearly demonstrate that spontaneous breathing can improve gas exchange without any further increase in airway pressures during lung protective mechanical ventilation. Moreover, pulmonary compliance in this range of airway pressures is greatest meaning that spontaneous breathing is efficient even with minimal ventilatory effort [60].

Maintaining Spontaneous Breathing

Based on available data, it has to be suggested that spontaneous breathing during ventilatory support should not be suppressed even in patients with severe pulmonary dysfunction if no contraindications (e.g., increased intracranial pressure) are present. Improvement in pulmonary gas exchange, systemic blood flow, and oxygen supply to the tissue which were observed when spontaneous breathing was allowed during ventilatory support are reflected in the clinical improvement in the patient's condition. Compared with an initial period of controlled mechanical ventilation for 72 hours followed by weaning, maintained spontaneous breathing with APRV/BIPAP is associated with significantly fewer days on ventilatory support, earlier extubation, and a shorter stay in the ICU [33].

However, the positive effects of spontaneous breathing have only been documented for some of the available partial ventilatory support modalities. If one limits oneself to ventilatory modalities whose positive effects have been documented, then partial ventilatory support can be used as a primary modality even in patients with severe pulmonary dysfunction. Whereas controlled mechanical ventilation followed by weaning with partial ventilatory support modalities used to be the standard in ventilation therapy, this approach should be reconsidered in view of the available data. Today's standard practice should be to maintain spontaneous breathing from the very beginning of ventilatory support and to continuously adapt ventilatory support to the patient's individual needs.

References

1. Marini JJ (1993) New options for the ventilatory management of acute lung injury. New Horiz 1:489–503
2. Downs JB, Klein EF Jr, Desautels D, Modell JH, Kirby RR (1973) Intermittent mandatory ventilation: a new approach to weaning patients from mechanical ventilators. Chest 64:331–335
3. Esteban A, Frutos F, Tobin MJ, et al (1995) A comparison of four methods of weaning patients from mechanical ventilation. Spanish Lung Failure Collaborative Group. N Engl J Med 332:345–350
4. Tobin MJ (2001) Advances in mechanical ventilation. N Engl J Med 344:1986–1996
5. Marini JJ, Rodriguez RM, Lamb V (1986) The inspiratory workload of patient-initiated mechanical ventilation. Am Rev Respir Dis 134:902–909
6. Hansen J, Wendt M, Lawin P (1984) A new weaning procedure (inspiratory flow assistance). Anaesthesist 33:428–432
7. MacIntyre NR (1986) Respiratory function during pressure support ventilation. Chest 89:677–683
8. Younes M (1992) Proportional assist ventilation, a new approach to ventilatory support. Theory. Am Rev Respir Dis 145:114–120
9. Fabry B, Guttmann J, Eberhard L, Wolff G (1994) Automatic compensation of endotracheal tube resistance in spontaneously breathing patients. Technol Health Care 1:281–291
10. Stock MC, Downs JB (1987) Airway pressure release ventilation. Crit Care Med 15:462–466
11. Downs JB (1987) Airway pressure release ventilation: a new concept in ventilatory support. Crit Care Med 15:459–461
12. Baum M, Benzer H, Putensen C, Koller W (1989) Biphasic positive airway pressure (BIPAP)—a new form of augmented ventilation. Anaesthesist 38:452–458
13. Wrigge H, Zinserling J, Hering R, et al (2001) Cardiorespiratory effects of automatic tube compensation during airway pressure release ventilation in patients with acute lung injury. Anesthesiology 95:382–389
14. Räsänen J, Downs JB (1991) Are new ventilatory modalities really different? Chest 100:299–300
15. Froese AB (1974) Effects of anesthesia and paralysis on diaphragmatic mechanics in man. Anesthesiology 41:242–255
16. Reber A, Nylund U, Hedenstierna G (1998) Position and shape of the diaphragm: implications for atelectasis formation. Anaesthesia 53:1054–1061
17. Patroniti N, Foti G, Cortinovis B, et al (2002) Sigh improves gas exchange and lung volume in patients with acute respiratory distress syndrome undergoing pressure support ventilation. Anesthesiology 96:788–794
18. Rommelsheim K, Lackner K, Westhofen P, Distelmaier W, Hirt S (1983) Respiratory distress syndrome of the adult in the computer tomograph. Anasth Intensivther Notfallmed 18:59–64
19. Gattinoni L, Presenti A, Torresin A, et al (1986) Adult respiratory distress syndrome profiles by computed tomography. J Thorac Imaging 1:25–30
20. Tokics L, Hedenstierna G, Strandberg A, Brismar B, Lundquist H (1987) Lung collapse and gas exchange during general anesthesia: effects of spontaneous breathing, muscle paralysis, and positive end-expiratory pressure. Anesthesiology 66:157–167
21. Bernard GR, Artigas A, Brigham KL, et al (1994) Report of the American-European consensus conference on ARDS: definitions, mechanisms, relevant outcomes and clinical trial coordination. Intensive Care Med 20:225–232
22. Puybasset L, Cluzel P, Chao N, Slutsky AS, Coriat P, Rouby JJ (1998) A computed tomography scan assessment of regional lung volume in acute lung injury. The CT Scan ARDS Study Group. Am J Respir Crit Care Med 158:1644–1655
23. Putensen C, Zech J, Zinserling J (1998) Effect of early spontaneous breathing during Airway Pressure Release Ventilation on cardiopulmonary function. Am J Respir Crit Care Med 157:A45 (abst)

24. Putensen C, Mutz NJ, Putensen-Himmer G, Zinserling J (1999) Spontaneous breathing during ventilatory support improves ventilation- perfusion distributions in patients with acute respiratory distress syndrome. Am J Respir Crit Care Med 159:1241–1248
25. Hedenstierna G, Tokics L, Lundquist H, Andersson T, Strandberg A (1994) Phrenic nerve stimulation during halothane anesthesia. Effects of atelectasis. Anesthesiology 80:751–760
26. Wrigge H, Neumann P, Zinserling J, Magnusson A, Putensen C, Hedenstierna G (2001) Gas distribution during spontaneous breathing with airway pressure release ventilation in oleic acid lung injury. Am J Respir Crit Care Med 164:A682 (abst)
27. Putensen C, Räsänen J, Lopez FA (1995) Interfacing between spontaneous breathing and mechanical ventilation affects ventilation-perfusion distributions in experimental bronchoconstriction. Am J Respir Crit Care Med 151:993–999
28. Putensen C, Räsänen J, Lopez FA (1994) Effect of interfacing between spontaneous breathing and mechanical cycles on the ventilation-perfusion distribution in canine lung injury. Anesthesiology 81:921–930
29. Putensen C, Räsänen J, Lopez FA (1994) Ventilation-perfusion distributions during mechanical ventilation with superimposed spontaneous breathing in canine lung injury. Am J Respir Crit Care Med 150:101–108
30. Sydow M, Burchardi H, Ephraim E, Zielmann S (1994) Long-term effects of two different ventilatory modes on oxygenation in acute lung injury. Comparison of airway pressure release ventilation and volume-controlled inverse ratio ventilation. Am J Respir Crit Care Med 149:1550–1556
31. Cereda M, Foti G, Marcora B, et al (2000) Pressure support ventilation in patients with acute lung injury. Crit Care Med 28:1269–1275
32. Marini JJ, Crooke PS, III, Truwit JD (1989) Determinants and limits of pressure-preset ventilation: a mathematical model of pressure control. J Appl Physiol 67:1081–1092
33. Putensen C, Zech S, Wrigge H, et al (2001) Long-term effects of spontaneous breathing during ventilatory support in patients with acute lung injury. Am J Respir Crit Care Med 164:43–49
34. Pinsky MR (1984) Determinants of pulmonary arterial flow variation during respiration. J Appl Physiol 56:1237–1245
35. Kirby RR, Perry JC, Calderwood HW, Ruiz BC (1975) Cardiorespiratory effects of high positive.end-expiratory pressure. Anesthesiology 43:533–539
36. Downs JB, Douglas ME, Sanfelippo PM, Stanford W (1977) Ventilatory pattern, intrapleural pressure, and.cardiac output. Anesth Analg 56:88–96
37. Falkenhain SK, Reilley TE, Gregory JS (1992) Improvement in cardiac output during airway pressure release ventilation. Crit Care Med 20:1358–1360
38. Putensen C, Leon MA, Putensen-Himmer G (1994) Timing of pressure release affects power of breathing and minute ventilation during airway pressure release ventilation. Crit Care Med 22:872–878
39. Räsänen J, Downs JB (1988) Cardiovascular effects of conventional positive.pressure ventilation and airway pressure release ventilation. Chest 93:911–915
40. Lemaire F, Teboul JL, Cinotti L, et al (1988) Acute left ventricular dysfunction during unsuccessful weaning from mechanical ventilation. Anesthesiology 69:171–179
41. Räsänen J, Heikkila J, Downs J, Nikki P, Vaisanen I, Viitanen A (1985) Continuous positive airway pressure by face mask in acute cardiogenic pulmonary edema. Am J Cardiol 55:296–300
42. Räsänen J, Nikki P (1982) Respiratory failure arising from acute myocardial infarction. Ann Chir Gynaecol Suppl 196:43–47
43. Nikki P, Räsänen J, Tahvanainen J, Makelainen A (1982) Ventilatory pattern in respiratory failure arising from acute myocardial infarction. I. Respiratory and hemodynamic effects of IMV4 vs IPPV12 and PEEP0 vs PEEP10. Crit Care Med 10:75–78
44. Nikki P, Tahvanainen J, Räsänen J, Makelainen A (1982) Ventilatory pattern in respiratory failure arising from acute myocardial infarction. II. PtcO2 and PtcCO2 compared to Pao2 and PaCO2 during IMV4 vs IPPV12 and PEEP0 vs PEEP10. Crit Care Med 10:79–81

45. Steinhoff H, Falke K, Schwarzhoff W (1982) Enhanced renal function associated with intermittent mandatory ventilation in acute respiratory failure. Intensive Care Med 8:69-74
46. Steinhoff HH, Kohlhoff RJ, Falke KJ (1984) Facilitation of renal function by intermittent mandatory ventilation. Intensive Care Med 10:59–65
47. Hering R, Peters D, Zinserling J, Wrigge H, von Spiegel T, Putensen C (2002) Effects of spontaneous breathing during airway pressure release ventilation improves renal perfusion and function in patients with acute lung injury. Intensive Care Med 28:1426–1433
48. Hering R, Viehöfer A, Zinserling J, et al (2001) Effects of spontaneous breathing with airway pressure release ventilation on intestinal blood flow in experimental lung injury. Intensive Care Med 27:A567 (abst)
49. Hudson LD, Hurlow RS, Craig KC, Pierson DJ (1985) Does intermittent mandatory ventilation correct respiratory alkalosis in patients receiving assisted mechanical ventilation? Am Rev Respir Dis 132:1071–1074
50. Domino KB, Lu Y, Eisenstein BL, Hlastala MP (1993) Hypocapnia worsens arterial blood oxygenation and increases VA/Q heterogeneity in canine pulmonary edema. Anesthesiology 78:91–99
51. Culpepper JA, Rinaldo JE, Rogers RM (1985) Effect of mechanical ventilator mode on tendency towards respiratory alkalosis. Am Rev Respir Dis 132:1075–1077
52. Wheeler AP (1993) Sedation, analgesia, and paralysis in the intensive care unit. Chest 104:566–577
53. Hsiang JK, Chesnut RM, Crisp CB, Klauber MR, Blunt BA, Marshall LF (1994) Early, routine paralysis for intracranial pressure control in severe head injury: is it necessary? Crit Care Med 22:1471–1476
54. Hansen-Flaschen JH, Brazinsky S, Basile C, Lanken PN (1991) Use of sedating drugs and neuromuscular blocking agents in patients requiring mechanical ventilation for respiratory failure. A national survey. JAMA 266:2870–2875
55. Rossiter A, Souney PF, McGowan S, Carvajal P (1991) Pancuronium-induced prolonged neuromuscular blockade. Crit Care Med 19:1583–1587
56. Burchardi H, Rathgeber J, Sydow M (1995) The concept of analgo-sedation depends on the concept of mechanical ventilation. In: Vincent JL (ed) Yearbook of Intensive Care and Emergency Medicine. Springer-Verlag, Heidelberg, pp:155–164.
57. Rathgeber J, Schorn B, Falk V, Kazmaier S, Spiegel T (1997) The influence of controlled mandatory ventilation (CMV), intermittent mandatory ventilation (IMV) and biphasic intermittent positive airway pressure (BIPAP) on duration of intubation and consumption of analgesics and sedatives. A prospective analysis in 596 patients following adult cardiac surgery. Eur J Anaesthesiol 14:576–582
58. Amato MB, Barbas CS, Medeiros DM, et al (1998) Effect of a protective-ventilation strategy on mortality in the acute respiratory distress syndrome. N Engl J Med 338:347–354
59. The Acute Respiratory Distress Syndrome Network (2000) Ventilation with lower tidal volumes as compared with traditional tidal volumes for acute lung injury and the acute respiratory distress syndrome.. N Engl J Med 342:1301–1308
60. Katz JA, Marks JD (1985) Inspiratory work with and without continuous positive airway pressure in patients with acute respiratory failure. Anesthesiology 6:598–607

Pressure Support Ventilation in Patients With ALI/ARDS

N. Patroniti, B. Cortinovis, and A. Pesenti

Introduction

Pressure support ventilation (PSV) was introduced into clinical practice in the early 1980s [1, 2], and it quickly became the most commonly used partial ventilatory support technique in intensive care units (ICUs) [3]. Originally devised to improve patient-ventilator interaction and comfort over other popular ventilatory modes such as assist-control ventilation or synchronized intermittent mandatory ventilation (SIMV) [2, 3], PSV gained its popularity as a weaning technique. Although PSV probably still finds its main application in weaning, growing attention is being paid to the use of PSV as a stand-alone major ventilatory mode in acute lung injury/acute respiratory distress syndrome (ALI/ARDS). After a short general introduction, we will discuss some recent aspects of PSV use in patients with ALI/ARDS.

What is PSV?

PSV is a pressure-targeted mode of ventilation, that provides breath-by-breath patient-triggered support, synchronized with the patient's inspiratory effort [4]. Following the detection of patient's inspiratory effort, a demand valve allows the airway pressure to rise to a pre-set level, which is maintained until the detection of the patient's wish to expire. At this stage an expiratory trigger system stops the support and allows the airway pressure to drop down to the expiratory level. Expiration is therefore passive in principle, while a selected level of positive end-expiratory pressure (PEEP) can be applied. Thus, PSV requires a patient's intact drive to breathe. As increasing levels of pressure support are used, the inspiratory muscles progressively unload and the patient's inspiratory work of breathing (WOB) and the pressure time product (PTP) decrease [5–7]. These changes are commonly associated with a decrease in respiratory rate (RR), in respiratory neural drive and in P0.1 [6, 8], while tidal volume (V_T) shows a tendency to increase [2, 7]. Indeed, the clinician can set the ventilator to obtain a target patient effort by simply adjusting the pressure support level. However, despite these major features, and the claimed better synchronization and patient comfort compared to other popular weaning modes such as SIMV [2, 7], the advantages of PSV in weaning patients from the ventilator are non univocal [9, 10]. Moreover, new ventilatory modes promising better patient ventilator synchronization [11] and comfort [12, 13] have partially overcome the advantages of PSV. Still, as recently reported, PSV alone (36% of patients) or in combination with SIMV (28% of patients), is the most frequent weaning ventilatory mode [4] in North America, South America, Portugal and Spain.

Why Assisted rather than Controlled Mechanical Ventilation in ALI/ARDS Patients?

In the last 10 years, various studies investigated the beneficial effects of maintaining spontaneous breathing activity during mechanical ventilation. Indeed, spontaneous breathing yields the benefits of preserving diaphragmatic activity [14], preventing muscle atrophy, decreasing the need for sedative drugs [15], and (obviously) avoiding the use of muscle relaxants [16]. Moreover, during partial ventilatory support, the spontaneous inspiratory effort decreases pleural pressure, and increases venous return, stroke volume and cardiac output [17–19].

Both in animals [17] and in ARDS patients [18], Putensen at al. showed a better ventilation-perfusion (V/Q) distribution during airway pressure release ventilation (APRV) with spontaneous breathing compared to APRV alone. The proposed mechanism for the beneficial effect of spontaneous breathing is an improved ventilation of dependent lung regions [20]. During controlled mechanical ventilation, the dependent lung regions in ALI/ARDS patients are indeed perfused, but poorly aerated. Therefore, diaphragmatic contraction during spontaneous inspiration, enhancing the ventilation of dependent collapsed areas, results in an improved V/Q distribution. Multiple trauma patients at risk for ALI/ARDS in whom spontaneous breathing was maintained during APRV, benefited from a better cardiopulmonary function, a shorter duration of ventilatory support, and a shorter ICU stay [21].

Very few studies however, have up to now investigated the feasibility of maintaining spontaneous breathing through PSV during ALI/ARDS [18, 22, 23]. This is somehow strange, since PSV is frequently and successfully used to deliver non-invasive ventilation (NIV) in patients with acute respiratory failure [24, 25].

Monitoring Respiratory Mechanics in ALI/ARDS During PSV

The hallmark of ALI/ARDS is altered gas exchange combined with impaired respiratory system mechanics. While monitoring respiratory mechanics is important during controlled mechanical ventilation, it becomes essential to the success of PSV. The main purpose of this section is to explain the measurement and discuss the clinical value of respiratory mechanics parameters, in setting the ventilator and monitoring patient's response to PSV. Assessment of respiratory function during PSV may guide physicians in setting the level of ventilatory support, optimizing sedation, and in making therapeutic decisions.

Respiratory Drive

Since during PSV the patient controls the respiratory rate and contributes actively to the ventilatory output, integrity and preservation of spontaneous neural activity are essential. The pressure support level and the patient-ventilator synchrony may greatly affect a patient's neural drive [8], therefore information concerning neural drive may be very useful in setting and monitoring PSV function.

To investigate the respiratory drive during PSV, many authors use the pressure drop developed during the first 100 ms following the onset of an expiratory occlusion (P0.1). P0.1 is widely accepted as an index of respiratory drive [8, 26, 27], though it is worth remembering that the patient's neural drive, and thus P0.1, are affected also by drugs, gas exchange, respiratory muscle function [27], and lung volume [28]. Since the measurement of P0.1 could be limited by the need of special equipment, a simplified technique has been proposed [29]. Automatic measurements implemented on many ventilators make P0.1 easily available in clinical settings [30].

As an alternative, the patient's respiratory drive and control of breathing may be inferred from output ventilatory variables such as V_T, RR, and mean inspiratory flow. The ratio of RR to V_T, named shallow breathing index (SBI), has been used as a predictor of weaning outcome [31]. The combination of P0.1 with SBI has shown comparable sensitivity but better specificity as a weaning predictor than either P0.1 or SBI alone [32].

Respiratory Muscle Function

By adjusting the pressure support level it is possible to modulate the relative contribution of the patient and of the ventilator to the total WOB [33]. This is certainly a major advantage of PSV: indeed, aside from the mandatory presence of an intact neural drive, an effective muscular function is necessary to initiate the PSV breath and at least participate in inspiratory WOB. A relatively simple method to assess muscular strength is the maximal absolute pressure that is generated against an occluded airway [34].

Respiratory Mechanics

Respiratory system compliance (Crs)

The widespread notion that complete relaxation of respiratory muscles is not reliably achievable in spontaneously breathing patients has limited the measurement of respiratory mechanics during partial ventilatory support.

A clinically reliable measurement of respiratory system compliance may be most commonly obtained by performing the classic occlusion maneuvers [35, 36], according to the simple equation:

$$Crs = V_T/(Pel,rsi-Pel,rse)$$

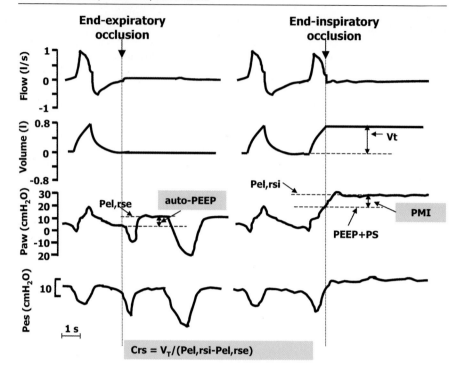

Fig. 1. Tracing of flow, volume, airway pressure (Paw), and esophageal pressure (Pes), of an end-expiratory (left side), and end-inspiratory (right side) airway occlusion during pressure support ventilation (PSV). Main parameters obtained during occlusions are displayed. V_T: tidal volume; Pel,rse: elastic recoil pressure of respiratory system at the end of expiration; Pel,rsi: elastic recoil pressure of respiratory system at the end of inspiration; PMI: pressure muscle index; Crs, respiratory system compliance. See text for details.

where Pel,rsi = elastic recoil pressure of respiratory system at the end of inspiration, and Pel,rse = elastic recoil pressure of respiratory system at the end of expiration, which amounts to the sum of PEEP plus auto-PEEP (Fig. 1).

In most modern ventilators, end-inspiratory and end-expiratory occlusion maneuvers are possible also during partial ventilatory support modes. We have shown that, during PSV, the plateau pressure relaxation following an inspiratory occlusion is a clinically acceptable estimate of the elastic recoil pressure of the respiratory system [36]. Assessment of the occlusion method in ALI patients who had been shifted from continuous positive pressure ventilation (CPPV) to PSV, showed a good correlation between Crs measured during PSV and during CPPV ($Crs_{PSV} = 1.4+0.98*Cpl_{CPPV}$, r=0.945, p<0.001) [37]. However, it is important to underline that in patients with a very high respiratory drive the occlusion method could be limited by insufficient time to achieve a reliable muscle relaxation, and, thus, the measurement should not be trusted.

Respiratory system resistance (Rrs)

Measurement of Rrs during PSV is particularly critical, since it requires the use of esophageal pressure [38]. A method to estimate Rrs, avoiding esophageal pressure measurement, is based on the use of the interrupter technique [39] that has been successfully applied in patients undergoing to PSV [35]. Alternatively, Iotti et al. have proposed an approach based on a least square fitting technique, which allows contemporaneous measurement of Rrs and Crs, avoiding any occlusion maneuver [40]. It is important to note however, that, while airway resistance evaluation is most important in chronically obstructed patients, its clinical relevance in the management of ALI /ARDS is certainly more limited.

Auto-PEEP

The measurement of auto-PEEP is of great importance, since aside from the well known detrimental effects on hemodynamics and dynamic hyperinflation, it may profoundly affect the feasibility and effectiveness of PSV. Auto-PEEP represents a threshold load the patient must overcome to trigger the ventilator, and constitutes an adjunctive ineffective effort. Auto-PEEP can be easily measured by means of the end-expiratory occlusion technique (Fig. 1) [41, 42]. It is important to underline that, at variance with the measurement of P0.1 and maximal inspiratory pressure (MIP), the measurement of auto-PEEP requires that the patient relaxes during the occlusion. Patients with very high respiratory drive may not allow enough time for muscle relaxation to reach a plateau.

Work of Breathing and Related Measurements.

Assessment of respiratory muscle activity during PSV, can be achieved by measurements of WOB [43] and PTP [44]. However, both WOB and PTP require the correct positioning of an esophageal balloon to estimate pleural pressure, and, although extensively used in investigational studies, neither is commonly used in clinical practice. $P_{0.1}$ has shown good correlation with WOB during PSV [6], and may estimate the respiratory effort. Alternatively, an index of muscular activity, which we have named pressure muscle index (PMI), can be easily obtained during PSV. PMI is measured as the difference between the end-inspiratory occlusion plateau pressure and the airway pressure before the occlusion (PEEP + pressure support), obtained from the ventilator display during an end-inspiratory occlusion (Fig. 1) [36]. PMI has shown a good correlation with PTP ($p < 0.01$). Despite the underlying assumptions and many simplifications required, PMI may be a sensitive estimation of respiratory effort and could be a useful parameter in setting the level of pressure support.

Clinical Application of PSV In ALI/ARDS

Recent data support the possibility of using PSV safely and effectively in the course of acute respiratory failure. Cereda et al. demonstrated that PSV could be used

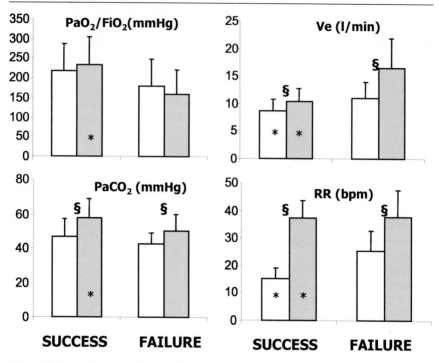

Fig. 2. Main ventilatory and gas exchange parameters during continuous positive pressure ventilation (CPPV) (white bars) and pressure support ventilation (PSV) (gray bars) in the PSV success (left histograms) and failure (right histograms) groups. PaO_2/FiO_2: oxygen arterial tension to inspiratory oxygen fraction ratio; $PaCO_2$: carbon dioxide arterial tension; Ve: minute ventilation; RR: respiratory rate. * $p<0.05$ success vs failure for CPPV or PSV; § $p<0.05$ PSV vs CPPV in success or failure groups. Modified from [23].

rather early in ALI/ARDS patients [23]. Forty-eight intubated, sedated and paralyzed patients were studied: all subjects had been receiving CPPV for at least 24 hours, and had PaO_2 >80 mmHg, at any FiO_2, with PEEP <15 cmH2O. Before switching the ventilator to PSV mode, muscle relaxants were withdrawn and sedative drugs reduced in order to obtain arousal on verbal command, while still relieving patients' pain and anxiety. The pressure support level was initially set to fully unload the patient respiratory muscles. The pressure support level was then adjusted to maintain RR and $PaCO_2$ roughly constant. Switching to PSV was characterized by a decrease in $PaCO_2$ (Fig. 2) with a corresponding increase in pH, with non-substantial changes in PaO_2/FiO_2 (Fig. 2), despite significantly lower FiO_2 and mean airway pressure. Minute ventilation (Ve) and RR increased during PSV (Fig. 2), while V_T decreased. Ten patients (21%) failed the PSV trial, and CPPV was reinstituted. Return to CPPV was based on the occurrence of the following conditions: high RR in seven patients, increased $PaCO_2$ in three, decreased PaO_2 in one, and hemodynamic instability in three (Fig. 2). Patients who showed lower Crs, higher Ve, and longer time since intubation were more prone to fail the PSV trial.

Most ALI patients were successfully managed by means of PSV (79%), even if partial ventilatory support seemed more likely to fail in sicker patients.

A few aspects of this study require some comments. First, the authors may not have exploited all PSV features to full advantage, since the pressure support level was not targeted to enhance the patient's respiratory activity, but rather to maintain a constant $PaCO_2$ level and RR. Second, prolonged use of CPPV might have caused respiratory muscle atrophy, and therefore some decrease in muscle function, particularly in the group of patient who failed the trial. Unfortunately, this issue was insufficiently investigated. Moreover, although a low V_T ventilation strategy actually represents a proven advantage in the management of ARDS patients, the collapse that may result from a strategy based on a low V_T, both in assisted and controlled modes, could further impair gas exchange and respiratory mechanics, thus affecting PSV effectiveness [45].

Tejeda et al. compared PSV with assist-control ventilation in 45 patients with various causes of respiratory failure. PSV showed comparable efficacy to treat patients, with lower peak and mean airway pressure, in spite of a higher minute ventilation and dead space to tidal ventilation ratio [22].

Zeravik et al. investigated the effect of extravascular lung water (EVLW) on PSV efficacy [46]. PSV was successful in 29 of 32 patients with moderate acute respiratory failure. The effect of PSV on oxygenation was dependent on the EVLW: patients who failed the PSV trial showed higher basal levels of EVLW.

In a study by Putensen et al., PSV was compared with APRV with and without spontaneous breathing delivered at equal pressure limits (10 patients) or at equal minute ventilation (10 patients). The authors reported that in ARDS patients APRV with spontaneous breathing resulted in better cardiovascular function and V/Q distribution compared both to PSV and APRV alone. They could not demonstrate, however, any improvement with PSV compared to APRV alone [18]. The authors concluded that the spontaneous activity associated with PSV was not sufficient to reverse the V/Q mismatch caused by the alveolar collapse in ARDS patients. It is worth considering, however, whether the patients were somehow over-assisted during PSV; if this was the case then the patient's own contribution to inspiration was so limited to minimize the beneficial effects of PSV. Unfortunately, though Putensen et al. measured the esophageal pressure, no information about patient effort was reported. In COPD patients with ALI, in whom PSV and APRV were applied at equal pressure limits, APRV did not result in decreased WOB, or diaphragm electromyographic activity, while PSV determined a stable reduction of patient's effort [47]. This result suggested that the interface of spontaneous breathing during PSV and APRV is different and interpretation of results comparing these ventilatory modalities may be difficult.

Beside factors related to respiratory load (ventilatory needs and respiratory mechanics), another important aspect to consider during PSV is patient-ventilator interaction. An increased WOB, and a worse synchronization, likely associated to an increased respiratory drive, may more likely lead to PSV failure. We assessed the effects of short-term oxygenation changes on respiratory drive (P0.1, Ve and RR) on 12 ALI patients undergoing PSV [48]. We investigated three different levels of oxygenation (PaO_2 was respectively 155±68, 75±12, and 55±6 mmHg) and found that decreased oxygenation level resulted in significant increases in Ve, RR, and

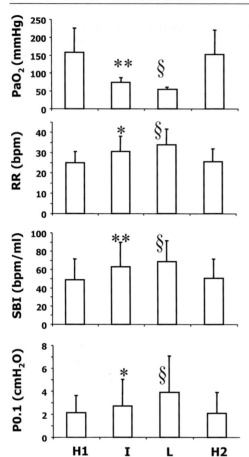

Fig. 3. Oxygen arterial tension (PaO_2), respiratory rate (RR), rapid shallow breathing index (SBI), and inspiratory occlusion pressure in the first 100 ms (P0.1), at different level of inspiratory oxygen fraction (FiO_2): H1, high FiO_2 ($SatO_2 > 95\%$); I, intermediate FiO_2 ($SatO_2$ between 90 and 95%); L, low FiO_2 ($SatO_2$ between 85 and 90%); H2, return to high FiO_2 ($SatO_2 > 95\%$). *, ** $p<0.05$ or $p<0.01$ for the comparison I vs H1; § $p<0.05$ for the comparison of L vs H1+I. Modified from [48].

$P_{0.1}$ (Fig. 3). An important result of this study was that at PaO_2 levels considered clinically adequate, patients still present an important residual hypoxic drive (Fig. 3). Since hypoxia is the main clinical feature of patients with ALI/ARDS, this suggests that acting on FiO_2 to decrease respiratory drive and ventilatory needs (Ve and RR) may improve PSV tolerability and success.

Combining PSV with other Ventilatory Modes

One of the advantages of PSV is the possibility, implemented in most new ventilators, of combining PSV with other ventilatory modes. It is surprising that, despite scanty supporting evidence, PSV in combination with SIMV is one of the most used ventilatory strategies in ICU [3].

The use of periodical recruitment maneuvers (sigh) proved effective during CPPV [49, 50] to promote alveolar recruitment and improve gas exchange in ARDS

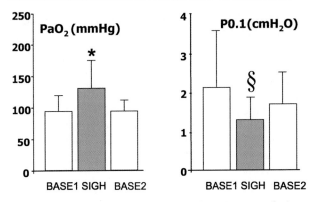

Fig. 4. Oxygen arterial tension (PaO2), and inspiratory occlusion pressure in first 100 ms (P0.1) during PSV alone (BASE1) (white bars), PSV with addition of one sigh per minute (SIGH) (gray bars), and return to PSV alone (PSV2) (white bars). * p<0.01 SIGH vs BASE1; § p<0.05 SIGH vs BASE1. Modified from [51].

patients. In order to improve the efficacy of PSV and to extend its application in ARDS patients, Patroniti at al. [51] tested the use of sigh in 13 ARDS patients undergoing PSV. All patients were studied within 5 days from the diagnosis of ARDS, and none of them received CPPV before the study. Patroniti et al. combined PSV with APRV/BiPAP and delivered the sigh by applying the higher CPAP level of APRV/BiPAP ventilation at pressure higher than 35 cmH2O for at least 3 seconds once per minute. Use of sigh produced an increase in PaO2 (Fig. 4), lung volumes and Crs. Moreover the introduction of sigh resulted in a decreased respiratory drive as indicated by the significant reduction in P0.1 (Fig. 4). The authors concluded that the association of PSV and sigh could extend the use of PSV itself and that the introduction of sigh may enhance feasibility and tolerability of partial ventilatory techniques in ALI/ARDS patients.

PSV For Non-invasive Ventilation

PSV has been extensively used as a first line intervention for NIV delivered via oro-facial or nasal masks (N-PSV) in patients with acute respiratory failure [24, 25, 52–54]. The physiological effects of N-PSV are comparable to those commonly observed during invasive ventilation.

Future Developments

PSV may greatly benefit by technological improvement. Most innovations are being introduced in the patient-ventilator synchronization. Messinger et al. performed a tracheal pressure triggered CPAP, demonstrating that by moving the triggering site at the carinal end of endotracheal tube, WOB is reduced. This result is achieved by avoiding the additional work to overcome the resistance of the circuitry and tube. Indeed an added respiratory load due to tubes (airways, endotracheal tube, circuit) and tissue barriers (alveolar walls and pleura) may exceed the physiological capabilities of respiratory muscles, thus determining a relative inefficiency of the trigger system. Taking into account the *true* airway pressure, at the carina, patient-machine interaction may be improved [55, 56].

Esophageal pressure triggered support ventilation was performed by Bernard et al. in normal volunteers to reduce the possibility of ineffective inspiratory attempt and dyssynchrony due to auto-PEEP. Triggering the inspiratory PSV from the esophagus lead to earlier detection of patient effort, to decreased response time to initiation of gas flow and to lower WOB, when compared to conventionally triggered PSV [57].

An exciting innovation has been proposed by Sinderby et al.: an electrode array, mounted on a nasogastric tube (routinely used for enteral feeding) is positioned in the lower part of the esophagus at the level of the diaphragm. The active muscle generates an electric signal (digitized and filtered to reduce the influence of cardiac electrical activity, motion artifacts and common electrical noise) which, amplified, is used to control both inspiratory and expiratory timing as well as the level of ventilatory assist [58]. This approach proved effective in improving patient-ventilator interactions and patient's comfort. Moreover, this represents the first form of assisted ventilation, fully controlled by respiratory centers, and is independent from integrity of muscles function and auto-PEEP.

Other investigators have directed their attention on inspiratory termination criteria [59, 60]. Yamada and Du, proposed an automatic system of expiratory trigger sensitivity regulation, which is based on a mathematical model description of the PSV inspiratory flow profile [60].

PSV is particularly suited for closed loop control systems. Closed-loop controls of pressure support level based on P0.1 (61), or on RR, V_T, and end-tidal CO_2 pressure [62] have been investigated. An automatic control of pressure support level by means of fuzzy logic has also been tested [63].

Finally, new promising possibilities could come from the use of ventilatory strategies, which combine different modes and may integrate the different advantages and benefits within a single approach [51, 64].

Conclusion

Several data indicate that PSV may be safely and successfully used during the early phase of acute respiratory failure in most ALI/ARDS patients. Various associations with other ventilatory modes finalized to improve lung recruitment and oxygenation, promise to extend the use of PSV in ALI/ARDS. Further clinical investigations and experience are needed to better define indications and limitations of PSV in patients with ALI/ARDS.

References

1. Fahey PJ, Vanderwarf C, David A (1985) Comparison of oxygen costs of breathing during weaning with continuous positive airway pressure versus pressure support ventilation. Am Rev Respir Dis 131 suppl:A130 (abst)
2. MacIntyre N (1986) Respiratory function during pressure support ventilation. Chest 89:677–683
3. Esteban A, Anzueto A, Alia I, et al. for the Mechanical Ventilation International Study Group (2000) How is mechanical ventilation employed in the intensive care unit? Am J Respir Crit Care Med 161:1450–1458
4. Brochard L (1994) Pressure support ventilation. In: Martin J, Tobin MD (eds) Principles and Practice of Mechanical Ventilation. 1st edn. McGraw-Hill, New York 239–257
5. Brochard L, Harf A, Lorino H, Lemaire F (1989) Inspiratory pressure support prevents diaphragmatic fatigue during weaning from mechanical ventilation. Am Rev Respir Dis 139:513–521
6. Berger KI, Sorkin B, Norman RG (1996) Mechanism of relief of tachypnea during pressure support ventilation. Chest 109:1320–1327
7. Van de Graaff WB, Gordey K, Dornseif SE, et al (1991) Pressure support: changes in ventilatory pattern and components of the work of breathing. Chest 100:1082–1089
8. Alberti A, Gallo F, Fongaro A, Valenti S, Rossi A (1995) P0.1 is a useful parameter in setting the level of pressure support ventilation. Intensive Care Med 21:547–553
9. Brochard L, Rauss A, Benito S, et al (1994) Comparison of three methods of gradual withdrawal from ventilatory support during weaning from mechanical ventilation. Am J Respir Crit Care Med 150:896–903
10. Esteban A, Frutos F, Tobin MJ et al (1995) A comparison of four methods of weaning patients from mechanical ventilation. N Engl J Med 332:345–350
11. Younes M, Puddy A, Roberts D, et al (1992) Proportional assist ventilation: results of an initial critical trial. Am Rev Respir Dis 145:121–129
12. Mols G, von Ungern-Stenberg B, Rohr E, Haberthur C, Geiger K, Guttmann J (2000) Respiratory comfort and breathing pattern during volume proportional assist ventilation and pressure support ventilation: A study on volunteers with artificially reduced compliance. Crit Care Med 28:1940–1946
13. Mols G, Rohr E, Benzing A, Haberthur C, Geiger K, Guttmann J (2000) Breathing pattern associated with respiratory comfort during automatic tube compensation and pressure support ventilation in normal subjects. Acta Anaesthesiol Scand 44:223–230
14. Le Bourdelles G, Viires N, Boczkowski J, Seta N, Pavlovic D, Aubier M (1994) Effects of mechanical ventilation on diaphragmatic contractile properties in rats. Am J Respir Crit Care Med 149:1539–1544
15. Stewart KG (1989) Clinical evaluation of pressure support ventilation. Br J Anaesth 63:362–364
16. Rossiter A, Souney PF, McGowan S (1991) Pancuronium induced prolonged neuromuscular blockade. CritCare Med 19:1583–1587
17. Putensen C, Räsänen J, Lopez FA (1994) Ventilation-perfusion distributions during mechanical ventilation with superimposed spontaneous breathing in canine lung injury. Am J Respir Crit Care Med 150:101–108
18. Putensen C, Mutz N, PutensenHimmer G, Zinserling J (1999) Spontaneous breathing during ventilatory support improves ventilation-perfusion distributions in patients with acute respiratory distress syndrome. Am J Respir Crit Care Med 159:1241–1248
19. Downs JB, Douglas ME, Sanfelippo PM et al (1977) Ventilatory pattern, intrapleural pressure, and cardiac output. Anesth Analg 56:88–96
20. Froese AB, Bryan AC (1974) Effects of anesthesia and paralysis on diaprhagmatic mechanics in man. Anesthesiology 38:242–255
21. Putensen C, Zech S, Wrigge H, et al (2001) Long-term effects of spontaneous breathing during ventilatory support in patients with acute lung injury. Am J Respir Crit Care Med 164:43–49

22. Tejeda M, Boix JH, Alvarez F, Balanzà R, Morales M (1997) Comparison of pressure support ventilation and assist-control ventilation in the treatment of respiratory failure. Chest 111:1322–1325
23. Cereda M, Foti G, Marcora B, et al (2000) Pressure support ventilation in patients with acute lung injury. Crit Care Med 28:1269–1275
24. Kramer N, Meyer TJ, Meharg J, et al (1995) Randomized prospective trial of non-invasive positive pressure ventilation in acute respiratory failure. Am J Respir Crit Care Med 151:1799–1806
25. Brochard L, Mancebo J, Wysocki M, et al (1995) Noninvasive ventilation for acute exacerbations of chronic obstructive pulmonary disease. N Engl J Med 333:817–822.
26. Whitelaw WA, Derenne JP, Milic-Emili J (1975) Occlusion pressure as a measure of respiratory centers output in conscious man. Respir Physiol 23:181–199
27. Fernandez R, Cabrera J, Calaf N, Benito S (1990) P0.1/PIMax an index for assessing respiratory capacity in acute respiratory failure. Intensive Care Med 16:175–179
28. Marshall R (1962) Relationship between stimulus and work of breathing at different lung volumes. J Appl Physiol 17:917–919
29. Conti G, Cinnella G, Barboni E, Lemaire F, Harf A, Brochard L (1996) Estimation of occlusion pressure during assisted ventilation in patients with intrinsic PEEP. Am J Respir Crit Care Med 154:907–912
30. Kuhlen R, Hausmann S, Pappert D, Slama K, Roissant R, Falke K (1995) A new method for P0.1 measurement using standard respiratory equipment. Intensive Care Med 21:554–560
31. Yang KL, Tobin MJ (1991) A prospective study of indexes predicting the outcome of trials of weaning from mechanical ventilation. N Engl J Med 324:1445–1450
32. Sassoon CSH, Mahutte CK (1993) Airway occlusion pressure and breathing pattern as predictors of weaning outcome. Am Rev Respir Dis 148:860–866
33. Brochard L, Harf A, Lorino H, Lemaire F (1989) Inspiratory pressure support prevents diaphragmatic fatigue during weaning from mechanical ventilation. Am Rev Respir Dis 139:513–521
34. Marini JJ, Smith TC, Lamb V (1986) Estimation of inspiratory muscle strength in mechanically ventilated patients: the measurement of maximal inspiratory pressure. J Crit Care 1:32–38
35. Pesenti A, Pelosi P, Foti G, D'Andrea L, Rossi N (1992) An interrupter technique for measuring respiratory mechanics and the pressure generated by respiratory muscles during partial ventilatory support. Chest 102:918–923
36. Foti G, Cereda M, Banfi G, Pelosi P, Fumagalli R, Pesenti A (1997) End-inspiratory airway occlusion: a method to assess the pressure developed by inspiratory muscles in patients with acute lung injury undergoing pressure support. Am J Respir Crit Care Med 156:1210–1216
37. Foti G, Patroniti N, Cereda M, Sparacino ME, Giacomini M, Pesenti A (1995) Assessment of the airway occlusion method to estimate respiratory system compliance (Cpl,rs) during pressure support ventilation. Intensive Care Med 21 (suppl 1):S133 (abst)
38. Truwit JD, Marini JJ (1988) Evaluation of thoracic mechanics in ventilated patients (pt. 2). J Crit Care 3:133–150
39. Bates JHT, Milic-Emili J (1991) The flow interruption technique for measuring respiratory resistance. J Crit Care 6:227–238
40. Iotti GA, Braschi A, Brunner JX, et al (1995) Respiratory mechanics by least squares fitting in mechanically ventilated patients: applications during paralysis and during pressure support ventilation. Intensive Care Med 21:406–413
41. Smith TC, Marini JJ (1988) Impact of PEEP on lung mechanics and work of breathing in severe airflow obstruction. J Appl Physiol 65:1488–1499
42. Gottfried SB, Reissman H, Ranieri VM (1992) A simple method for the measurement of intrinsic positive end-expiratory pressure during controlled and assisted modes of mechanical ventilation. Crit Care Med 20:621–628
43. Kacmarek RM (1988) The role of pressure support ventilation in reducing work of breathing. Respir Care 33:99–120

44. Sassoon CSH, Light RW, Lodia R, Sieck GC, Mahutte K (1991) Pressure-time product during continuous positive airway pressure, pressure support ventilation, and T-Piece during weaning from mechanical ventilation. Am Rev Respir Dis 143:469–475

45. Cereda M, Foti G, Mush G, Sparacino ME, Pesenti A (1996) Positive end-expiratory pressure prevents the loss of respiratory compliance during low tidal volume ventilation in acute lung injury patients. Chest 109:480–485

46. Zeravik J, Borg U, Pfeiffer UJ (1990) Efficacy of pressure support ventilation dependent on extravascular lung water. Chest 97:1412–19

47. Viale JP, Duperret S, Mahul P, et al (1998) Time course evolution of ventilatory responses to inspiratory unloading in patients. Am J Respir Crit Care Med 157:428–434

48. Pesenti A, Rossi N, Calori A, Foti G, Rossi GP (1993) Effects of short oxygenation on acute lung injury patients undergoing pressure support ventilation. Chest 103:1185–1189

49. Pelosi P, Cadringher P, Bottino N, et al (1999) Sigh in acute respiratory distress syndrome. Am J Respir Crit Care Med 159:872–880

50. Foti G, Cereda M, Sparacino ME, De Marchi L, Villa F, Pesenti A (2000) Effects of periodic lung recruitment maneuvers on gas exchange and respiratory mechanics in mechanically ventilated acute respiratory distress syndrome patients. Intensive Care Med 26:501–507

51. Patroniti N, Foti G, Cortinovis B, et al (2002) Sigh improves gas exchange and lung volume in ARDS patients undergoing pressare support ventilation. Anesthesiology 96:788–94.

52. Antonelli M, Conti G, Rocco M, et al (1998) A comparison of noninvasive positive-pressure ventilation and conventional mechanical ventilation in patients with acute respiratory failure N Engl J Med 339:429–435

53. Wysocki M, Tric L, Wolff MA, et al (1995) Noninvasive pressure support ventilation in patients with acute respiratory failure: a randomized comparison with conventional therapy. Chest 107:761–768

54. Keenan SP, Kernermann PD, Cook DJ, et al (1997) The effect of non invasive positive pressure ventilation on mortality in patients admitted with acute respiratory failure: a meta-analysis. Crit Care Med 25:1685–1692

55. Messinger G, Banner MJ (1996) Tracheal pressure triggering a demand-flow continuous positive airway pressure system decreases patient work of breathing. Crit Care Med 24:1829–1834

56. Messinger G, Banner MJ, Blanch PB, Layon AJ (1995) Using tracheal pressure to trigger the ventilator and control airway pressure during continuous positive airway pressure decreases work of breathing. Chest 108:509–514

57. Barnard M, Shukla A, Lovell T, Goldstone J (1999) Esophageal-directed pressure support ventilation in normal volunteers. Chest 115:482–489

58. Sinderby C, Navaöeso P, Beck J, et al (1999) Neural control of mechanical ventilation in respiratory failure. Nature Med 5:1433–1436

59. Yamada Y, Du H (1998) Effects of different pressure support termination on patient-ventilator synchrony. Respir Care 43:1048–1057

60. Yamada Y, Du H (2000) Analysis of the mechanisms of expiratory asynchrony in pressur support ventilation: a mathematical approach. J Appl Physiol 88:2143–2150

61. Iotti GA, Brunner JX, Braschi A, et al (1996) Closed-loop control of airway pressure at 0.1 second (P0.1) applied to pressure support ventilation: algorithm and application in intubated patients. Crit Care Med 24:771–779

62. Dojat M, Harf A, Touchard D, Lemaire F, Brochard L (2000) Clinical evaluation of a computer-controlled pressure support mode. Am J Respir Crit Care Med 161:1161–1166

63. Nemoto T, Hatzakis GE, Thorpe CW, Olivenstein R, Dial S, Bates JHT (1999) Automatic control of pressure support mechanical ventilation using fuzzy logic. Am J Respir Crit Care Med 160:550–556

64. Takeda S, Nakanishi K, Takano T, et al (1997) The combination of external high-frequency oscillation and pressure support ventilation in acute respiratory failure. Acta Anesthesiol Scand 41:670–674

Prone Ventilation

R. K. Albert

Introduction

Patients hospitalized in intensive care units (ICUs) are generally positioned supine. This approach disregards the adverse effects of the supine position on the lung which have been recognized for over 2500 years. Hippocrates noted in 500 BC that:

> "It is well when the patient is …reclining upon either his right or left side…and the whole body lying in a relaxed state, for thus the most of persons of health recline. But to lie on one's back, with the hands, neck and the legs extended is far less favorable" [1].

The first study providing a scientific base for this observation appeared in 1922 when Christie and Beams [2] noted that lying supine reduced the vital capacity from that measured in the upright posture. In 1933, Hurtado and Frey [3]) noted that functional residual capacity (FRC) was similarly diminished by lying supine.

Moreno and Lyons [4] observed that the FRC was higher prone versus supine in 1961. This observation was cited by Mellins in 1974 when he suggested that body position could be an important determinant of airspace closure [5]. Finally, Bryan [6] seems to have been the first to propose that ventilating patients in the prone position might be the only way to expand areas of dorsal lung that are collapsed as a result of the adverse mechanical effects attributable to lying supine.

This chapter will review the literature investigating the effects of position on regional ventilation and perfusion in the setting of acute lung injury (ALI) and summarize the results of clinical studies in ALI and/or the acute respiratory distress syndrome (ARDS).

Effects of Posture on Determinants of Regional Ventilation and Perfusion

Perfusion

The zonal theory proposed to explain regional perfusion heterogeneity in the lung ascribes differences in perfusion to the effects of gravity on pulmonary vascular pressures (which increase in a linear fashion going from non-dependent to depend-

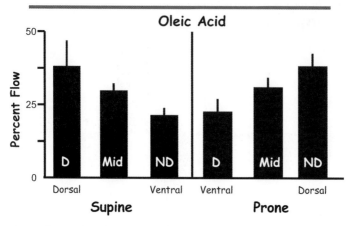

Fig. 1. Effect of prone position on regional perfusion. Radiolabeled microspheres injected into the pulmonary circulation of a lung with the animal positioned supine and prone. Lungs were excised, fixed at total lung capacity and divided into thirds in the ventral-dorsal orientation. Data are presented for dependent (D), mid (Mid) and non-dependent (ND) lung regions. From [7] with permission.

ent lung regions) while the pressure surrounding pulmonary capillaries (i.e., alveolar pressure) is constant throughout the lung. If this were true, dependent lung regions would receive a greater fraction of the total pulmonary blood flow regardless of body position. Recent studies show, however, that gravity is only a minor determinant of perfusion heterogeneity (Fig. 1), explaining no more than 7% of the variation observed [7–9]. The remainder seems to result from anatomic differences in vessel number, diameter and/or branching pattern. Accordingly, although regional perfusion will vary somewhat with changes in posture, dorsal caudal lung regions will always receive a majority of the pulmonary blood flow, regardless of whether they are in the dependent or the non-dependent position (Fig. 1).

Ventilation

Regional ventilation, on the other hand, is markedly altered by the effects of gravity. Milic-Emili and colleagues [10] first demonstrated a vertical gradient in alveolar size in 1966, and a vertical gradient in ventilation was demonstrated by Engel and colleagues in 1974 [11]. In the upright, supine, and right and left lateral decubitus positions there is a gravitational gradient in end-expiratory lung volume with dependent lung regions being less well-expanded than non-dependent regions [12]. These heterogeneities occur in conjunction with regional differences in pleural pressure (Ppl, and accordingly, with regional differences in transpulmonary pressure), and from differences in lung compliance that result from differences in alveolar volume.

The situation is considerably different in the prone position because the lung fits better inside the thorax such that there is less lung deformation in this posture.

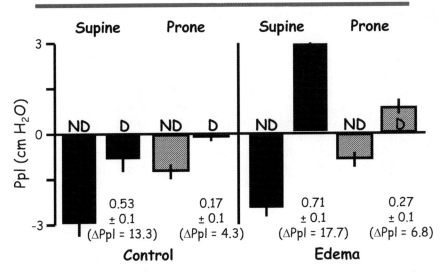

Fig. 2. Pleural pressure gradient (ΔPpl) in normal and edematous lung. Pleural pressure gradients are presented from non-dependent (ND) to dependent (D) lung regions, and expressed for the example of a subject with a ventral-dorsal chest diameter of 25 cm.

This difference results in a much more uniformly distributed Ppl, such that the end-expiratory lung volume is much more uniformly distributed from non-dependent to dependent regions (Fig. 2). This, in turn, allows most of the lung to be at approximately the same place on the pressure-volume (PV) curve [13, 14]. Accordingly, regional ventilation during tidal breathing is much more uniform. In addition, in the supine position, the dependent portions of the lung are exposed to a positive Ppl in the setting of lung injury (Fig. 2). On turning prone, this positive pressure is markedly reduced, i.e., the compressive forces on the dependent region are diminished [13].

History and Clinical Utility of the Prone Position

Piehl and Brown [15] and Douglas and colleagues [16] first noted the marked improvement in oxygenation that occurs when ventilating patients with ARDS in the prone position. Their observation has subsequently been reproduced by numerous other groups including the largest single series to date published by Gattinoni and colleagues [17]. These reports indicate that from 50 to 75% of patients have an improvement in their oxygenation on turning prone that is sufficient to allow a reduction in the level of positive end-expiratory pressure (PEEP) and/or the inspired oxygen fraction (FiO$_2$). Contrary to predictions and assertions made by some, none of the studies indicate that the improvement is transient and, in fact, many reports indicate quite the opposite. Chatte and colleagues [18] and others have noted that some patients maintain most or all of the improvement on returning to the supine position.

Mechanism by which the Prone Position Improves Oxygenation

The mechanism by which the prone position improves oxygenation relates directly to the effect of body position on how the lung fits into the thoracic. This, in turn, is a function of both lung and chest wall anatomy and physiology, and is manifested by regional Ppl and the Ppl gradient. Regional Ppl is generally considered to be an *independent* variable determining regional lung distension, but, in fact, it is a *dependent* variable, changing as a result of lung deformations that develop as a result of the lung having to fit into the thorax. The ability of the lung to fit into the thorax depends on lung distensibility and on chest wall distensibility (Table 1). It is important to recognize that the diaphragm and, accordingly, abdominal pressure is an important contributor to chest wall anatomy and physiology, as was first suggested in 1939 [19].

Factors affecting the lung are straightforward - lungs are more distensible at lower, compared with higher, volumes, and when lungs are air- as opposed to fluid-filled.

Factors affecting the chest wall (which includes the abdomen as these affect the diaphragm) are more complex. The ventral region of the rib cage is more distensible than the dorsal region. Accordingly, when patients are positioned prone a given tidal volume (V_T) produces a greater plateau pressure [20]. This could have important effects with regard to airspace opening, recruitment, and shunt reduction in patients with ARDS. The mass of the abdomen is unchanged by position, but distensibility is greater in the supine compared with the prone position. More importantly, one vector resulting from abdominal pressure (1 cmH$_2$O/cm distance

Table 1. Factors determining the pleural pressure gradient.

Lung Distensibility	Chest Wall Distensibility
Lung volume*	Chest wall mass
Air- or liquid-filling*	Chest wall compliance*
	Abdominal mass
	Abdominal compliance*
	Heart size and mass
	Amount of lung affected by heart mass*
	Mediastinum mass
	Amount of lung affected by mediastinum mass*
	Diaphragm curvature*
	Diaphragm anatomy

* Factors affected by gravity and, therefore, by body position.

in the dependent-to-non-dependent direction) compresses a sizeable portion of the dorsal lung in supine patients. Because of differences in the anatomy and curvature of the diaphragm relative to the ventral vs the dorsal thoracic wall, a similar compression does not result in the ventral regions when patients are prone. In supine patients, the mass of the heart is, in part, supported by the dorsal lung regions (left > right). When patients are prone the heart sits on the sternum and the lung is displaces laterally and subjected to less compressive force [21].

A relatively steep Ppl gradient exists in the supine position (Fig. 2). We [13], and several others, have found that the gravitational gradient of Ppl is more uniform in the prone compared with the supine position. As above, this translates into there being a more uniform distribution of end-expiratory lung volume, and therefore more uniform distribution of alveolar ventilation. Several investigators have demonstrated a flatter slope of phase III in the single-breath oxygen test given to normal human subjects when they are prone as opposed to when they are supine. In addition, we and others have demonstrated a redistribution of ventilation to dorsal lung regions in prone versus supine animals with ALI [22].

Because regional perfusion is relatively unaffected by a change from supine to prone (particularly in the setting of lung injury, Fig. 1), the effect of a prone position-induced improvement in dorsal ventilation will reduce shunt and improve ventilation-perfusion homogeneity.

Approach to Turning Patients Prone

Some argue that turning patients prone is difficult and risky. This is not supported by any published series, and most centers experienced in turning patients feel quite the opposite. Detailed algorithms describing a step-by-step approach to the mechanics of turning patients from supine to prone have been published [23].

Factors determining which patients will respond have not yet been elucidated. The data from Chatte and colleagues [18] suggest that improvement does not relate to the duration of ARDS but may be limited in those with the most severe degrees of shunt. Their observation that over 50% of responding patients maintain their improvement when returned supine is particularly interesting and suggests either that some patients have marked differences between their airspace opening and closing pressures, and/or that drainage of airspace secretions may be playing a role in this improvement. Others suggest that patients in the late stage of ARDS are less likely to improve.

Recruitment Maneuvers

Cakar and colleagues [24] found that a recruiting maneuver (a 30 sec period of static inflation to 60 cmH_2O) employed in an animal model of ALI resulted in a more sustained improvement in oxygenation when the animals were prone compared to when they were supine. The effect of a positive end-expiratory pressure (PEEP) level of 15 cmH_2O on oxygenation in the supine position could be reproduced in the prone position by only 8 cmH2O. Lim and colleagues [25] used a different type of recruiting maneuver (a stepwise increase in PEEP to 30 cmH2O with a concomitant decrease in tidal volume from 8 to 2 ml/kg when the peak pressure exceeded 40 cmH2O) and found a greater response in patients who were supine. Of note was the fact that the oxygenation pre-recruitment was considerably higher in those who were prone. Pelosi and colleagues [26] produced the highest PaO_2, and the greatest improvement in recruited volume, using a recruitment maneuver consisting of three consecutive sighs to a plateau pressure of 45 cmH2O in patients who were prone compared with those supine.

Clinical Implications

It is now clear that gas exchange can and does improve in a large fraction of patients with ARDS when they are turned prone, that the improvement is frequently of sufficient magnitude that PEEP and/or the FiO_2 can be reduced, and that managing patients in the prone position does not seem to be associated with any undue risks or complications. In addition, recent limited studies suggest the response to a recruitment maneuver may be better when patients are prone.

Although a number of questions remain, of greatest importance is whether prone ventilation reduces the morbidity and mortality of patients with ARDS.

There are two mechanisms by which this might occur and they are not mutually exclusive. First, the improvement in oxygenation seen with prone ventilation frequently allows a reduction in the FiO_2. If oxygen toxicity occurs in the setting of ALI, if it contributes to the morbidity or mortality of ARDS, and if it can be reduced by using slightly lower FiO_2s, then prone ventilation might save lives.

Second, lung overdistension and/or cyclic airspace opening and closing are thought to cause ventilator-induced lung injury (VILI) and the results of the recently published ARDS Network study on low-stretch ventilation indicates that VILI contributes to the mortality of ARDS [27]. Since prone positioning should reduce lung overdistension in non-dependent regions, and should reduce cyclical airspace opening and closing in dependent regions, it may also reduce VILI [28].

The first attempt to study the effects of prone ventilation on mortality was published by Gattinoni and colleagues [17]. While they found that the patients randomized to the prone position had better oxygenation, no survival benefit was observed. Unfortunately, the study had numerous methodological problems:

1. Patients randomized to prone ventilation only received it an average of seven hours/day. This is of concern because of the data from a number of experimental studies reporting that an injurious ventilatory strategy could produce VILI in a matter of minutes or hours.
2. The study was too small for mortality to be a valid end-point.
3. Prone ventilation was not instituted early in the course of ALI/ARDS.
4. Standard ventilation and weaning protocols were not used
5. The study only lasted 10 days.
6. There were numerous breaks in protocol.

A recently completed study from Spain found that mortality was reduced 25% in patients with ARDS who were randomized to receive prone ventilation [29]. Unfortunately, only 138 patients were enrolled and this difference in mortality was not statistically significant (p = 0.12). Accordingly, the effect of prone ventilation on outcome in patients with ARDS must await additional studies.

Conclusion

The physiologic rationale supporting the idea that prone ventilation improves oxygenation in patients with ARDS is strong, but there is, at present, no convincing data that this intervention reduces morbidity or mortality. On the other hand, there is no evidence in the literature that prone ventilation is associated with any major side-effects or adverse outcomes. Many turn to prone ventilation, with frequent success, when oxygenation cannot be improved by other means. On the basis of a number of laboratory investigations, however, it is possible that prone ventilation should be used as early as possible when treating patients with ARDS as there is also a strong rationale supporting the hypothesis that it may reduce the incidence of VILI.

Such a major change in the routine care of patients with ALI/ARDS is met with the criticism that the inconvenience of caring for patients in the prone position, together with the increase in nursing time that likely results from the need to turn patients prone and position them appropriately cannot be justified with a prospective randomized trial showing that this approach improves outcomes. Although it is difficult to argue with this position, Hippocrates might have thought otherwise and he was the first to recognize that the supine position is, in itself, not without risk to the patient.

References

1. Adams F (1939) The Genuine Works of Hippocrates. Williams & Wilkins, Baltimore
2. Christie CD, Beams AJ (1922) The estimation of normal vital capacity with special reference to the effect of posture. Arch Intern Med 30:34–39
3. Hurtado A, Frey WW (1933) Studies of total pulmonary capacity and its subdivisions. III: Changes with body posture. J Clin Invest 12:825–31
4. Moreno F, Lyons HA (1961) Effect of body posture on lung volumes. J Appl Physiol 16:27–29
5. Mellins RB (1974) Pulmonary physiotherapy in the pediatric age group. Am Rev Respir Dis 110 (suppl):137–142
6. Bryan AC (1974) Comments of a devil's advocate. Am Rev Respir Dis 110 (suppl):143–144
7. Wiener CM, Kirk W, Albert RK (1990) The prone position revderses the gravitational distribution of perfusion in dog lungs with oleic acid-induced injury. J Appl Physiol 68:1386–1392
8. Glenny RW, Robertwon HT (1990) Fractal properties of pulmonary blood flow: Characterization of spatial heterogeneity. J Appl Physiol 69:532–545
9. Glenny RW, Lamm WJE, Albert RK, Robertson HT (1991) Gravity is a minor determinant of pulmonary blood flow distribution. J Appl Physiol 71; 620–629
10. Milic-Emili J, Henderson JAM, Dolovich MB, Trop D, Kaneko K (1966) Regional distribution of inspired gas in the lung. J Appl Physiol 21:749–759

11. Engel LA, Utz G, Wood LDH, Macklem PT (1974) Ventilation distribution in anatomical lung units. J Appl Physiol 22:760–766
12. Milic-Emili J (1986) Static distribution of lung volumes. In: Macklem PT, Mead J (eds) Handbook of Physiology. The Respiratory System, vol 3. Mechanics of Breathing. Am Physiol Soc, Bethesda, pp:561–579
13. Mutoh T, Guest RJ, Lamm WJE, Albert RK (1992) Prone position alters the effect of volume overload on regional pleural pressures and improves hypoxemia in pigs in-vivo. Am Rev Respir Dis 146:300–306
14. Lai-Fook S, Rodarte JR (1991) Pleural pressure distribution and its relationship to lung volume and interstitial pressure. J Appl Physiol 70: 967–978
15. Piehl MA, Brown RS (1976) Use of extreme position changes in acute respiratory failure. Crit Care Med 4:13–14
16. Douglas WW, Rehder K, Beynen RM, Sessler AD, Marsh HM (1977) Improved oxygenation in patients with acute respiratory failure: the prone position. Am Rev Respir Dis 115: 559–566
17. Gattinoni L, Tognoni G, Pesenti A, et al (2001) Effect of prone positioning on the survival of patients with acute respiratory failure. N Engl J Med 345:568–573
18. Chatte G, Sab J-M, Dubois J-M, Sirodot M, Gaussorgues P, Robert D (1996) Prone position in mechanically ventilation patients with severe acute respiratory failure. Am J Respir Crit Care Med 155:473–478
19. McMichael J, McGibbon JP (1939) Postural changes in the lung volume. Clin Sci 4:175–183
20. Pelosi P, Tubiolo D, Mascheroni D, et al (1998) Effects of the prone position on respiratory mechanics and gas exchange during acute lung injury. Am J Respir Crit Care Med 157:387–393
21. Albert, RK, Hubmayr, RD (2000) The prone position eliminates compression of the lungs by the heart. Am J Respir Crit Care Med 161:1660–1665
22. Lamm WJE, Graham MM, Albert RK (1994) Mechanism by which the prone position improves oxygenation in acute lung injury. Am J Respir Crit Care Med 150:184–193
23. Messerole E, Peine P, Wittkopp S, Marini JJ, Albert RK (2002) The pragmatics of prone positioning. Am J Respir Crit Care Med 165:1359–1363
24. Cakar N, de Kloot TV, Youngblood M, Adams A, Nahum A (2000) Oxygenation response to a recruitment maneuver during supine and prone positions in an oleic acid-induced lung injury model. Am J Respir Crit Care Med 161:1949–1956
25. Lim CM, Jung H, Koy Y, et al (2003) Effect of alveolar recruitment maneuver in early acute respiratory distress syndrome according to antiderecruitment strategy, etiological category of diffuse lung injury and body position of the patient. Crit Care Med 31:411–418
26. Pelosi P, Bottino N, Chiumello D, et al (2003) Sigh in supine and prone position during acute respiratory distress syndrome. Am J Respir Crit Care Med 167:521–527
27. The ARDS Network (2000) Ventilation with lower tidal volumes as compared with traditional tidal volumes for acute lung injury and the acute respiratory distress syndrome. N Engl J Med 342:1301–1308
28. Broccard AF, Shapiro RS, Schmitz LL, Ravenscraft SA, Marini JJ (1997) Influence of prone position on the extent and distribution of lung injury in a high tidal volume oleic acid model of acute respiratory distress syndrome. Crit Care Med 25:16–27
29. Mancebo J, Rialp G, Fernández R, Gordo F, Albert RK and the Spanish ARDS Randomized Control Trial Group to study Prove vs Supine Ventilation (2003) Prone vs Supine position in ARDS patients. Results of a randomized multicenter trial. Am J Respir Crit Care Med 167:A180 (abst)

Adjuncts to Mechanical Ventilation for ARDS Including Biological Variability

R. M. Kacmarek

Introduction

Over the last 15 years it has been clearly established in numerous animal models that some approaches to mechanical ventilation can induce lung injury [1] and clinical data have demonstrated improved mortality when a lung protective ventilatory strategy is employed [2, 3]. However, overall mortality in acute respriratory distress syndrome (ARDS) is still about 40% [4, 5]. As a result, investigations focusing on approach and adjuncts to ventilatory support are still ongoing. Throughout this text, data on alternate modes of ventilation, such as high frequency oscillatory ventilation (HFOV), airway pressure release ventilation (APRV) and bilevel ventilation, as well as prone positioning have been presented. In this chapter, a review of the current status of tracheal gas insufflation (TGI), partial liquid ventilation (PLV), inhaled nitric oxide (NO), and the less well developed concept of integrating biological variability into ventilatory support are presented.

Tracheal Gas Insufflation

The injection of a secondary flow of gas at the level of the carina during conventional mechanical ventilation has been referred to as TGI [6]. This concept was first introduced by Stresemann and Sattler [7] in 1969 who proposed TGI as an adjunct to mechanical ventilation. Ideally, this secondary gas flow is independent of the actual tidal volume (V_T) delivered by the mechanical ventilator. The role of the TGI gas flow is to flush carbon dioxide (CO_2) from the anatomic deadspace of the trachea and proximal mainstem bronchi as well as the endotracheal tube and mechanical deadspace of the ventilator circuit (Fig. 1) [6]. Since CO_2 only accumulates in anatomic and mechanical deadspace at end expiration, TGI flow is only necessary at end exhalation. The secondary mechanism by which CO_2 elimination is enhanced, is the turbulence generated at the tip of the TGI catheter by the high velocity gas flow. This causes CO_2 movement from the airways distal to the catheter tip [8].

No TGI   **TGI**

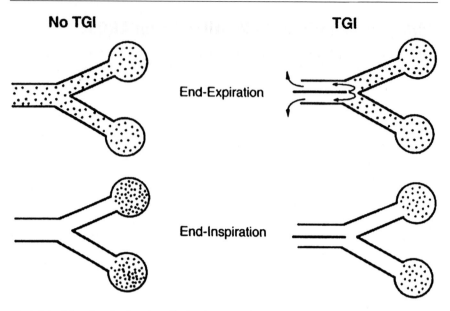

End-Expiration

End-Inspiration

Fig. 1. Principles of tracheal gas insufflation (TGI). With no TGI (left) the gas in the central airways is laden with CO_2 (black dots) at end expiration. This gas is then rebreathed into the alveoli at the onset of the next inspiration. With TGI (right), the gas in the central airways is replaced with fresh gas during expiration, and less CO_2 is rebreathed during the next inspiration, effectively lowering the deadspace. From [6] with permission.

TGI Systems

A number of different approaches to the establishment of TGI have been described [9]. Essentially, the TGI catheter can be directed toward the carina or toward the ventilator circuit [10]. There appears to be little difference in gas exchange enhancement between these approaches, but each effect has a different influence on the development of positive end-expiratory pressure (PEEP) [10, 11]. TGI flow directed toward the carina creates an additional threshold to prevent exhalation, increasing total PEEP [10, 11], whereas TGI directed toward the ventilator circuit creates a jet drag effect in the airway, decreasing the total PEEP [10, 11].

The ideal TGI system flushes the airway of CO_2 but does not alter gas delivery during tidal breathing [6, 9]. Therefore, TGI should only be active during the expiratory phase. If TGI flow is maintained continuously, V_T and peak alveolar pressure will increase thus potentially negating the beneficial lung protective effect of TGI. Continuous flow TGI can be modified by decreasing the delivered V_T equivalent to the TGI flow [12, 13]. This, however, is limited by the size of the V_T versus the TGI flow and it is impossible to adjust V_T during pressure ventilation. The addition of a flow relief or pressure relief valve during continuous TGI and pressure ventilation can also avoid increases in airway pressure and V_T [14, 15]. Many of the newest generation mechanical ventilators incorporate exhalation valves that remain active during the inspiratory phase of pressure ventilation, effectively dissipating excessive flow and avoiding increased plateau pressure.

An additional concern with continuous flow TGI is integration with the mechanical ventilator. As indicated above, increased V_T and plateau pressure can be avoided with TGI, but inactivation of the TGI flow if an airway obstruction occurs proximal to the tip of the TGI catheter is impossible if the TGI system is unable to interface with the ventilator. This is a critical safety issue since the ventilator alarm systems and pressure release mechanisms, will not affect the TGI system unless the system is capable of 'talking' to the ventilator [9].

Two additional approaches to tracheal CO_2 removal have been proposed in the last few years: tracheal gas exsufflation (TGE) [16] and coaxial ventilation [17]. With TGE, a negative pressure is applied to the insufflation catheter during expiration removing gas from the lungs. As expected, this does not affect inspiratory pressure or volume, but does decrease PEEP [16]. The effect on PEEP depends on catheter design, catheter exsufflation velocity, and flow. When a similar catheter is used for expiratory TGI directed toward the carina and TGE with the same insufflating and exsufflating velocities, the increase and decrease in PEEP are of similar magnitudes [18].

A coaxial ventilating system has been recently described by Lethvall et al. [17]. With this system, a 5 mm outer diameter Teflon tube is inserted into a standard 8 mm inner diameter endotracheal tube. As a result of the configuration of the two tubes, inspiration occurs via the inner Teflon tube and expiration around the inner tube via the 8 mm endotracheal tube. This system effectively eliminates ventilator and endotracheal deadspace all the way to the tip of the 5 mm Teflon tube because it essentially moves the y piece of the ventilator circuit to the tip of the endotracheal tube. All functions of the ventilator are maintained and there is no need for a secondary gas delivery system, but a potential for the development of excessive PEEP does exist. Only preliminary lung model data have been presented using this system [17]. Animal and patient data are needed before this system can be recommended, however, it does have intriguing possibilities.

Clinical Utility

TGI has been used in the management of ARDS where CO_2 elimination has been a problem. Studies evaluating the efficacy of TGI have focused on the reduction or maintenance of V_T and plateau pressure while decreasing $PaCO_2$ [19–21] or the maintenance of $PaCO_2$ while reducing V_T and plateau pressure [22]. Figure 2 illustrates the finding of Kalfon et al. [21] who demonstrated that the addition of expiratory TGI to a series of patients with permissive hypercapnia resulted in a 20% decrease in $PaCO_2$. Similar data have been provided by Richecoeur et al. [22], who found that the combination of increasing respiratory rate to the limit of auto-PEEP, removing the tubing connecting the y piece to the endothracheal tube, and expiratory TGI of 15 l/min produced a reduction of $PaCO_2$ from 84 mmHg during conventional ventilation prior to these adjustments to 45 mmHg after the adjustments. In all of the studies to date PaO_2 is not affected provided total PEEP is kept constant [19–22].

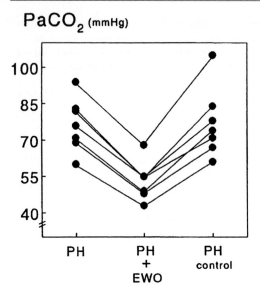

Fig. 2. Individual changes in $PaCO_2$ during permissive hypocapnia (pH) and pH plus expiratory tracheal gas insufflation (EWO) in seven patients with severe acute respiratory distress syndrome (ARDS). From [21] with permission.

A number of factors determine the efficiency of TGI systems. The volume of gas injected per breath is the most critical determinant of TGI efficiency [6]. The greater the injected volume the greater the CO_2 removal. TGI flows ranging from 4–15 l/min have been used on adult patients with ARDS [19–22]. The closer the tip of the TGI catheter to the carina, the greater the TGI efficiency [6]. A position about 1 cm above the carina seems ideal. Finally, TGI is more effective if total physiologic deadspace is primarily a result of anatomic deadspace. The greater the alveolar dead space, the lower the efficiency of TGI [6].

Complications and Monitoring

In order for TGI to be safely administered it must interface with the mechanical ventilator [9]. As indicated earlier, expiratory TGI eliminates problems with increasing V_T and plateau pressure during TGI. Appropriate system monitoring should be available, including measurement of total PEEP, peak inspiratory pressure and V_T. To insure patient safety, a method of identifying increased carinal pressure and deactivating the TGI system if an obstruction occurs must be incorporated into any TGI system. The TGI system must be appropriately humidified, not an easy task because of the small diameter of TGI catheters. Up to 15 psi driving pressure is required to establish a flow of 8 l/min though a 1 mm internal diameter TGI catheter [12]. Few humidifiers are designed to withstand this type of pressure. If patients are breathing spontaneously, TGI interferes with ventilator triggering. As a result, precise timing of activation and deactivation of the TGI system is critical.

Partial Liquid Ventilation (PLV)

The first successful use of liquid ventilation was performed by Kylstra et al. in 1966 [23]. In this experiment, dogs were maintained under hyperbaric conditions with saline used as the ventilating media. Total liquid ventilation required that the fluid 'ventilating' the lung be pumped into and out of the lung and a mechanism for adding oxygen to, and removing CO_2 from the fluid be established. To date, no total liquid ventilation system has been used on adults. The use of saline in this original experiment was also a major problem because of the poor capacity of saline to carry O_2 (2 ml/100 ml) and CO_2 (70 ml/100 ml).

The introduction of perfluorocarbons with their high capacity for carrying O_2 (63 ml/100 ml) and CO_2 (210 ml/100 ml), and the first successful use of PLV by Fuhrman et al. in 1991 made liquid ventilation a clinical reality [24]. With PLV, the lung is filled to a percentage of functional residual capacity (FRC) with a perfluoro-carbon and then conventionally ventilated. The only perfluorocarbon used to date in humans has been Perflubron (Alliance Pharmaceuticals, San Diego, CA, USA), chemical formula C_8F_{14} BR. Table 1 summarizes the physical properties of Per-flubron and its proposed mechanisms of action.

Oxygenation

PLV has been able to dramatically improve gas exchange in animal models of ARDS [25, 26]. Much of this oxygenation benefit is a result of perfluorocarbon recruitment of dependent lung units. PLV has been referred to by many as regional PEEP.

Table 1. Physical properties of Perflubron and proposed mechanism of action

Physical Properties	Mechanisms of Action
Colorless	Alveolar tamponade
Odorless	Anti-inflammatory effects
Insoluble in H_2O	Pulmonary lavage
Biologically inert	Redistribution of pulmonary blood flow
Chemically stable	Prevention of alveolar collapse
O_2 solubility 63 ml/100 ml	Lung recruitment
CO_2 solubility 210 ml/100 ml	
Surface tension 18 dynes/cm	
Density 1.92 g/ml	
Spreading coefficient + 2.7 dynes/cm	
Vapor pressure 11 mmHg	

However, because of the gravity dependent distribution of perfluorocarbons, three distinct regions of lung are established during PLV [27]: the most gravity dependent lung where little ventilation takes place is filled with the perfluorocarbon; the least gravity dependent lung where most ventilating volume is distributed; and the zone in between where gas and perfluorocarbon coexist. The weight of the perfluorocarbon redistributes blood flow from gravity dependent to nongravity dependent lung, improving ventilation/perfusion (V/Q) matching [28]. In addition, perfluorocarbons have a surfactant like quality, high spreading co-efficient and low surface tension [24]. As a result, along with an improvement in oxygenation is an improvement in lung compliance [25, 26].

Anti-Inflammation

Perfluorocarbons have an anti-inflammatory effect. Dickson et al. [29] demonstrated that PLV improved survival in rats infected with pneumococcal pneumonia. Rats (75–300 g) were intratracheally inoculated with *Streptococcus pneumoniae*. Twenty four hours after infection, the rats were allocated randomly to five treatment groups of 15 animals each. Group 1 received no treatment; Group 2, one intramuscular injection of penicillin G; Group 3 PLV with Perflubron; Group 4 PLV with Perflubron and a single intramuscular dose of penicillin G; and Group 5, only gas ventilation. After 10 days, a significantly greater number of rats survived in the PLV with penicillin group.

Additionally, perfluorocarbons lavage secretions from the lung. This occurs because perfluorocarbons do not mix with water. As a result of the density of perfluorocarbons, they move behind secretions, forcing them to the top of the perfluorocarbon column. However, this process requires that the clinician be alert to potential airway obstruction by the large volumes of secretions that can be mobilized. In some settings bronchoscopy is necessary to relieve obstruction of the airway.

Filling and Evaporation

Delivering perfluorocarbon to the lung is a tedious procedure. The drug must be slowly dripped into the airway to avoid obstruction by air locks in the distal lung. Hypoxemia, tachycardia, and hyper or hypotension are common during filling if care is not exercised. Since perfluorocarbons have a high vapor pressure, they readily evaporate [24] removing the drug from the lung within 48 hours of the last dose. Repeat dosing is required every 2 to 4 hours to maintain an appropriate drug level.

Mechanical Ventilation During PLV

Initially, it was felt that large V_{TS} were required to maintain oxygenation during PLV [24]. However, it has been clearly demonstrated that PLV does not protect the

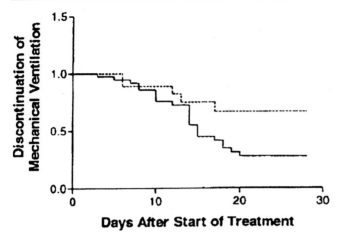

Fig. 3. Kaplan-Meier curves for the rate of discontinuation of mechanical ventilation in the conventional mechanical ventilation (dotted line) and partial liquid ventilation (solid line) groups among those patients with $PaO_2/FiO_2 < 300$ mmHg at $FiO2 = 1.0$ and age ≤ 55 years (p = 0.045 by log rank test). From [40] with permission.

lung from ventilator induced lung injury (VILI) [30]. Small (6–10 ml/kg) V_{TS} are now generally used during PLV. PEEP is also necessary during PLV to maintain oxygenation [31]. The use of PEEP does shift the lower inflection point on the PV curve to the left. PEEP levels of 12 to 15 cmH_2O are currently recommended during PLV. PEEP seems to improve oxygenation by two mechanisms: first, moving the perfluorocarbon out of central airways and second, stabilizing nondependent lung. As with conventional ventilation, plateau pressure during PLV should be kept ≤ 30 cmH_2O. However, the actual distending pressure on dependent lung is difficult to measure because of the added effect of the weight of the perfluorocarbon to the airway pressure.

Response in Humans

Overall data on the use of PLV in humans are limited [32–40]. Much of the early data regarding PLV is in neonates who were also receiving extracorporeal membrane oxygenation (ECMO) [32–34]. Two case series of adult ARDS patients receiving PLV who participated in a randomized trial have also been published [35, 37]. These studies demonstrated the ability of PLV to sustain adult ARDS patients, and focused on the ability of PLV to diminish the inflammatory response in trauma patients and evaluated the pulmonary and systemic distribution and elimination of Perflubron.

The most encouraging patient data during PLV are those of Leach et al. [34] who presented data on 13 premature infants in severe respiratory distress refractory to other therapy. When these infants received PLV, PaO_2 increased, $PaCO_2$ decreased, and lung compliance improved. Eight of the 13 babies survived. A phase II adult

ARDS randomized trial was performed in 1995 [40]. No differences in mortality or ventilator-free days were observed between groups, but there was a trend toward higher levels of adverse events (hypoxemia and hemodynamic compromise) during filling with Perflubron. In post hoc analysis, in patients < 55 years old with a $PaO_2/FiO_2 < 300$ mmHg at FiO_2 1.0, PLV reduced mortality and ventilator free days (Fig. 3). A phase II/III trial with three groups; low dose, (50% of FRC), high dose (100% of FRC) and control was completed in January of 2001. Patients who qualified for entry had a PaO_2/FiO_2 of < 300 mmHg on a PEEP ≥ 13 cmH$_2$O. All aspects of mechanical ventilation and weaning were carefully protocolized. The unpublished results of this study were presented by Dr. Herbert Wiedemann at the 2001 American Thoracic Society meeting. No differences in any outcome variable were observed among groups, but the PLV groups demonstrated a significantly greater number of adverse events during the study. A number of reasons can be speculated as to why this seemly well-designed trial failed to show differences: Over 50 centers participated, many with no prior laboratory experience with PLV. In the PLV groups, patients were disconnected from the ventilator every 3 hours for evaluation of the Perflubron level by suctioning, and finally the approach to ventilation during PLV may not have been optimal.

PLV and High Frequency Oscillatory Ventilation

It has been cogently argued that the combination of HFOV and PLV (HFOV-PLV) has a number of distinct advantages over conventional ventilation during PLV [27]. Perflubron reverses the atelectasis in the dependent lung and directs pulmonary blood flow to the nondependent lung [28], whereas HFOV ventilates the nondependent lung with sufficient mean airway pressure to avoid atelectasis and overdistension. In addition, HFOV minimizes the shear stress in the region of the lung where both gas and fluid reside. A number of laboratory trials have demonstrated the superiority of HFOV-PLV, in relation to gas exchange over conventional ventilation-PLV, [41,42,43] but no patient data are available on HFOV-PLV.

Nitric Oxide

NO is produced endogenously by the reaction of NO synthase and the amino-acid L-arginine [44]. Endogenous NO affects multiple organ systems and receptor sites. It inhibits platelet function, is involved in immune and enzyme regulation, is a neurotransmittor, and is cytotoxic, but most importantly for this discussion, NO is a potent dilator of vascular smooth muscle [44]. Inhaled NO selectively dilates pulmonary vascular beds that are ventilated. Since NO rapidly reacts with hemoglobin, at usual clinical doses (≤ 20 ppm) inhaled NO only has an effect on local vasculature in contact with ventilated lung, improving the ventilation perfusion relationship [44]. As a result, inhaled NO in ARDS increases PaO_2 and decreases intrapulmonary shunt, while decreasing pulmonary vascular resistance and pulmonary artery pressure [45].

Effect in ARDS

The beneficial effects of inhaled NO on oxygenation in ARDS patients was first demonstrated by Rossaint et al. [45], who showed that 18 ppm inhaled NO resulted in an increased PaO_2, decreased shunt function, and decreased pulmonary vascular resistance without any effect on systemic circulation. Numerous other case series support this initial finding that inhaled NO is a selective pulmonary vasodilator that improves oxygenation without system hemodynamic compromise [44].

Randomized Trials in ARDS

There have been a number of prospective randomized controlled trials of inhaled NO in ARDS [46–49] all of which have been negative, each showing an initial oxygenation benefit that was lost within 48 hours, but none demonstrating an improvement in outcome with the use of inhaled NO. The protocols used to manage the ventilator while patients received inhaled NO with each of these trials can be criticized. However, the fact that four trials by different groups were negative makes the conclusion that inhaled NO in ARDS does not result in improved outcome unavoidable.

Inhaled NO with Other Adjuncts

A number of groups are continuing to evaluate the role of inhaled NO in ARDS, but doing so by combining NO with other novel approaches to managing ARDS [50]. There is a body of literature that has evaluated combining inhaled NO with either prone positioning, HFOV or PLV [50]. Each of these combined approaches has resulted in better gas exchange in patients or animal models than conventional mechanical ventilation but no randomized controlled trials have been conducted demonstrating improved outcome.

Biological Variability

Our perspective on how a critically ill patient should ideally present is generally based on the concept of homeostasis or the assumption that variability in physiologic parameters is not good [51]. Walter B. Cannon indicated that homeostatic mechanisms are regulatory mechanisms engineered to reduce variability and maintain steady state [52]. Clearly, few are comfortable with a critically ill patient whose respiratory rate and V_T rapidly change or those whose heart rate and blood pressure fluctuate markedly over time. However, our preoccupation at the bedside with a lack of variability is being challenged. Current theory on biological systems emphasizes the fact that variability to the level of appearing chaotic is associated with health [51]. Much work regarding heart rate variability has been performed [53]. On closer observation, the seemingly regular resting sinus rhythm is highly variable with large complex fluctuations occurring over milliseconds to hours [54].

Loss of the body's ability to maintain complex arrays of highly variable rhythms has been associated with pathology [53, 55] and occurs with aging [55].

Should Ventilatory Support be Variable?

Recently, Suki et al. [56, 57] provided a theoretical argument for 'noise' during ventilatory support. Ventilatory variability according to Suki et al. [56] improves recruitment of lung in ARDS. Based on the concept of "avalanches and power-law behavior of lung inflation", Suki et al. hypothesized that airways open in bursts once a threshold pressure is reached. This occurs to a greater extent with a power law distribution than with a gaussian or exponential distribution. According to the concept of "stochastic resonance" applied to the respiratory system, V_Ts varying above and below the Pflex result in a mean peak airway pressure lower than that of the same average V_T delivered constantly [57]. As a result, breath to breath variability in V_T and respiratory rate about Pflex recruits and maintains greater lung volume and improves PaO_2 more than constant volume and rate ventilation. This concept has been experimentally tested by a number of groups [58–63]. Lefevre et al. [58] used a computer controlled ventilator capable of randomly varying V_T and respiratory rate, but maintaining minute ventilation to conventional control mode volume ventilation with the same minute volume in randomly assigned pigs injured with oleic acid. No PEEP was applied to either group. After 4 hours of ventilation, the biologically variable mechanical ventilation group had a significantly higher PaO_2, lower shunt fraction, higher compliance and a lower wet:dry lung weight ratio. In addition to mean rate and minute ventilation being the same, mean peak airway pressure and mean airway pressures were the same between groups. Mutch et al. [60] also used a porcine model of complete right lung atelectasis to compare the effect of biologically variable mechanical ventilation to conventional volume control ventilation and the impact of sighs during conventional volume controlled ventilation. As in the Lefevre et al. [58] study, minute ventilation was kept constant among groups and PEEP was not applied. After 5 hours of ventilation PaO_2 was much greater in the biologically variable mechanical ventilation group (502 ± 40 mmHg) than in the sigh group (381 ± 40 mmHg) and the non-sigh conventional mechanical ventilation group (309 ± 79 mmHg). Shunt fraction and PCO_2 were also lower and compliance was higher in the biologically variable mechanical ventilation group. Boker et al. [61] also showed improved PaO_2, shunt fraction and better compliance with biologically variable mechanical ventilation versus controlled mechanical ventilation. However, Nam et al. [59] in a canine model of oleic acid induced lung injury did not find any differences in PaO_2, shunt, or static compliance after 4 hours of ventilation.

In all of these studies, minute ventilation was kept constant between groups, but only two studies [59, 61] maintained V_T constant between groups throughout the protocol. Both Mutch et al. [60] and Lefevre et al. [58] allowed V_T in the biologically variable mechanical ventilation group to increase over the conventional ventilation group by the end of the trial. However, in the study by Nam et al. [59] PaO_2 (53 ± 10 vs 95 ± 28 mmHg), $PaCO_2$ (55 ± 5 vs 45 ± 3 mmHg), PvO_2 (36 ± 5 vs 47 ± 7 mmHg) and pH (7.24 ± 0.03 vs 7.33 ± 0.03) all trended to be better with biologically variable mechanical ventilation even with the V_T constant. Other factors that may have caused the different outcome in the study by Nam et al. [59] compared to the other three studies [58, 60, 61] include a difference in species studied (pigs [59] vs dogs [58, 60, 61]), the severity of injury (in the Nam [59] study the level of injury was much greater resulting in 33% mortality prior to the end of the study), and the type of ventilator used. In the two studies [58, 60] where V_T varied based on compliance change an Ohio 7000 anesthesia machine was used which alters delivered V_T as impedance changes, whereas, Nam et al. [59] and Boker et al. [61] used ICU ventilators in the volume mode. However, the most important difference may have been the algorithm establishing variability. The three studies demonstrating benefit of biologically variable mechanical ventilation established variability based on the peak to peak variability in systolic blood pressure of the anesthetized pig. This was based on the concept that variability in heart rate, peak to peak changes in systolic blood pressure and respiratory rate are similar and share a common centering frequency equal to respiratory rate [64]. Thus, Lefevre et al. [58], Mutch et al. [60] and Boker et al. [61] used 369 respiratory rate and V_T combinations over 1089 seconds with a coefficient of variation equal to 11.5%. However, Nam et al. [59] used 784 respiratory rate and V_T combinations over 3,138 seconds with a coefficient of variation equal to 26.2%. As defined by Suki et al. [56, 57] there is a specific level of variation where biologically variable ventilation will be maximally effective with effectiveness decreasing as variability increases or decreases about this point. As a result, the level of variability used by Nam et al. [59] may have simply been too great.

Conclusion

TGI does reduce CO_2 without increasing V_T and plateau pressure, but before it can be recommended on a routine clinical basis appropriately monitored systems capable of interfacing with the mechanical ventilator must be developed and clinical trials conducted. In laboratory models, PLV outperforms conventional mechanical ventilation. All human data have failed to identify a benefit from PLV. It is unlikely that PLV with conventional mechanical ventilation will ever be used as an approach to manage ARDS patients. Current research on perfluorocarbons has focused on the use of the fluid as a vehicle to deliver drugs or as an adjunct to lung recruitment and in combination with HFO. Inhaled NO cannot be recommended for the routine management of ARDS. Additional data combining NO with other adjuncts to ventilatory support is promising; however, there is a need for clinical trials before these techniques can be recommended except as rescue therapy. Based on the animal data with biologically variable mechanical ventilation, it is interesting to speculate the effects of this approach on humans. However, we must await human trials before recommendations can be made, as we know animal and human data can be very different.

References

1. Dreyfuss D, Saumon G (1998) Ventilator induced lung injury: lessons from experimental studies. Am J Respir Crit Care Med 157:294–323
2. Amato MBP, Barbas CSV, Medeiros DM, et al (1998) Effect of protective-ventilation strategy on mortality in the acute respiratory distress syndrome. N Engl J Med 338:347–354
3. ARDSnet (2000) Ventilation with lower tidal volumes compared with traditional tidal volume for acute lung injury and the acute respiratory distress syndrome. N Engl J Med 342:1301–1308
4. Gattinoni L, Tognoni G, Pesenti A, et al (2001) Effect of prone positioning on the survival of patients with acute respiratory failure. N Engl J Med 345:568–573
5. Esteban A, Anzueto A, Frutos F, et al (2002) Characteristics and outcomes in adult patients receiving mechanical ventilation: A 28-day international study. JAMA 287:345–355
6. Ravencraft SA (1996) Tracheal gas insufflation: Adjunct to conventional mechanical ventilation. Respir Care 41:105–111
7. Streseman E and Sattler FP (1969) Effects of washout of anatomical deadspace on ventilation, pH, and blood gas composition in anesthetized dogs. Respiration 26:116–121
8. Nahum A, Shapiro RS, Ravenscraft SA, Adams AB, Marini JJ (1995) Efficacy of expiratory tracheal gas insufflation in a canine model of lung injury. Am J Respir Crit Care Med 152:489–495
9. Kacmarek RM (2001) Complications of tracheal gas insufflation. Respir Care 46:167–176
10. Nahum A, Ravenscraft SA, Nakos G, Adams AB, Burke WC, Marini JJ (1993) Effect of catheter flow direction on CO_2 removal during tracheal gas insufflation in dogs. J Appl Physiol 75:1238–1246
11. Imanaka H, Kirmse M, Mang H, Hess D, Kacmarek RM (1999) Expiratory phase tracheal gas insufflation and pressure control in sheep with permissive hypercapnia. Am J Respir Crit Care Med 159:49–54
12. Imanaka H, Kacmarek RM, Riggi V, Ritz R, Hess D (1998) Expiratory phase and volume-adjusted tracheal gas insufflation: A lung model study. Crit Care Med 126:939–946
13. Burke WC, Nahum A, Ravenscraft SA, et al (1993) Modes of tracheal gas insufflation. Comparison of continuous and phase-specific gas injection in normal dogs. Am Rev Respir Dis 148:562–568
14. Kirmse M, Fujino Y, Hromi J, Mang H, Hess D, Kacmarek RM (1999) Pressure release tracheal gas insufflation reduces airway pressures in lung-injured sheep maintaining eucapnia. Am J Respir Crit Care 160:1462–1467
15. Gowski DT, Delgado E, Miro AM, Tasota FJ, Hoffman LA, Pinsky MR (1997) Tracheal gas insufflation during pressure-control ventilation: effect of using a pressure relief valve. Crit Care Med 25:145–152
16. De Robertis E, Serville G, Jonson B, Tufano R (1999) Aspiration of deadspace allows normocapnic ventilation at low tidal volumes in man. Intensive Care Med 25:674–679
17. Lethvall S, Sondergaard S, Karason S, Lundin S, Stenquist O (2002) Deadspace reduction and tracheal pressure measurement using a coaxial inner tube in an endotracheal tube. Intensive Care Med 28:1042–1048
18. Takahashi T, Bugedo G, Adams AB, Bliss PL, Marini JJ (1999) Effects of tracheal gas insufflation and tracheal gas exsufflation on intrinsic positive end-expiratory pressure and carbon dioxide elimination. Respir Care 44:918–924
19. Ravenscraft SA, Burke WC, Nahum A, et al (1993) Tracheal gas insufflation augments CO_2 clearance during mechanical ventilation. Am Rev Respir Dis 148:345–351
20. Saura P, Lucangelo Blanch L, Artigas A, Mas A, Fernandez R (1996) Factores determinantres de la reduccion de la $PaCO_2$ con la insuflacion de gas traqual en pacientes con lesion pulmonar aguda. Med Intensiva 20:246–251
21. Kalfon P, Rao GS, Gallart L, Puybasset L, Coriat P, Rouby JJ (1997) Permissive hypercapnia with and without expiratory washout in patients with severe acute respiratory distress syndrome. Anesthesiology 87:6–17

22. Richecoeur J, Lu Q, Vieira SRR, et al (1999) Expiratory washout versus optimization of mechanical ventilation during permissive hypercapnia in patients with severe acute respiratory distress syndrome. Am J Respir Crit Care Med 160:77–85
23. Kylstra JA, Paganelli CV, Lanphier EH (1966) Pulmonary gas exchange in dogs ventilated with hyperbarically oxygenated liquid. J Appl Physiol 21:177–184
24. Fuhrman BP, Paczan PR, DeFrancisis M (1991) Perfluorocarbon-associated gas exchange. Crit Care Med 19:712–722
25. Tutuncu AS, Faithful NS, Lachmann B (1993) Intratracheal perfluorocarbon administration combined with mechanical ventilation in experimental respiratory distress syndrome dose-dependent improvement of gas exchange. Crit Care Med 21:962–969
26. Hirschl RD, Tooley R, Parent AC, Johnson K, Barlett RH (1995) Improvement of gas exchange, pulmonary function, and lung injury with partial liquid ventilation: a study model in the setting of severe respiratory failure. Chest 108:500–508
27. Arnold JH (2000) High-frequency oscillatory ventilation and partial liquid ventilation: Liquid breathing to a different beat (frequency). Crit Care Med 28:2660–2662
28. Doctor A, Ibla JC, Grenier BM, et al (1998) Pulmonary blood flow distribution during partial liqid ventilation. J Appl Physiol 84:1540–1550
29. Dickson EW, Heard SO, Chu B, Fraire A, Brueggemann AB, Doern GV (1998) Partial liquid ventilation with perfluorocarbon in the treatment of rats with lethal pneumococcal pneumonia. Anesthesiology 88:218–223
30. Cox PN, Frndova H, Tan PSK, et al (1997) Concealed air leak associated with large tidal volumes in partial liquid ventilation. Am J Respir Crit Care Med 156:992–997
31. Kirmse M, Fujino Y, Hess D, Kacmarek RM (1998) Positive end-expiratory pressure improves gas exchange and pulmonary mechanics during partial liquid ventilation. Am J Respir Crit Care Med 158:1550–1556
32. Hirschl RB, Pranikoff T, Gauger P, Schreiner RJ, Dechert R, Bartlett RH (1995) Liquid ventilation in adults, children, and full-term neonates. Lancet 346:1201–1202
33. Hirschl RB, Pranikoff T, Wise C, et al (1996) Initial experience with partial liquid ventilation in adult patients with the acute respiratory distress syndrome. JAMA 275:383–389
34. Leach CL, Greenspan JS, Rubenstein SD, Shaffer TH, Wolfson MR, Jackson JC (1996) Partial liquid ventilation with Perflubron in premature infants with severe respiratory distress syndrome. N Engl J Med 335:761–7
35. Croce MA, Fabian TC, Patton JH, Melton SM, Moore M, Trenthem LL (1998) Partial liquid ventilation decreases the inflammatory response in the alveolar environment of trauma patients. J Trauma 45:273–282
36. Tsai WC, Lewis D, Nasr SZ, Hirschl RB (1998) Liquid ventilation in an infant with pulmonary alveolar proteinosis. Pediatr Pulmonol 26:283–286
37. Reickett CA, Pranikoff T, Overbeck MC, et al (2001) The pulmonary and systemic distribution and elimination of Perflubron from adult patients treated with partial liquid ventilation. Chest 119:515–522
38. Greenspan JS, Wolfson MR, Rubenstein D, Shaffer TH (1990) Liquid ventilation of human preterm neonates. J Pediatr 117:106–111
39. Hirschl RB, Tooley R, Parent A, Johnson K, Bartlett RH (1995) Partial liquid ventilation improves gas exchange in the setting of respiratory failure during extracorporeal life support. Chest 108:500–508
40. Hirschl RB, Croce M, Gore D, et al (2002) Prospective, randomized, controlled pilot study of partial liquid ventilation in adult acute respiratory distress syndrome. Am J Respir Crit Care Med 165:781–787
41. Baden HP, Mellema JD, Bratton SL, O'Rourke PO, Jackson JC (1997) High-frequency oscillatory ventilation with partial liquid ventilation in a model of acute respiratory failure. Crit Care Med 25:299–302

42. Sukumar M, Bommaraju M, Fisher JE, Morin FC, Papo MC, Fuhrman BP (1998) High-frequency partial liquid ventilation in respiratory distress syndrome hemodynamics and gas exchange. J Appl Physiol 84:327–334
43. Doctor A, Mazzoni MC, DelBalzo U, DiCanzio J, Arnold JH (1999) High-frequency oscillatory ventilation of the perfluorocarbon-filled lung: Preliminary results in an animal model acute lung injury. Crit Care Med 27:2500–2507
44. Hurford WE (1997) The biologic basis for inhaled nitric oxide. Respir Care Clin N Am 3:357–369
45. Rossaint R, Falke KJ, Lopez F, Slama K, Pison U, Zapol WM (1993) Inhaled nitric oxide for the adult respiratory distress syndrome. N Engl J Med 328:399
46. Dellinger RP, Zimmerman JL, Taylor RW, et al (1998) Effects of inhaled nitric oxide in patients with acute respiratory distress syndrome: Results of a randomized phase II trial. Crit Care Med 26:15–23
47. Michael JR, Barton RG, Saffle JR, et al (1998) Inhaled nitric oxide versus conventional therapy. Effect on oxygenation in ARDS. Am J Respir Crit Care Med 157:1372–1380
48. Troncy E, Collet JP, Shapiro S, et al (1998) Inhaled nitric oxide in acute respiratory distress syndrome. Am J Respir Crit Care Med 157:1483–1488
49. Lundin S, Mang H, Smithies M, Stenqvist O, Frostell (1999) Inhalation of nitric oxide in acute lung injury: results of a European multicentre study. Intensive Care Med 25:911–919
50. Kacmarek RM (2001) Combination therapy. Respir Care Clin N Am 7:663–681
51. Goldberger AL (2001) Heartbeats, hormones, and health. Is variability the spice of life? Am J Respir Crit Care Med 163:1289–1296
52. Cannon WB (1927) Organization for physiological homeostasis. Physiol Rev 9:399–431
53. Kleiger RE, Miller JP, Bigger JT, Moss AJ (1987) Decreased heart rate variability and its association with increased mortality after acute myocardial infarction. Am J Cardiol 59:256–262
54. Goldberger AL (1996) Non-linear dynamics for clinicians: chaos theory, fractals, and complexity at the bedside. Lancet 347:1312–1314
55. Goldberger AL, Amaral LAN, Hausdorff JM, Ivanov P, Pend CK, Stanely HE (2002) Fractal dynamics in physiology: Alterations with disease and aging. Proc Natl Acad Sci USA 99:2466–2472
56. Suki B, Barabasl AL, Hantos Z, Petak F, Stanley HE (1994) Avalanches and power-law behaviour in lung inflation. Nature 368:615–618
57. Suki B, Alencar AM, Sujeer MK, et al (1998) Life support systems benefit from noise. Nature 393: 127–128
58. Lefevre, GR, Kowalski SE, Girling LG, Thiessen DB, Mutch AC (1996) Improved arterial oxygenation after oleic acid lung injury in the pig using a computer-controlled mechanical ventilator. Am J Respir Crit Care Med 154:1567–1572
59. Nam AJ, Brower RG, Fessler HE, Simon BA (2000) Biologic variability in mechanical ventilation rate and tidal volume does not improve oxygenation or lung mechanics in canine oleic acid lung injury. Am J Respir Crit Care Med 161:1797–1804
60. Mutch WAC, Harms S, Graham MR, Kowalski SE, Girling LG, Lefevre GR (2000) Biologically variable or naturally noisy mechanical ventilation recruits atelectatic lung. Am J Respir Crit Care Med 162:319–323
61. Boker A, Graham MR, Walley KR, et al (2002) Improved arterial oxygenation with biologically variable or fractal ventilation using low tidal volumes in a porcine model of acute respiratory distress syndrome. Am J Respir Crit Care Med 165:456–462
62. Mutch WAC, Eschun GM, Kowalski SE, Graham MR, Girling LG, Lefevre GR (2000) Biologically variable ventilation prevents deterioration of gas exchange during prolonged anaesthesia. Br J Anesth 84:197–203
63. Arold SP, Mora R, Lutchen KR, Ingenito EP, Suki B (2002) Variable tidal volume ventilation improves lung mechanics and gas exchange in a rodent model of acute lung injury. Am J Respir Crit Care Med 165:366–371

64. Rimoldi OS, Pierini A, Ferrari S, Cerutti M, Pagani M, Malliani A (1990) Analysis of short-term oscillations of R-R and arterial pressure in conscious dogs. Am J Physiol 258:H967–H976

Summary of Clinical Trials of Mechanical Ventilation in ARDS

R. G. Brower and G. D. Rubenfeld

Introduction

Acute respiratory distress syndrome (ARDS) is characterized pathophysiologically by increased intrapulmonary shunt and ventilation-perfusion imbalances, increased intrapulmonary dead space, and decreased respiratory system compliance. Most ARDS patients experience hypoxemia while ventilating spontaneously, even with high fractions of inspired oxygen (FiO_2). Many patients cannot sustain adequate ventilation, leading to hypercapnia, respiratory acidosis, and worsening hypoxemia. Without mechanical ventilation, death may occur within a short time. With mechanical ventilation, adequate ventilation and oxygenation can be sustained in most patients, providing more time for administration of specific treatments such as antibiotics for infections and for natural healing. However, mechanical ventilation may also cause acute lung injury (ventilation-associated or ventilator-induced lung injury, VILI). Thus, our primary means of respiratory support, which is critical for survival of most patients with ARDS, may paradoxically prevent recovery of some patients.

Many studies in experimental animal models suggested that some specific aspects of mechanical ventilation techniques are responsible for VILI, and that modifications of mechanical ventilation approaches could decrease or prevent VILI [1–9]. However, these modifications could also have adverse effects on respiratory or circulatory function which could be detrimental to recovery of ARDS patients. Therefore, clinical trials were necessary to demonstrate the value of different mechanical ventilation strategies for improving important clinical outcomes. This chapter summarizes the rationale for the modified mechanical ventilation strategies and the results of several randomized clinical trials designed to compare clinical outcomes among patients who received different mechanical ventilation approaches.

Traditional Approach to Mechanical Ventilation in ARDS

Positive pressure ventilation techniques were developed by anesthesiologists in the first half of the 20th century to support general anesthesia during thoracic surgery [10]. Ventilation with small, physiologic tidal volumes (V_T) led to progressive hypoxemia during several hours of volume-cycled ventilation, presumably from progressive atelectasis. Ventilation with generous V_T of 10-15 ml/kg was adopted because this approach was associated with lower alveolar-arterial oxygen gradients and decreased intrapulmonary shunt [11, 12].

Positive pressure ventilation was used with increasing frequency in patients with acute respiratory failure in the 1950s. Many aspects of the techniques developed by anesthesiologists for support of general anesthesia were adopted for use in critically ill patients. Two aspects of these techniques probably contributed to VILI.

VILI from Ventilation with High Volumes and High Pressures

Because dead space is increased in ARDS, the generous V_T approach was useful for maintaining near-normal $PaCO_2$ and pH. Moreover, the generous V_T approach was also useful for preventing or decreasing atelectasis and reversing some of the intrapulmonary shunt caused by atelectasis or intraalveolar filling [13, 14]. However, much of the ARDS lung is not available for ventilation because of consolidation, atelectasis, and alveolar filling [15, 16]. Therefore, most of the V_T is delivered to the less diseased or normal lung regions. This may cause overdistention in the aerated lung tissue. Numerous studies in experimental animal models have demonstrated that overdistention can cause increased pulmonary vascular permeability, decreased surfactant function, hemorrhage, inflammation, and hypoxemia [1, 4, 7, 17, 18]. Ventilation with smaller V_T may decrease mechanical stresses in the aerated lung regions and attenuate this form of acute lung injury (ALI). However, the smaller V_T approach is less effective for maintaining gas exchange than the traditional approach that used generous V_T. Some ARDS patients experience hypercapnia and acidosis while receiving ventilation with small V_T [19, 20]. Therefore, it was not clear that the smaller V_T approach would lead to improved clinical outcomes in ARDS patients.

VILI from Ventilation with Low End-Expiratory Volume and Pressure

VILI occurred in experimental animal models of ALI when positive pressure ventilation was delivered with low end-expiratory volumes and airway pressures [1, 8, 9]. At least three mechanisms for this form of VILI have been suggested:
1. Low volume/low pressure VILI may occur if there is some atelectasis at end-expiration, which is more likely when low end-expiratory airway pressures are applied. This may allow repeated opening and closing of small bronchioles and alveoli, which could involve injurious mechanical stresses [8].
2. Low volume/low pressure VILI may occur from excessive stress in the parenchymal attachments between atelectatic and aerated lung units [21].
3. Low volume/low pressure VILI may occur if there is substantial atelectasis or alveolar filling, leading to maldistribution of the V_T to the aerated lung units, causing overdistention[22, 23]. Several studies in experimental models demonstrated decreased VILI when higher levels of positive end-expiratory pressure (PEEP) were applied, to raise end-expiratory lung volume by recruiting atelectasis or flooded alveoli [1, 8, 9]. Higher levels of PEEP were recommended by some investigators to prevent this form of VILI in ARDS patients [24, 25]. However,

higher levels of PEEP may cause higher levels of end-inspiratory pressure and volume, which could cause VILI from overdistention. Moreover, higher levels of PEEP may cause circulatory depression [26, 27]. Therefore, it was not clear that modifying traditional mechanical ventilation approaches with higher PEEP would improve clinical outcomes.

Schemes for Prioritizing Competing Clinical Objectives

Surveys of physicians' use of mechanical ventilation in ARDS demonstrated great variability in practices [28–30]. Some physicians used generous V_T with higher airway pressures. This approach gave high priority to traditional goals of maintaining gas exchange and breathing comfort; it gave lower priority to preventing VILI from overdistention. Other physicians used moderate or small V_T with lower airway pressures. This approach gave higher priority to preventing VILI from overdistention; it gave lower priority to maintaining gas exchange and breathing comfort. There was also great variability in physicians' use of PEEP [28]. These differences in physicians' practices reflect disparity in physicians' estimations of the risks and benefits of the different approaches to setting V_T and levels of PEEP. Randomized clinical trials were necessary to provide clinically relevant information to guide clinician practice.

Clinical Trials of Mechanical Ventilation Strategies

Clinical Trials Using Conventional Mechanical Ventilation

Five different randomized trials were conducted in the 1990s to test modified mechanical ventilation strategies in ARDS patients (Table 1). One of these trials compared clinical outcomes in ARDS patients randomized to receive either a conventional approach with generous V_T and relatively low levels of PEEP to those randomized to receive small V_T and relatively high levels of PEEP [31]. Patients in the small V_T/higher PEEP group also received recruitment maneuvers (continuous positive pressure airway pressure [CPAP] of 40 cmH2O for 40 seconds) to reverse atelectasis. Oxygenation was substantially improved with the small V_T/high PEEP approach. Thus, higher levels of PEEP can compensate for the deleterious effects of the small V_T approach on oxygenation. The small V_T/higher PEEP approach was also associated with respiratory acidosis, as expected. However, the small V_T/higher PEEP approach was associated with substantially improved survival. These striking results demonstrated that the approach to mechanical ventilation could alter clinical outcomes and suggested that mechanical ventilation approaches should be modified from those that were used in the past. However, it was not clear if the improved outcomes were attributable to the use of smaller V_T, higher PEEP, recruitment maneuvers, or the possibility of some unrecognized imbalances between the study groups [32]. Moreover, because this was a relatively small trial that involved many patients with causes of ARDS that are uncommon in other intensive care environments, it was important to confirm the findings.

Table 1. Clinical trials of lung-protective mechanical ventilation strategies in patients with ARDS. Values shown for tidal volumes are as reported in the studies.

Study	Tidal volumes (ml/kg)		Mortality (%)	
	Higher	Lower	Higher	Lower
Amato et al.[31] [a]	~12	~6	71	38
Brochard et al. [33] [b]	~10	~7	38	47
Stewart et al. [35] [c]	~11	~7	47	50
Brower et al. [34] [d]	~10	~7	46	31
NIH Network [36] [d]	~12	~6	40	31

Tidal volumes expressed in ml/kg of [a] measured body weight, [b] dry body weight, [c] ideal body weight, or [d] predicted body weight.

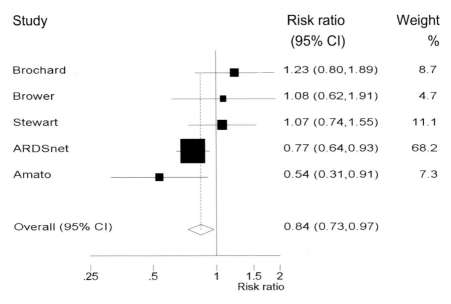

Fig. 1. Relative risks of mortality (± 95% confidence intervals) for the study groups that received lung-protective mechanical ventilation strategies relative to those that received conventional, standard, or traditional mechanical ventilation strategies. The mortality estimates from the two trials that stopped early for efficacy [31, 36] may be biased in favor of beneficial effects. The two studies that stopped early for futility [33–35] may be biased against beneficial effects of the lung protective approach. The confidence intervals shown overlap, suggesting that the differences could be from chance variation.

Four of the clinical trials summarized in Table 1 tested the value of ventilation with small V_T with limited inspiratory airway pressures [33–36]. Three of these trials did not demonstrate improved clinical outcomes with the volume and pressure limited approach [33–35]. However, the trial conducted by the NIH ARDS Network demonstrated improved mortality, more ventilator-free days, and more organ failure-free days with the volume and pressure limited approach [36]. There are several possible explanations for the different results among the four trials.

Chance variation

Risk ratios for mortality for each of the five clinical trials summarized in Table 1 are shown in Figure 1. The 95% confidence intervals for the mortality estimates are inversely proportional to the sizes of the clinical trials. In other words, we have less confidence in the mortality estimates from the smaller clinical trials.

Mortality estimates for some of the trials shown in Figure 1 may also be biased because the trials stopped earlier than had been originally planned. Two of the studies that did not show a beneficial effect of lower V_T ventilation [33, 34] were stopped early at an interim analysis because it was very unlikely that a beneficial effect of the lower V_T approach could be demonstrated if the trial continued to its original planned enrollment (futility). The NIH trial [36] and also the trial of combined lower V_T/higher PEEP [31] stopped earlier than was originally planned because there was convincing evidence for efficacy of the modified ventilation approaches. The mortality estimates from clinical trials that stop early tend to be biased in favor of the early stopping rules [37]. The two studies that stopped early for futility are more likely to be biased towards over-estimating harmful effects or underestimating beneficial effects of the lower V_T approach. The two studies that stopped early for efficacy are more likely to be biased in favor of the beneficial effects of the small V_T approach. These biases, if present, tend to be proportional to the fraction of the planned enrollment that was actually enrolled in the studies. The NIH trial enrolled a greater proportion (86%) of the planned enrollment than the two trials that stopped early for futility. Moreover, the NIH trial was the largest of the trials, and, therefore, the confidence intervals around the mortality estimate from this study are the smallest. These considerations support a higher level of confidence in the mortality estimate from the NIH trial than in the other trials. Most importantly, the confidence intervals for all of the trials overlap. Thus, one plausible explanation for the differences in outcomes among these trials is variation by chance alone.

Differences in the V_T used in the study groups

The mean difference in V_T between the two study groups in the NIH trial was 5.6 ml/kg of predicted body weight [36]. This difference was probably greater than the difference in V_T between the study groups in the three other trials that tested low V_T ventilation [33–35]. Direct comparisons of the V_T used in the NIH trial and those used in two of the other studies are possible because these studies used explicit formulae for setting V_T [34–36]. In the fourth trial that tested ventilation with low V_T, the V_T were set according to dry body weight, which required a clinical estimation of weight gain from extravascular fluid accumulation [33]. To compare the V_T in this study to those in the other studies requires some estimations and assumptions regarding the relationships of dry body weight to the body weights and V_T that were set according to explicit formulae [38].

The values for V_T for the three studies that did not show a beneficial effect of V_T reduction [33–35] suggest that the separation between the study groups was smaller than 5.6 ml/kg, as used in the NIH study (Table 1). The greater separation in V_T between study groups in the NIH study appears to be due to both the use of lower V_T in the lower V_T study group of the NIH study and higher V_T in the higher V_T study group of the NIH study.

Other differences in the study protocols

There were several other methodologic differences between the study protocols used in the trials. One difference between the NIH study and the three studies that did not show a beneficial effect was in the management of respiratory acidosis. The NIH trial utilized higher respiratory rates to maintain near-normal arterial $PaCO_2$ and pH. There may be deleterious effects of respiratory acidosis [39–42]. Beneficial effects of V_T reduction could be counteracted by adverse effects of respiratory acidosis. On the other hand, respiratory acidosis has been shown to reduce ALI in experimental animal models [43,44]. The net effect of respiratory acidosis on important clinical outcomes in ARDS patients remains to be demonstrated.

High Frequency Ventilation

High frequency ventilation uses very small V_T at very high rates [45, 46]. The rationale for using very small V_T is, as explained earlier, to prevent lung injury from overdistention. With very high respiratory rates, adequate CO_2 clearance can be achieved despite V_T that are smaller than traditional estimations of dead space. Moreover, with this approach, lung volumes can be maintained at higher levels to achieve greater recruitment and aeration; to prevent VILI from low volume/low pressure ventilation [47].

An early trial of high frequency jet ventilation in ARDS patients was not associated with improved clinical outcomes [48]. However, using refined high frequency ventilation approaches (high frequency oscillatory ventilation, HFOV), some clinical trials demonstrated modest improvements in clinical outcomes in infants with neonatal respiratory distress [49–52]. In other studies there were no apparent beneficial effects of HFOV in neonates [53,54].

In a recent clinical trial, ARDS patients were randomized to receive HFOV or a conventional mechanical ventilation approach [55]. Mortality was lower in the study group that received HFOV, although this difference was not statistically significant. Patients randomized to receive the conventional mechanical ventilation approach received V_T of approximately 10 ml/kg predicted body weight. These V_T were not as small as those used in the NIH trial, and they were associated with inspiratory airway pressures that were higher than those used in the lower V_T approach as in the NIH study [36]. Therefore, although the results of this trial were promising for HFOV, the investigators acknowledged that additional studies were needed to compare important clinical outcomes among patients who receive HFOV to those that receive the best conventional ventilator-based lung protective strategies.

Summary

Each of the clinical trials summarized in this chapter compared clinical outcomes among ARDS patients who received mechanical ventilation according to different schemes for prioritizing competing clinical objectives. The NIH trial demonstrated that a prioritization scheme that gave higher priority to preventing high volume/high pressure VILI would yield better clinical outcomes than a prioritization scheme that gave higher priority to maintaining traditional goals with respect to gas exchange and comfort.

The NIH trial was not designed to demonstrate the best mechanical ventilation strategy. However, the results of this trial strongly suggest that V_T of 12 ml/kg predicted body weight and higher should be avoided unless there are compelling reasons to use this approach in some patients. Some investigators have suggested that the use of V_T that are intermediate between 6 and 12 ml/kg will yield better clinical outcomes than the use of 6 ml/kg [56]. Also, it has been suggested that an inspiratory plateau pressure of 3032 cmH2O may be a safe limit [56, 57]; that reductions of V_T to achieve lower inspiratory plateau pressures are not necessary. However, subset and multiple logistic regression analyses of the NIH study database suggest that better outcomes result from V_T reduction to achieve lower inspiratory plateau pressures [58].

Numerous studies in experimental animals strongly suggest that higher levels of end-expiratory lung volume are beneficial to prevent low volume/low pressure VILI. The clinical trial in which improved clinical outcomes were associated with the "open-lung approach" [31] is consistent with the animal studies. However, it is not yet clear that higher levels of end-expiratory lung volume can improve clinical outcomes in patients already receiving mechanical ventilation with small V_T and limited inspiratory airway pressures. Three multi-center clinical trials were initiated between 1999 and 2002 to assess the value of higher levels of end-expiratory pressure and recruitment maneuvers in patients with ARDS receiving small V_T. Preliminary analysis of one of the trials, which concluded in 2002, suggests that raising PEEP may not alter clinical outcomes. The other two trials continue to enroll patients. We do not yet know the answer to this question.

Conclusion

Mechanical ventilation is necessary for the survival of most ARDS patients. However, traditional approaches to mechanical ventilation may have prevented recovery of some patients. Mechanical ventilation with a volume and pressure limited approach appears to improve clinical outcomes relative to a mechanical ventilation approach that utilizes generous V_T and inspiratory airway pressures. Further improvements in clinical outcomes may result from mechanical ventilation approaches designed to prevent low volume/low pressure VILI. This may be possible using conventional mechanical ventilation, but definitive evidence for this approach awaits conclusion of the current clinical trials. HFOV is a promising lung-protective approach that must be further developed and proven in relation to conventional mechanical ventilation lung protective approaches.

Acknowledgement. Supported in part by National Institutes of Health/National Heart, Lung, and Blood Institute grants NO1-HR 46054–64 and HLR0167939

References

1. Webb HH, Tierney DF (1974) Experimental pulmonary edema due to intermittent positive pressure ventilation with high pressures. Am Rev Respir Dis 110:556–565
2. Tsuno K, Prato P, Kolobow T (1990) Acute lung injury from mechanical ventilation at moderately high airway pressures. J Appl Physiol 69:956–961
3. Parker JC, Hernandez LA, Longenecker GL, Peevy K, Johnson W (1990) Lung edema caused by high peak inspiratory pressures in dogs. Am Rev Respir Dis 142:321–328
4. Parker JC, Hernandez LA, Peevy KJ (1993) Mechanisms of ventilator-induced lung injury. Crit Care Med 21:131–143
5. Dreyfuss D, Saumon G (1992) Barotrauma is volutrauma but which volume is the one responsible? Intensive Care Med 18:139–141
6. Dreyfuss D, Saumon G (1993) Role of tidal volume, FRC, end-inspiratory volume in the development of pulmonary edema following mechanical ventilation. Am Rev Respir Dis 136:730–736
7. Dreyfuss D, Saumon G (1998) State of the Art: Ventilator-induced lung injury; lessons from experimental studies. Am J Respir Crit Care Med 157:294–323
8. Muscedere JG, Mullen JBM, Gan K, Slutsky AS (1994) Tidal ventilation at low airway pressures can augment lung injury. Am J Respir Crit Care Med 149:1327–1334
9. Corbridge TC, Wood LDH, Crawford GP, Chudoba MJ, Yanos J, Sznajder JI (1990) Adverse effects of large tidal volume and low PEEP in canine acid aspiration. Am Rev Respir Dis 142:311–315
10. Colice GL (1994) Historical perspective on the development of mechanical ventilation. In: Tobin M (ed) Principles and Practice of Mechanical Ventilation. McGraw-Hill, Inc, New York, pp 1–35
11. Benedixen HH, Hedley-Whyte J, Laver MB (1963) Impaired oxygenation in surgical patients during general anesthesia with controlled ventilation. N Engl J Med 269:991–997
12. Hedley-Whyte J, Laver MB, Benedixen HH (1964) Effect of changes in tidal ventilation on physiologic shunting. Am J Physiol 206:891–897
13. Cheney FW, Burnham SC (1971) Effect of ventilatory pattern on oxygenation in pulmonary edema. J Appl Physiol 31:909–912
14. Hedley-Whyte J, Pontoppidan H, Morris MJ (1966) The response of patients with respiratory failure and cardiopulmonary disease to different levels of constant volume ventilation. J Clin Invest 45:1543–1554
15. Maunder RJ, Shuman WP, McHugh JW, Marglin SI, Butler M (1986) Preservation of normal lung regions in the adult respiratory distress syndrome. JAMA 255:2463–2465
16. Gattinoni L, Pesenti A, Avalli L, Ross F, Bomino M (1987) Pressure-volume curve of total respiratory system in acute respiratory failure: computed tomographic scan study. Am Rev Respir Dis 136:730–736
17. Tsuno K, Miura K, Takeya M, Kolobow T, Morioka T (1991) Histopathologic pulmonary changes from mechanical ventilation at high peak airway pressures. Am Rev Respir Dis 143:1115–1120
18. Parker JC, Townsley MI, Rippe B, Taylor AE, Thigpen J (1984) Increased microvascular permeability in dog lungs due to high peak airway pressures. J Appl Physiol 57:1809–1816

19. Hickling KG, Walsh J, Henderson S, Jackson R (1994) Low mortality rate in adult respiratory distress syndrome using low-volume, pressure-limited ventilation with permissive hypercapnia: a prospective study. Crit Care Med 22:1568–1578

20. Hickling KG, Henderson SJ, Jackson R (1990) Low mortality associated with low volume pressure limited ventilation with permissive hypercapnia in severe adult respiratory distress syndrome. Intensive Care Med 16:372–377

21. Mead J, Takishima T, Leith D (1970) Stress distribution in lungs: A model of pulmonary elasticity. J Appl Physiol 28:596–608

22. Martynowicz MA, Minor TA, Walters BJ, Hubmayr RD (1999) Regional expansion of oleic acid-injured lungs. Am J Respir Crit Care Med 160:250–258

23. Hubmayr RD (2002) Perspective on lung injury and recruitment: A skeptical look at the opening and collapse story. Am J Respir Crit Care Med 165:1647–1653

24. Lachman B (1992) Open up the lung and keep the lung open. Intensive Care Med 18:319–321

25. Amato MBP, Barbas CSV, Medeiros DM, et al (1995) Beneficial effects of the "open lung approach" with low distending pressures in acute respiratory distress syndrome. Am J Respir Crit Care Med 152:1835–1846

26. Pinsky MR (1993) Heart-lung interactions. In: Pinsky MR, Dhainaut JF (eds) Pathophysiologic Foundations of Critical Care. Williams & Wilkins, Baltimore, pp: 472–490

27. Scharf SM (1998) Mechanical cardiopulmonary interactions in critical care. In: Dantzker DR, Scharf SM (ed) Cardiopulmonary Critical Care. W.B. Saunders Company, Philadelphia, pp: 75–91

28. Carmichael LC, Dorinsky PM, Higgins SB, et al (1996) Diagnosis and therapy of acute respiratory distress syndrome in adults: an international survey. J Crit Care 11:9–18

29. Esteban A, Anzueto A, Alia I, et al (2000) How is mechanical ventilation employed in the Intensive Care Unit? An international utilization review. Am J Respir Crit Care Med 161:1450–1458

30. Esteban A, Anzueto A, Frutos F, et al (2002) A 28-day international study of the characteristics and outcomes in patients receiving mechanical ventilation. JAMA 287:345–355

31. Amato MBP, Barbas CSV, Medeiros DM, et al (1998) Effect of a protective-ventilation strategy on mortality in the acute respiratory distress syndrome. N Engl J Med 338:347–354

32. Hudson LD (1998) Protective ventilation for patients with acute respiratory distress syndrome. N Engl J Med 338:385–387

33. Brochard L, Roudot-Thoraval F, Roupie E, et al (1998) Tidal volume reduction for prevention of ventilator-induced lung injury in the acute respiratory distress syndrome. Am J Respir Crit Care Med 158:1831–1838

34. Brower RG, Shanholtz CB, Fessler HE, et al (1999) Prospective randomized, controlled clinical trial comparing traditional vs. reduced tidal volume ventilation in ARDS patients. Crit Care Med 27:1492–1498

35. Stewart TE, Meade MO, Cook DJ, et al (1998) Evaluation of a ventilation strategy to prevent barotrauma in patients at high risk for acute respiratory distress syndrome. N Engl J Med 338:355–361

36. Acute Respiratory Distress Syndrome Network (2000) Ventilation with lower tidal volumes as compared with traditional tidal volumes for acute lung injury and the acute respiratory distress syndrome. N Engl J Med 342:1301–1308

37. Whitehead J (1986) On the bias of maximum likelihood estimation following a sequential test. Biometrika 73:573–581

38. Brower R (1990) Mechanical ventilation in acute lung injury and ARDS. Crit Care Clin 18:1–13

39. Walley KR, Lewis TH, Wood LDH (1990) Acute respiratory acidosis decreases left ventricular contracticility but increases cardiac output in dogs. Circ Res 67:628–635

40. Manley ES, Nash CB, Woodbury RA (1964) Cardiovascular responses to severe hypercapnia of short duration. Am J Physiol 207:634–640

41. Feihl F, Perret C (1994) Permissive hypercapnia - How permissive should we be? Am J Respir Crit Care Med 150:1722–1737

Subject Index